Expert System Techniques in Biomedical Science Practice

Prasant Kumar Pattnaik
KIIT University, India

Aleena Swetapadma
KIIT University, India

Jay Sarraf
KIIT University, India

A volume in the Advances in Bioinformatics and Biomedical Engineering (ABBE) Book Series

IGI Global
DISSEMINATOR OF KNOWLEDGE

Published in the United States of America by
IGI Global
Medical Information Science Reference (an imprint of IGI Global)
701 E. Chocolate Avenue
Hershey PA, USA 17033
Tel: 717-533-8845
Fax: 717-533-8661
E-mail: cust@igi-global.com
Web site: http://www.igi-global.com

Library of Congress Cataloging-in-Publication Data

Names: Pattnaik, Prasant Kumar, 1969- editor. | Swetapadma, Aleena, 1983- editor. | Sarraf, Jay, 1989- editor.
Title: Expert system techniques in biomedical science practice / Prasant Kumar Pattnaik, Aleena Swetapadma, and Jay Sarraf, editors.
Description: Hershey, PA : Medical Information Science Reference, [2018] | Includes bibliographical references.
Identifiers: LCCN 2017035748| ISBN 9781522551492 (hardcover) | ISBN 9781522551508 (ebook)
Subjects: | MESH: Expert Systems | Medical Informatics Applications
Classification: LCC R855.3 | NLM W 26.55.A7 | DDC 610.285--dc23 LC record available at https://lccn.loc.gov/2017035748

This book is published in the IGI Global book series Advances in Bioinformatics and Biomedical Engineering (ABBE) (ISSN: 2327-7033; eISSN: 2327-7041)

British Cataloguing in Publication Data
A Cataloguing in Publication record for this book is available from the British Library.

Advances in Bioinformatics and Biomedical Engineering (ABBE) Book Series

ISSN:2327-7033
EISSN:2327-7041

Editor-in-Chief: Ahmad Taher Azar, Benha University, Egypt

MISSION

The fields of biology and medicine are constantly changing as research evolves and novel engineering applications and methods of data analysis are developed. Continued research in the areas of bioinformatics and biomedical engineering is essential to continuing to advance the available knowledge and tools available to medical and healthcare professionals.

The **Advances in Bioinformatics and Biomedical Engineering (ABBE) Book Series** publishes research on all areas of bioinformatics and bioengineering including the development and testing of new computational methods, the management and analysis of biological data, and the implementation of novel engineering applications in all areas of medicine and biology. Through showcasing the latest in bioinformatics and biomedical engineering research, ABBE aims to be an essential resource for healthcare and medical professionals.

COVERAGE

- Structural Biology
- Dental Engineering
- Bayesian Methods
- Prosthetic Limbs
- Protein Engineering
- Data Mining
- Molecular Engineering
- Molecular Simulations
- Robotics and Medicine
- Computational Biology

IGI Global is currently accepting manuscripts for publication within this series. To submit a proposal for a volume in this series, please contact our Acquisition Editors at Acquisitions@igi-global.com or visit: http://www.igi-global.com/publish/.

Titles in this Series

For a list of additional titles in this series, please visit:
https://www.igi-global.com/book-series/advances-bioinformatics-biomedical-engineering/73671

Applying Big Data Analytics in Bioinformatics and Medicine
Miltiadis D. Lytras (Deree - The American College of Greece, Greece) and Paraskevi Papadopoulou (Deree - The American College of Greece, Greece)
Medical Information Science Reference • ©2018 • 465pp • H/C (ISBN: 9781522526070) • US $245.00

Comparative Approaches to Biotechnology Development and Use...
Tomas Gabriel Bas (University of Talca, Chile) and Jingyuan Zhao (University of Toronto, Canada)
Medical Information Science Reference • ©2017 • 592pp • H/C (ISBN: 9781522510406) • US $205.00

Computational Tools and Techniques for Biomedical Signal Processing
Butta Singh (Guru Nanak Dev University, India)
Medical Information Science Reference • ©2017 • 415pp • H/C (ISBN: 9781522506607) • US $225.00

Handbook of Research on Computational Intelligence Applications in Bioinformatics
Sujata Dash (North Orissa University, India) and Bidyadhar Subudhi (National Institute of Technology, India)
Medical Information Science Reference • ©2016 • 514pp • H/C (ISBN: 9781522504276) • US $230.00

Applying Business Intelligence to Clinical and Healthcare Organizations
José Machado (University of Minho, Portugal) and António Abelha (University of Minho, Portugal)
Medical Information Science Reference • ©2016 • 347pp • H/C (ISBN: 9781466698826) • US $165.00

For an entire list of titles in this series, please visit:
https://www.igi-global.com/book-series/advances-bioinformatics-biomedical-engineering/73671

IGI Global
DISSEMINATOR OF KNOWLEDGE

701 East Chocolate Avenue, Hershey, PA 17033, USA
Tel: 717-533-8845 x100 • Fax: 717-533-8661
E-Mail: cust@igi-global.com • www.igi-global.com

To my wife, Bismita, and my daughter, Prasannakshi.
Prasant Pattnaik

To my guide and mentor, Dr. Anamika Yadav, NIT Raipur, India. The process of how you do research and made the research work simple and very much interesting if you learn the rules of research. I learn from her. Dr. Yadav has been always my source of motivation, inspiration, and as a wonderful mentor, guide, advisor, philosopher, and supporter to be remembered all times.
Aleena Swetapadma

To my parents.
Jay Sarraf

Table of Contents

Detailed Table of Contents

Soft tissues are non-homogeneous deformable structures having varied structural arrangements, constituents, and composition. This chapter explains the design of a capacitance sensor array for analyzing and imaging the non-homogeneity in biological materials. Further, tissue mimicking phantoms are developed using Agar-Agar and Polyacrylamide gels for testing the developed sensor. Also, the sensor employs an unsupervised learning algorithm for automated analysis of non-homogeneity. The reconstructed capacitance image can also be sensitive to topographical and morphological variations in the sample. The proposed method is further validated using a fiberoptic-based laser imaging system and the Jaccard index. In this chapter, the design of the sensor array for smart analysis of non-homogeneity along with significant results are presented in detail.

The disorders of the digestive tract lead to various problems such as bleeding, bloating, nausea, etc. In order to diagnose various digestive abnormalities, the electrogastrograms (EGG) can serve as an efficient tool. In an EGG, several electrodes are placed onto the abdomen over the stomach and the electrical signals originating from the stomach muscles are recorded. By analyzing these electrical patterns, the abnormalities in digestive system can be analyzed. This chapter describes the developed system for measuring EGG signals along with the decision support system developed for automated classification of digestive disorders. The normal and abnormal EGG signals were acquired at Balaji Medical Hospital, Chennai. Further, the features were extracted using descriptive statistics and empirical mode decomposition (EMD) algorithm. Finally, an automated classification system was developed using k-means algorithm. This chapter explains the recording of electrogastrograms and a method for classification of normal and abnormal EGG signals.

Preface

INTRODUCTION

In Biomedical Science and Artificial Intelligence (AI), an expert system is designed to solve complex problems which usually requires human expertise; it automates the decision making by representing mainly if-then-else rule rather than using conventional procedural methods. Inference engine and Knowledge base are mainly the two subsystems that an expert system can divide into. Knowledge base basically represents facts and rules whereas inference engine applies to the rules to the known facts. Expert system mainly implicates the increase in productivity via quick diagnoses and allowing the expert knowledge to be extracted when there is no ready access to human expert.

ABOUT THE BOOK

This book will aim to provide relevant theoretical frameworks and the latest empirical research findings in the area. It will be written for professionals who want to improve their understanding of the strategic role of trust at different levels of the information and knowledge society, that is, trust at the level of the global economy, of networks and organizations, of teams and work groups, of information systems and, finally, trust at the level of individuals as actors in the networked environments.

Key Features

1. Overview of biomedical signal and image processing
2. Address different levels of the information and knowledge society
3. Explore trust at the level of the global economy
4. Based performance analysis of expert system based methods in medical science
5. Feature selection methods for biomedical signals

ORGANIZATION OF THE BOOK

This book is organised into an introduction, eight chapters, and a conclusion.

In the introduction, biomedical science, expert system and application of expert system in various fields of engineering has been discussed.

Chapter 1 addressed the strategy of this research is dependent kind of surveying tools of collecting data standard questionnaire about SI. The dual aspects of spiritual intelligence as "self-knowledge" and then "Theology " correlated with commitment organization. Also, the main hypothesis of this study is to examine the relationship between organizational commitment and spiritual intelligence is concerned, remains the highest correlation with intellectual intelligence and emotional commitment.

Chapter 2 aimed in this study to improve the performance of classification in computer-aided medical diagnosis. Within the scope of the study, experiments have been performed on three different datasets, which include heart disease, hepatitis and BUPA liver disorders datasets. First, all features obtained from these datasets were converted into complex-valued number format using phase encoding method. After complex-valued feature set was obtained, these features were then classified by an ensemble of complex-valued radial basis function (^{E}CVRBF) method. In order to test the performance and the effectiveness of the medical diagnostic system; ROC analysis, classification accuracy, specificity, sensitivity, kappa statistic value and f-measure were used. Experimental results show that the developed system gives better results compared to other methods described in the literature. The proposed method can then serve as a useful decision support system for medical diagnosis.

Chapter 3 introduced a novel kernel based fuzzy clustering approach to enhance the contrast of masses. Novelty of the proposed technique is incorporation of two important features of mammograms that convey the properties of masses. Local entropy and intensity mean of each kernel position play the key role to enhance masses. A kernel is moved across the mammograms to collect all possible values of those features and hence they are exploited as the input data of fuzzy clustering technique. Performance of the proposed approach is compared with two other conventional contrast enhancement techniques. Both subjective and objective evaluations of the proposed technique show an evidence of improvement in compare to other methods. Moreover, unwanted enhancement of obscured tissues is also suppressed in our approach.

Chapter 4 explained the design of a capacitance sensor array for analyzing and imaging the non-homogeneity in biological materials. Further, tissue mimicking phantoms are developed using Agar-Agar and Polyacrylamide gels for testing the developed sensor. Also, the sensor employs an unsupervised learning algorithm for automated analysis of non-homogeneity. The reconstructed capacitance image can also be sensitive to topographical and morphological variations in the sample. The proposed method is further validated using a fibber optic based laser imaging system and the Jacquard index. In this chapter, the design of the sensor array for smart analysis of non-homogeneity, along with significant results are presented in detail.

Chapter 5 describes the developed system for measuring EGG signals along with the decision support system developed for automated classification of digestive disorders. The normal and abnormal EGG signals were acquired at Balaji Medical Hospital, Chennai. Further, the features were extracted using descriptive statistics and Empirical Mode Decomposition (EMD) algorithm. Finally, an automated classification system was developed using k-means algorithm. This chapter explains the recording of electrogastrograms and a method for classification of normal and abnormal EGG signals.

Chapter 6 describes the effect of an old generation romantic music (stimulus) on the autonomic nervous system (ANS) activity and the cardiac electrophysiology of Indian male volunteers were investigated. Electrocardiogram (ECG) signals were acquired and the corresponding RR intervals (RRIs) were extracted. The recurrence analysis of the RRI time series suggested a more stable heart rate in the post-stimulus condition. Heart rate variability (HRV) analysis detected a dominant parasympathetic activity in the post-stimulus condition. The time- domain and the wavelet transform analyses of the ECG signals predicted an alteration in the electrical activity of the heart because of the exposure to the music stimulus. The classification of the HRV and the ECG parameters was performed using artificial neural network (ANN), which resulted in an accuracy of ≥80%.

Chapter 7 aimed to estimate the HbA1c value with high accuracy. Follow-up data of diabetic patients were used as data. The Orange data mining software is used because it is easy to use in the modelling phase and contains many methods. In this context, it is aimed to develop an effective prediction model by using a large number of feature selection and classification methods. The results show that the proposed model successfully predicts the HbA1c parameter. In addition, determination of the parameters which are effective in the diagnosis of diabetes has been carried out with the feature selection methods.

Chapter 8 investigated the effect of a motivational song (acting as a stimulus) on the electrical activity of the heart using wavelet packet analysis of electrocardiogram (ECG) signals. ECG signals were acquired from 18 healthy male volunteers during the pre- and the post-stimulus conditions. Wavelet packet decomposition of the ECG signals was performed up to level 3 using db04 wavelet, which resulted in the formation of 8 wavelet packet coefficients. Linear (t-test) and nonlinear (classification and regression tree (CART), boosted tree (BT) and random forest (RF)) methods were used to identify the statistically significant parameters. The statistically significant parameters were used as categorical inputs for Multilayer Perceptron (MLP)-based artificial neural network (ANN) classification of the ECG signals. A classification efficiency of $\geq 80\%$ was obtained, suggesting an alteration in the cardiac electrophysiology of the volunteers caused by the music stimulus.

Lastly, the conclusion of the book is given. The application of expert system in various fields of biomedical science has been discussed.

Prasant Kumar Pattnaik
KIIT University, India

Aleena Swetapadma
KIIT University, India

Jay Sarraf
KIIT University, India

Acknowledgment

The editors would like to acknowledge the help of all the people involved in this project and, more specifically, to the authors and reviewers that took part in the review process. Without their support, this book would not have become a reality.

First, the editors would like to thank each one of the authors for their contributions. Our sincere gratitude goes to the chapters' authors who contributed their time and expertise to this book. They are all models of professionalism, responsiveness and patience with respect to my cheerleading and cajoling. The group efforts that created this book are much larger, deeper and of higher quality than any individual could have created. Each and every chapter in this book has been written by a carefully selected distinguished specialist, ensuring that the greatest depth of understanding be communicated to the readers. We have also taken time to read each and every word of every chapter and have provided extensive feedback to the chapter authors in seeking to make the book perfect. Owing primarily to their efforts I feel certain that this book will prove to be an essential and indispensable resource for years to come.

As editors would like to thank the Expert System and Biomedical Science community for recognizing the quality, effort and care that has been made (by many) in creating such a successful, wonderful and useful product.

Second, the editors wish to acknowledge the valuable contributions of the reviewers regarding the improvement of quality, coherence, and content presentation of chapters. Most of the authors also served as referees; we highly appreciate their double task.

There have been several influences from our family and friends who have sacrificed lot of their time and attention to ensure that we are kept motivated to complete this crucial project.

Last but not least the editors would like to thank all members of IGI Global publication for their timely help; constant inspiration and encouragement with friendly support to publish the book in time.

Prasant Kumar Pattnaik
KIIT University, India

Aleena Swetapadma
KIIT University, India

Jay Sarraf
KIIT University, India

Introduction

In bio-medical science, the size of the data has been grown drastically during last two to three decades. The growing data does not seem to be linearly dependent on the characteristics of the data. Hence there is a requirement of good analysis tool for biomedical data. One such system that exists now days is expert system. Expert system is designed to solve complex problems by reasoning through bodies of knowledge, represented mainly as if–then rules. Expert system has two components, inference engine and knowledge base. Knowledge base generally represents facts and rules. Inference engine applies those rules to the known facts and derive the results for new facts. The expert system tools have extensive use of fuzzy logic to express inexactness and connections to neural networks. In biomedical science many of the expert system methods has been used in various research areas. Some of the topics are discussed below.

Artificial neural network (ANN) is one of the expert system tools which have been successfully used in biomedical science. One of the methods for detecting emboli in the cerebral circulation is trans-cranial Doppler ultrasound. There are two types of emboli, gaseous and particulate emboli in cerebral blood flow. These two embolies need to be distinguished. In Kemény et al. (1999), ANN has been used for emboli classification from trans-cranial Doppler ultrasound signals after pre-processing the signals with Fourier Transforms. In Sérgio Matos et al. (2001), wavelet transform is used for signal processing using Morlet wavelet. After that multi-layer perceptron for identifying emboli within the blood flow signal. In Teixeira et al. (2004), a radial basis function ANN has been used to distinguish among solid emboli and liquid emboli. In Teixeira et al. (2006), a black-box modelling scheme is proposed for temperature prediction in a homogeneous medium subjected to therapeutic ultrasound. In this work radial basis functions neural networks has been used where the best-fitted models were selected from the space of model structures using a genetic multi-objective strategy. In Teixeira et al. (2008a), the temporal echo-shifts of backscattered ultrasound signals are collected from a gel-based phantom. These are then given as input to the radial basis functions neural networks. The inputs and the number of neurons were selected using the multi-objective genetic algorithm.

In Teixeira et al. (2010), non-invasive temperature estimation scheme is proposed using soft-computing methods. Although magnetic resonance imaging has acceptable temperature resolutions it has high instrumentation cost. Computerised tomography is an imaging equipment for diagnosis of various diseases. Ischaemic cerebral vascular accident can be detected using encephalon image analysis. In Ribeiro et al. (2007), ischaemic cerebral vascular accidents are identified using tissue density images obtained by CT with the help of artificial neural networks. Authors claim that automatic identification of ischaemic lesions has been performed with no false negatives and very few false positives. In Teixeira et al (2007, performance assessment of non-invasive temperature models based on radial basis functions neural networks has been proposed. The models build without the intermediate data has a maximum absolute error. In Teixeira et al. (2008b), employed models were radial basis functions neural networks with external dynamics induced by their inputs. The set of model inputs and number of neurons in the network were found using the multi-objective genetic algorithm. The new data addressed two new spatial locations and a new intensity level, assessing the intensity and space prediction capacity of the proposed model.

The challenges in biomedical science also includes limited sample size and high-dimensionality of the dataset used for analysis. The problems arise due to less data samples are over-fitting of data, reliability, generalizability, applicability and class imbalance. In Dougherty, Hua, and Bitner (2007), it was suggested that validation of a model is not easy when the sample size is limited and the variables have high-dimensionality. In Lee and Lee (2006), it was suggested that the issue of high dimensionality of data can be overcome by feature selection. As suggested in Galar et al (2012), when the samples representing one class is much lower than those representing other classes the class imbalance problem may occur. In Tantra et al. (2015) and Oksel et al. (2015), several challenges that face the development of nanotechnology and other predictive models has been discussed.

In Koprowski et al. (2012), the ultrasound images together with other clinical data and features from images are discussed. Ten features for the images are obtained such as average image power spectrum, regional minimum value on the image, smoothness of the image, the minimum value of brightness of the image, the position of the center of Gray-Level Co-occurrence matrix gravity, range of contrast in different values and three parameters obtained from square-tree decomposition of the image. The images are analysed using SVM with a linear kernel with Matlab's Statistics Toolbox. In Cyran et al. (2013), a classifier using SVMs classification technique has been developed. The processes of classification includes several steps such as choosing a method of analysis, choosing a set of features or attributes that will be used to classify the subjects, training the classifier, validating the classifier and evaluating potential errors in the classification.

In biomedical science the use of expert system is more frequent now days. Various types of applications of expert system in bio-medical have been given in the next chapters of the book.

REFERENCES

Cyran, K. A., Kawulok, J., Kawulok, M., Stawarz, M., Michalak, M., Pietrowska, M., & Polańska, J. (2013). Support Vector Machines in Biomedical and Biometrical Applications. Emerging Paradigms in Machine Learning, 13, 379–417. doi:10.1007/978-3-642-28699-5_15

Dougherty, E. R., Hua, J., & Bittner, M. L. (2007). Validation of computational methods in genomics. *Current Genomics*, *8*(1), 1–19. doi:10.2174/138920207780076956 PMID:18645624

Galar, M., Fernandez, A., Barrenechea, E., Bustince, H., & Herrera, F. (2012). A review on ensembles for the class imbalance problem: Bagging-, boosting-, and hybrid-based approaches. *IEEE Transactions on Systems, Man, and Cybernetics*, *42*(4), 463–484. doi:10.1109/TSMCC.2011.2161285

Kemény, V., Droste, D. W., Hermes, S., Nabavi, D. G., Schulte-Altedorneburg, G., Siebler, M., & Ringelstein, B. (1999). Automatic embolus detection by a neural network. *Stroke*, *30*(4), 807–810. doi:10.1161/01.STR.30.4.807 PMID:10187883

Koprowski, R., Zieleźnik, W., Wróbel, Z., Małyszek, J., Stepien, B., & Wójcik, W. (2012). Assessment of significance of features acquired from thyroid ultrasonograms in Hashimoto's disease. *Biomedical Engineering Online*, *11*(1), 48. doi:10.1186/1475-925X-11-48 PMID:22898180

Lee, C., & Lee, G. G. (2006). Information gain and divergence-based feature selection for machine learning-based text categorization. *Information Processing & Management*, *42*(1), 155–165. doi:10.1016/j.ipm.2004.08.006

Oksel, C., Ma, C. Y., Liu, J. L., Wilkins, T., & Wang, X. Z. (2015). (Q) SAR modelling of nano-material toxicity: A critical review. *Particuology*, *21*, 1–19. doi:10.1016/j.partic.2014.12.001

Ribeiro, L., Ruano, A. E., Graça Ruano, M., & Pedro, M. (2007). Neural networks assisted diagnosis of ischemic CVA's through CT scan. *Proceedings of the IEEE International Symposium on Intelligent Signal Processing*, 223–227. 10.1109/WISP.2007.4447507

Sérgio Matos, A. E., Ruano, M., Ruano, G., & Evans, D. H. (2001). Neural network classification of cerebral embolic signals. *23rd Annual International Conference of the IEEE Engineering in Medicine and Biology Society.*

Tantra, R., Oksel, C., Puzyn, T., Wang, J., Robinson, K. N., Wang, X. Z., ... Wilkins, T. (2015). Nano(Q)SAR: Challenges, pitfalls and perspectives. *Nanotoxicology*, *9*(5), 636–642. doi:10.3109/17435390.2014.952698 PMID:25211549

Teixeira, C. A., Graça Ruano, M., & Ruano, A. E. (2004). Emboli classification using RBF neural networks. *Proceedings of CONTROL 2004*, 630–635.

Teixeira, C. A., Graça Ruano, M., Ruano, A. E., & Pereira, W. C. A. (2008a). A soft-computing methodology for non-invasive time-spatial temperature estimation. *IEEE Transactions on Biomedical Engineering*, *55*(2), 572–580. doi:10.1109/TBME.2007.901029 PMID:18269992

Teixeira, C. A., Graça Ruano, M., Ruano, A. E., & Pereira, W. C. A. (2008b). Neuro-genetic non-invasive temperature estimation: Intensity and spatial prediction. *Artificial Intelligence in Medicine*, *43*(2), 127–139. doi:10.1016/j.artmed.2008.03.008 PMID:18468870

Teixeira, C. A., Pereira, W. C. A., Ruano, A. E., & Graça Ruano, M. (2010). On non-invasive multi-layer temperature estimation using soft-computing methods. *Ultrasonics*, *50*(1), 32–43. doi:10.1016/j.ultras.2009.07.005 PMID:19695653

Teixeira, C. A., Ruano, A. E., Graça Ruano, M., & Pereira, W. C. A. (2007). Generalization assessment of non-invasive data-driven temperature estimators from therapeutic ultrasound. *Brazilian Journal of Biomedical Engineering*, *23*(2), 143–151.

Teixeira, C. A., Ruano, A. E., Ruano, M. G., Pereira, W. C. A., & Negreira, C. (2006). Non-invasive Temperature prediction of in-vitro therapeutic ultrasound signals using neural networks. *Medical & Biological Engineering & Computing*, *44*(1-2), 111–116. doi:10.100711517-005-0004-2 PMID:16929928

Chapter 1
Spiritual Intelligence and Organizational Commitment:
A Case Study of the Iranian Social Security Organization (ISSO)

Mohammad Abdolshah
Islamic Azad University, Iran

Narges Tarahhomi
Industrial Management Institute, Iran

Ali Hossein Nejad
Industrial Management Institute, Iran

Amirmohammad Khatibi
University of Isfahan, Iran

ABSTRACT

Denoting individual life along organizational commitment (OC) is one of the strategical programs in an organization. Although there are many researches about considering the meaning of organizational commitment and its relationship with other elements, but spiritual intelligence is an effective element of individual and behavior in organizations. The goal of this chapter is the investigation of the relationship between organizational spiritual intelligence (SI) and organizational commitment (OC) in Iranians' social security organization (ISSO). Base on this factor, during reviewing theatrical literature and relevant variable of scaling, the outline of research is made. The strategy of this research is a dependent kind of surveying tool for collecting data standard questionnaire about SI. The dual aspects of spiritual intelligence, self-knowledge and theology, correlated with commitment organization. Also, the main hypothesis of this study is to examine the relationship between organizational commitment and spiritual intelligence.

DOI: 10.4018/978-1-5225-5149-2.ch001

INTRODUCTION

The goal of any organization is to get success and growth. Human resource (HR) is a significant part which helps to attain the goal of the organization. Organization wants to achieve competitive advantage; for this organization need highly fulfilled satisfied, innovative, dedicated and creative employees. In the current era, spiritual intelligence (SI) has become important for the success of any organization (Kalantarkousheh, 2013). Spirituality builds values and culture in the organization; it is the understanding of oneself as spirit/soul. Intelligence is one of the important privileges of the human being distinguishing him from other creatures (Ghabaribanab, 2007). SI is the expression of innate spiritual qualities through attitudes, behaviours and thoughts of the individual (Kalantarkousheh, 2013).

SI is the mind's capacity to handle substantial and spiritual aspects of life. According to previous studies, SI can be effective in the promotion of different variables. One such variable is an organizational commitment (OC) may have potentially serious effects on an organization's function and can be a major influence on its effectiveness. SI is the most important concept in the management (Yazdani & Parsa, 2014). Employees, who are loyal to their organizations, they contribute in activities and enjoy collaboration in their organizations. Committed employees give more benefit to their organizations and put additional attention to fulfil their job, connect into extra-role behaviour, and help the organization to function competently. Spiritually intelligent people will be committed to their organizations only when they are satisfied with their jobs.

Therefore, considering the role of the Iranian social security organization (ISSO) as a serving organization with the highest and most sacred with aims of the massive generous society and the high-income retirees, it has led us to examine this paper. Hope that the results will be effective in defining the mission and organizational vision. This study explores the relationship between SI and OC in the staff of ISSO. The hypotheses in this paper are:

The main hypothesis is the semantic relationship between employ's SI and their emotional OC. And the other hypothesizes are:

1. There is a semantic relationship between employ's spiritual intelligence (SI) and their commitment (EC).
2. There is a semantic relationship between employ's spiritual intelligence (SI) and their rational commitment (RC).
3. There is a semantic relationship between employ's SI and their normal commitment (NC).

In the following, theoretical foundations, research background, methodology and findings of the research will be presented.

THEORETICAL FUNDAMENTALS OF RESEARCH

Gardner (1999) describes intelligence as a compound of ability to show the problem and creation of new prudent that is valuable in a culture Hayward garner`s multiple intelligence theory that shown in Table 1.

Spiritual Intelligence (SI)

There are so many descriptions of SI but all these flexibility of these against changes and learning form faults, meaning & targets in work, self-awareness, creation and developing the organization. Zohar (1997) for the first time introduced the concept of SI. By using this intelligence, people can expand their vision of lives and perform competently in their lives. It is the most essential kind of intelligence that has the influence to alter our history, society and life. SI is defined as the conformity application of spiritual information that aims to facilitate solving daily issues and attainment of goals (Emmons, 2000). In recent years, the intelligence is not considered only as cognitive ability and is extended to other fields as emotional intelligence, natural intelligence, existential intelligence and SI (Zare, 2011). Zohar and Marshall (2000) believed that SI causes that a person has the deep attitude to the life events

Table 1. Kind of the intelligence

Intelligence	Definition
Lingual intelligence	The ability of thimble abut word and using language to describe meanings
Logical-mathematical intelligence	The ability of doing mathematical actions
Special intelligence	The ability of 3d-thought
Body-action intelligence	The ability of manipulator & convert sense things
Musical intelligence	Sensitive to intonation & rhythm & voice tone
Inter subjective intelligence	Apprehensive ability of other & effective interaction
Subjectivism intelligence	Realizing ourselves
Natural intelligence	Observing natural pattern & realizing their natural & artificial relationship
Existence intelligence	Capacity of posing existence questions.
Spiritual Intelligence (SI)	*

and don't fear the hardship of life and cope up with patiently and find the logical and human solutions for them. SI requires the abilities and applies such spiritual issues for conformity and effective interaction and production of valuable products and outcomes (Hildebrant, 2011). Zohar (2001) stated 9 features for spiritual intelligence:

1. Self-Awareness,
2. Vision & Values Led (Idealism),
3. The Capacity to Face and USE Adversity,
4. To be Holistic,
5. Diversity,
6. Field Independence (braveness),
7. The Tendency to Ask WHY,
8. The Ability to Re-Frame,
9. Spontaneity.

Immense (2000) suggested that virtual intelligence is a framework of knowing & organizing skills & abilities that we need, that using spirituality increasing individual adaption. Amram (2007) suggested that virtual intelligence is the ability to use and appearing resources & values & virtual qualities can increase daily efficiency and comfort, King (2008) suggested that virtual intelligence is a collection of spiritual cupidity applied with conscious, solidarity & virtual & nonfinancial aspect of persons. And the outcome of that is a deep relation of persons. Increasing meaning & recognize self-transcendental and dominance of virtual property. Generally intelligence start with (IQ) the ability to control body and using things and based on that the neutral system specified. Zauhar and Marshal (2001) believe that other intelligence are a subset of these three (Figure 1).

- **IQ:** This kind of intelligence related to the skill of our linguistics & logic that now is more than other is a document of educational success & suitable for solving logical & mathematical questions.
- **EQ:** Helps people manage their emotions and it is very effective in the success of a professional and personal life and helps them in communicating to some extent.
- **SQ:** This kind of intelligence is specified for human,unlike intellect intelligence that applied in computers & emotional intelligence that seen in high-class mammals.

Zouharand Manshal (2001) describe this as a new dimension of human's intelligence and it finds intelligence in their idea. And used for solving recognition

Figure 1. The situation of IQ, EQ and SQ in the human brain

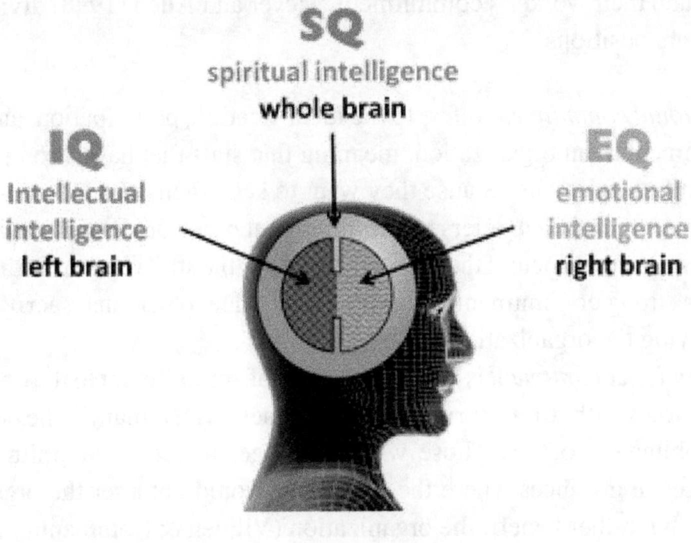

and valuable problems. Virtual intelligence is the background of all we believe in. Serious questions about where do we come form& where do we go & what is the main target of life is a sign of virtual intelligence.

Virtual intelligence connects various aspects of awareness, spiritual and mental life with actual life, work of a person and give an awareness about the whole of the word in a total form. Sidug and wiglours believe virtual intelligence is the ability to treat with sympathy and wisdom within natural and eternal comfort surrendering happenings and events. People with virtual intelligence treat fairly and sympathy when they judge. With virtual intelligence, we can see all things in the unreality and this is a kind of intelligence that conducts famous and beloved leaders of the world. Virtual leaders with having this intelligence can tolerate the biggest pressure. People with virtual intelligence are who know what to do and why to do. Usually, base on the same deputy they act. They live based on doing services to other and they don't blame others for something and usually responsible for their forgiveness and their act, for their self-content they don't need others minion. They don't want to depend others to have safely. Because they believe the safely is from their own and not from others. They know work a place for creativity self-confidence, leaving, the second place for money, benefits.

Organizational Commitment

Researchers show that organizational supporting for employs is clearly related to their commitment to the organization. On the other hand, there is a proof that indicates that organizational follow the strategy of human resources to increase efficiency and their worker's commitment. Meyer and Allen (1998) divide OC into three separate positions:

1. *Emotional commitment* refers to the identification, participation, and effective attachment to an organization, meaning that staff that have strong Emotional commitment remain because they want to keep their jobs.
2. *Rational commitment* refers to a commitment based on the staffs' awareness of the loss that they incur if they leave. Therefore, the staff remains in the company with a strong commitment either by force or due to personal sacrifices related to leaving the organization.
3. *Normative commitment* is based on a sense of commitment to the organization. Employees with strong normative commitment who remain in the organization feel obligated to stay. Those with a stronger affective commitment accept changes in instances where these changes would not alter the organization's goals, but rather benefit the organization (Viljoen & Rothmann, 2009).

The reason is that they feel their work is ethically good (Handlon, 2009) is a responsible person to the organization has an emotional attachment to the organization, takes part in organization & enjoy joining in the results of researches indicate that SI with results such as job content, being present in the workplace. Organizational behaviour, alter social and job efficiency have positive relation & with the trend of leaving job has a negative relationship. There are many researches done about SI such as: investing this value with defocusing (Shiuan et al. 2003-32), EQ (Gardner & Stough, 2003) organizational culture (Manetje & Martins, 2009).

Spirituality and Religion in Organization

Considering the complex and ambiguity of the concept of spirituality it's mentioned as black box describing spirituality is so delicate because it has various applies. Anderhill (1993) in the spiritual life book, when defining the difficulty of defining spirituality says: "we have no way except describing it, on the other hand, given up describing hastily because there is no word in humans language synonym and equal to the face of spirituality considering the difficulty of the concept of spirituality many of theorizations went to present a meaning of it (Meyers,1995). Spirituality is known us look in for finding the meaning and target of life deep realization the value of life, the extent of the universe, exist natural forces and the system of personal belief. Against his definition Helins (1995) emphasize on valuable interpersonal dimension and know the spirituality as art toward nurturing the self-sense, others and super force that utilize and coordinate this sensation and moving humans to accomplishment. Waggan`s (2003) suggested that spirituality a public case, the same as excitement it has levels and it is possible to be conscious or unconscious, growing or not growing, healthy or sick, simple or complex, useful or dangerous. Wiglens (2002) believe that spirituality is an internal requirement of human to be connected to a super creature that puts in tow levels.

- **Virtual Level:** At this level it indicates a holy Wight that knows his place & time extremely as a source of a superpower and extremely self-wars. & humans need to be guided by such as this person.

The second level or horizontal level includes all couple have the tendency of giving services to them. With the meaning similarity between the concepts of religion and spirituality, there are noticeable differences generally spiritual conducts begin out of religious orientation with an investigation about self-facts. Then there is the difference between religion and spirituality. Anderhill (1993) in the book of spiritual life, said spirituality is the heart of religion and spiritual life is an original and perfect life that creates for humans. Kale and Shivastava (2003) believe that religion includes ethics and loyalty to religious aim and religious ceremony, but spirituality connects with deep internal causes and their emotional relationship with their god. In fact, religion connects with answers and spirituality connects with questions. There are 2 points of view about the relationship between religion and spirituality. The first view believes in the relationship between religion and spirituality in 3 statements:

1. Covering and being equal considering concepts of religion & spiritualty
2. Spiritualty is form religion
3. Religion is form spiritualty

The second view emphasized the point that is no relationship between religion and spirituality. Totally there are 4 kinds of tendency about spirituality in the workplaces (Mitroff & Denton, 1999) regarding the person`s negative or positive view of religion and spirituality. It’s drawn 4 kinds of the matrix in Table 2. Regarding the positive persons view the only way of experiencing and nurturing the spirituality is religion. This group that contains 30 percent of total believes religion and spirituality have the same inseparable meaning and they are the main resource of belief and world value. People who have a positive view about spirituality and negative view about religion ascribe religions organized, dogmatic without an open mind and ascribe spirituality is an individual aspect and valuable for all. People have a positive view about religion and negative view about spiritually. These people focus all their power on religious life specially ethnics and a course of a particular religion. Finally, only 2 percent of people they have a negative viewabout religion and spirituality believe

Table 2. Grouping attitudes

Positive View	Positive View	Spirituality Negative View
Religion	Religion and spirituality have the same & inseparable meaning and both are main resources for word value and belief	Religion is prior to spirituality and is the main resource of belief and values
Negative View	Spirituality is better than religion and is the main resource of belief	Neither religion nor spirituality and worlds valve can be regardless and independently to them

that neither religion nor spirituality has foundation and world value can be described independently and regardless religion and spirituality. This group believes religion and spirituality have no application in an organization.

According to the presentations, the meaning of spirituality in the present article refers to two aspects of human super mental understanding and then human effort to apply this perception in life. It is also believed throughout the article that there is also a spiritual person, religion is also, so there is no difference between religion and spirituality.

LITERATURE OF RESEARCH

So many researches done on dimensions applications, individual and social of SI. Bagheri et al (2010) implies the relation between SI of nurses and merit. Also in organizational dimension the researches imply array in creativity, organizational, truth, confidence in working, evolution in character of employs through virtually self in Florence in capabilities. Tafreshi and Darbayegan (2011) have shown the presence of a meaningful relationship between job satisfaction and OC, job satisfaction and organizational citizenship behaviour, as well as OC and organizational citizenship behaviour. Padala (2011) studied occupation satisfaction and OC in an Indian fertilizer and chemical material production company. Akbarizadeh et al. (2012) have studied the relationship between SI, strong-willed characteristics and general health among nurses. The results showed a meaningful, positive relationship between SI and strong-willed characteristics, SI and general health, and strong-willed characteristics and general health. Nasel (2004) examined few characteristics of SI including Patience, love, sincerity, inner peace, sympathy. Emmons (2000) the spiritually intelligent people encompass the ability to resolve problems by utilizing spiritual resources. Chen (2006) an attitude toward a job is called job satisfaction. Job satisfaction is an effective reaction towards the definite parts of the job. Mottaz (1988) job satisfaction is an emotional response to the workplace. Robert (2000) says that job satisfaction is the distinction of the incentive obtains by a person and incentive which they believe to attain. Locke (1969) defined job dissatisfaction as: It is the unpleasant emotional condition of the individuals that is come from the assessment of their job as blocking the accomplishment of their job values. The six dimensions build up by Stamps and Piedmont (1986) for measuring job satisfaction are as follows: (1) Pay: Means the money received by employees, (2) Autonomy: Means that independence and liberty in the workplace, (3) Task requirements: Means actions that should be performed in a job, (4) Organizational policies: Means administrative and managerial strategies and practices, (5) Interaction: Means opportunities that employees are able to convey with each other, (6) Professional status: Means the overall significance of a job that is supposed by an employee himself or by others.

Balfour and Wechsler (1996) defined that OC is the employees wish to stay in the organization. Kaur (2013) studied the relationship between SI and job satisfaction of 100 secondary school teachers. The findings showed that SI has significant positive impact on job satisfaction. The result also reveals that gender has no impact on SI and job satisfaction. Torabi and Javadi (2013) studied the relationship between SI and job engagement. Nodehi and Nehardani (2013) investigate the association between job satisfaction and SI of 215 Mashhad high school teachers. They used five dimensions (coworker's relation, work itself, pay, supervision and promotional opportunity) for measurement of job satisfaction. There is little study done aboutSI and OC. Mohammaddi and Boroom (2014) studied the relationship between cultural intelligence and SI with OC of secondary schools' principals. The result indicates that cultural intelligence has a significant and positive influence on OC while there is no a significant correlation exists among SI and OC. They also fined those managers who used their own talents and skills to find the good causes for job and work performance and find importance and aims in life, they will fill find better solutions of the problems, will have a better understanding of themselves and others and perform their job efficiently. There is no direct relationship between among SI and OC considering the researches done in this course abroad. Considering exist empty point of this research tried to describe the importance of virtue in the organization and check the relationship between SI and OC in ISSO.

METHODOLOGY

Research is a descriptive study that used correlation for statistical analysis. The study population comprised all staff from universities in Iranians Social Security Organization (ISSO) in Iran. Research statistical society is the senior managers of Iranian Social Security Organization (ISSO) in 2017. Regarding the limitation of statistical society the whole considered as a statistical sample. The main aim of this paper is investigating the relationship between SI and OC and also the sub-goals based on the main target are consist of:

1. Scrutiny about SI and emotional commitment.
2. Scrutiny about SI and rational commitment.
3. Scrutiny about SI and normative commitment.

Main hypothesis:

1. There is a semantic relationship between employ's SI and their emotional commitment.
2. There is semantic relationship between employ's SI and their rational commitment.
3. There is semantic relationship between employ's SI and their normal commitment.

Using standard questionnaire of OC (Mayer & Allen, 1984) 24 questions and SI (Abdallahzadeh et al, 2006) 29 questions. Regarding the target this research is applicable because its outcome can be utilized in order to amplifying employs OC and regarding the way of research it is a kind of correlation and description. The way of collecting data is free and the kind of data are model. After collecting, coding and entering data into the computer, the SPSS statistical software was used to analyze the data.

The questionnaires validity was approved with reference to the related papers and also by professor's judgment. Reliability and validity of the standard questionnaire about OC (Rezaeian et al., 2006) subsequently 0.98 & 0.73. The cited questionnaire randomly was provided with 10 individuals to determine above questionnaire reliability and then reliability rate of the total questionnaire (0.69) and the dependent and independent variables (OC and SI) at the appropriate level of reliability was confirmed by using Cronbach's alpha coefficient. Based on the literature of research Dimensions of SI and OC and the conceptive pattern of study are shown in Figure 2 and Table 3. The independent variable is SI that consists of 2 dimensions of SI that definition gives below.

1. **Recognizing and Relationship With Existent (Theology):** Pointed to belief and, faith, and accepting the presence of God that measured by 12 questions.

Figure 2. Conceptive pattern of research

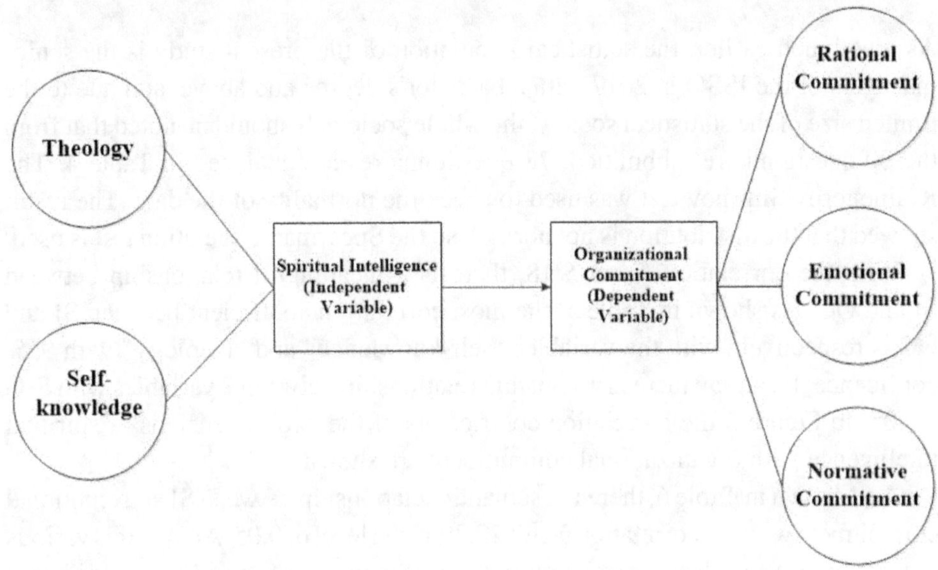

Table 3. Dimensions of SI and OC

Spiritual Intelligence	Organizational Commitment
Recognizing and relationship with existent (theology) **Spiritual life recognition internal kernel (self-knowledge)**	Rational Commitment Emotional Commitment Normative Commitment

2. **Spiritual Life Recognition Internal Kernel (Self-Knowledge):** Pointed to the sense of affect to god and utilizing the religious and belief that measured by 17 question the OC as a dependent variable consist of 3 dimensions of emotional, rational, normal (Abdollahzadeh et al., 2006).
    a. **Emotional Commitment:** Pointed to the correlation of a person to organizational that evaluated via 8 questions.
    b. **Rational Commitment:** The tendency to remain in the organization for the rests of learning organization or the rewards that pointed to remain in the organization and evaluated via 8 questions.
    c. **Normative Commitment:** Is a sense of duty to remain in the organization as a part the organization that evaluates via 8 questions (Allen &Mayer, 1990).

DATA ANALYSIS

As mentioned earlier, the statistical population of the present study is the senior managers of the ISSO in 2017 with a bachelor's degree and above, and due to the limited size of the statistical society, the whole society. It should be noted that from the 80 questionnaires submitted, 78 questionnaires are analyzed in Table 4. The Kolmogorov-Smirnov test was used to check the normality of the data. The result showed that the distribution is not normal, so the Spearman correlation test is used.

With the correlation factor %18, there is a meaningful relationship between SI and OC. As shown in Table 5, the most correlation coefficient between SI and OC is respectively with the variables "self-knowledge" and "theology" with 95% confidence. It can say there is a semantic relationship between 2 variables with SIG <0.05. In Figure 3 the correlation coefficients of the two dimensions of spiritual intelligence with organizational commitment are shown.

As it shown in Table 6, there is a semantic relationship between SI and emotional commitment with the correlation factor 22.3%in the level of 0.05. Among this various dimension of SI is also a correlation with the dimension of "self-knowledge" with "theology" with emotional commitment and also the correlation factor is 14.6% between SI and rational commitment. The correlation factor between SI and normal commitment with (sig >0.05) shows that there is no relationship between this two variable and rejected the hypothesis and also there isn't any relationship between these 2 dimensionss of SI, the "self-knowledge" and "theology" with normal commitment.

Table 4. Demographic characteristics of the statistical sample

Average Work Experience	Average Age	Frequency Percentage	Frequent	Sample
14.7	35.2	39.7%	31	Female
22.6	46.7	60.3%	47	Male
17.7	40.7	100%	78	Total

Table 5. The relationship between SI and OC

	Dimension of SI	Correlation
	Spiritual Intelligence	0.18
Organization Commitment	Self-Knowledge	0.199
	Theology	0.119

Figure 3. The Relationship between spiritual intelligence and organizational commitment

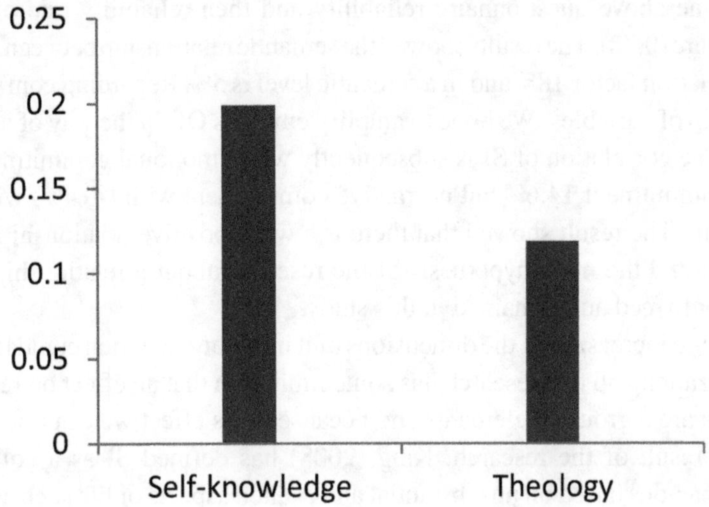

Table 6. The relationship between SI and emotional commitment

Correlation	Dimension of SI	
0.223	Spiritual Intelligence	
0.235	self-knowledge	**Emotional Commitment**
0.177	theology	
0.146	Spiritual Intelligence	
0.178	self-knowledge	**Rational Commitment**
0.063	theology	
-%0.4	Spiritual Intelligence	
-0.002	self-knowledge	**Normative Commitment**
-0.011	theology	

CONCLUSION

This research studied the relationship between SI and OC of ISSO. The results indicate meaningful relationship has been shown to exist between SI and OC of an organization's employees. In addition, positive effects of SI in the promotion of an organization's commitment; also the amount of SI and OC varied between males and females. When an individual's SI increases, the OC also increases. This relationship has been separately proven in both males and females. Questionnaire validity was approved with reference to the related papers, professors and appropriate alpha Cronbach. The cited questionnaire randomly was provided with 7 individuals to determine above questionnaire reliability and then reliability rate of the total questionnaire (0.78). The results showed the semantic relationship between SI and OC with correlation factor 18% and in a semantic level is 5%. Regarding confirming the relationship of variables. We hope to amplify employs OC in the way of amplifying their SI. The correlation of SI is subsequently with emotional commitment 22.3% rational commitment 14.6% but normative commitment with (-0.4%) without any relationship. The result showed that there is a weak positive relationship between. OC and SI and the main hypothesis of the research about a relationship between them is confirmed and remained in this study.

Then with increasing SI the dimensions of it in the organization could help pall in the organization and this research has some limitation that an effect on results. The limitations are a group of elements and because of its effect we can't be confident about the result of the research. King (2008) has defined SI as a collection of mental capacities based on unsubstantial and exalted aspects of life such as personal understanding, deep existential thinking, and expansion of meaning. Malik and Naeem (2011) concluded that dimensions of SI had a positive relationship with OC of university scientific board members. In addition, SI has a relationship with effective leadership components such as OC (Amram, 2009). The following solutions are also suggested:

1. Codify the main strategy of organization with regarding spiritual strategy in an organization.
2. Regarding confirmation the semantic relationship between SI and OC manager seen amplify their employs commitment by amplifying their SIs.
3. Based on the research results. Using people with high SI in guideline positions and guide their organization.
4. Using employs with low SI shows their lower commitment hence it recommends using this person in a career with lower commitment or in the form of part-time.
5. Regarding the most correlation between SI with OC it recommends. Figure out employs sensation in order to amplify their sprint-for example listen to their work problem. Their financial care to give them calmness.
6. Regarding that organizational is a part of world life that people spend much time init then it recommends to make employs to participate in drawing mission and organizational prospect in a suitable manner.
7. In order to make the spiritualities characteristic in organization codify a charter in organizations.

8. The level of employs SI must be considered when they employed.
9. Using the framework of holding religious ceremonies& in vacation and intend the culture of promotion of spiritual experiences in order to vacate the higher level of SI& amplifying employs OC.

FUTURE RESEARCH DIRECTIONS

Since the concept of SI has been raised recently in the science of organization and management the following is suggested as research areas:

1. Regarding that in this research all the effective elements on SI are not investigated hence we can't ignore this eventuality that the degree of correlation between this 2 factors with using structural pattern based on path analyzing is damped to some extent.
2. Responder to the question faced with cognition fault and answers with his special cognition. In the other hand they are inevitable give their opinion in the Questionnaire framework and it is possible that the questions answered with ignorance.

Suggestions of the research in order to nurtureSI and amplifying OC of employs the recommendations are proposed.

1. Examining the concept of SI, of effort into conceptualizing, designing theory of classification in order to consolidate the theoretical literature of the most basic research needs for the future.
2. Intellectual aptitude or other measurement is done using the comparative results.
3. Explaining the reasons for the deepening and retest results through research.
4. Study the relationship between SI with various types of corporate culture rational, hierarchical.
5. Relationship between SI with other concepts such as organizational justice, transformational leadership, emotional intelligence, organizational citizenship behaviour, organizational performance, products and services of the organization, dating agency.
6. Measure having SI in comparison with other religious organizations or religious organizations.
7. Assess the level of SI staff has high organizational commitment.

REFERENCES

Abdollahzade, H., Bagher Pour, M., BoujMehrani, S., & Lotfi, M. (2000). Spritual intelligence (Concepts, Assessment and Applications). Tehran: Psychometric Publications.

Akbarizadeh, F., Hajivandi, A., Bagheri, F., & Hatami, H. (2012). Relationship between nurses spiritual intelligence with hardiness and general health. *Majallah-i Danishgah-i Ulum-i Pizishki-i Kirmanshah, 15*(6).

Amram, J. Y. (2009). *The contribution of emotional and spiritual intelligence to effective business leadership*. Institute of Transpersonal Psychology.

Anderhill, E. (1993). The Spiritual Life. *Australian Journal of Psychology*, 23.

Bag heri, F., Akbarizadeh, F., & Hatami, H. (2010). The relationship between nurses' spiritual intelligence and happiness in Iran. *Procardia Social and Behavioral Sciences, 5*, 1556–1561.

Emmons, R. A. (2000). Spirituality and intelligence: Problems and prospects. *The International Journal for the Psychology of Religion, 10*(1), 57–64. doi:10.1207/S15327582IJPR1001_6

Emmons, R. A. (2000). *The Psychology of Ultimate Concerns: Motivation and Spirituality in Personality*. New York: Guilford Publication.

Emmons, R. A. (2000a). Is Spirituality an Intelligence? Motivation, Cognition, and the Psychology of Ultimate Concern. *The International Journal for the Psychology of Religion, 10*(1), 3–26. doi:10.1207/S15327582IJPR1001_2

Gardner, H. (1999). *Intelligence reframes: multiple intelligence for 21st century*. New York: Basic Books.

Gardner, L., & Stough, C. (2003). Assessing the Relationship between Workplace Emotional Intelligence, Job Satisfaction and Organizational Commitment. *Australian Journal of Psychology, 55*, 1–5.

Ghabaribanab, B, & Salim, M., Seliani, L., & NuriMoghadam, S. (2007). Spiritual intelligence. *Scientific-Research Journal of New Religious Thinking, 3*(10), 125–147.

Handlon, R. L. (2009). Departure Of The Insurance Agent: The Impact Organizational Commitment, Organizational Justice, And Job Satisfaction Have On Intent To Leave In The Insurance Industry (PhD thesis). Capella University.

HeydariTafreshi, G., & Darbayegan, A. (2011). Studying the Relationship between Job Satisfaction, Organizational Commitment and Organizational Citizenship Behavioral in the Employees of a Half-private Company in Hormozgan Province. *Scientific Journal of Educational Management Researches.*

Hildebrant, L. S. (2011). *Spiritual intelligence: Is it related to a leader's level of ethical development?* (Doctoral dissertation). Capella University.

Kalantarkousheha, S., Sharghib, N., Soleimanic, M., & Ramezanid, S. (2013). The Role of Spiritual Intelligence on Organizational Commitment in Employees of Universities in Tehran Province, Iran. *Social and Behavioral Sciences.*, *140*, 499–505.

Kale, S. H., & Shrivastava, S. (2003). The Enneagram System for Enhancing Workplace Spirituality. *Journal of Management Development*, *22*(4), 318–328. doi:10.1108/02621710310467596

Kaur, M. (2013). Spiritual intelligence of secondary school teachers in relation to their job satisfaction. *International Journal of Educational Research and Technology*, *4*(3), 104–109.

Kennedy, M. H. (2002). Spirituality in the Workplace: An Empirical Study of this Phenomenon. Nova Southeastern University.

King, D. B. (2007). The Spiritual Intelligence Project: Extracting Cognitive Ability from the Psycho Spiritual Realm. *Netherlands Journal of Happiness Studies*, *2*, 329–330.

King, U. (2008). *The search for spirituality: Our global quest for a spiritual life.* BlueBridge.

Locke, E. A. (1969). What is job satisfaction? *Organizational Behavior and Human Performance*, *4*(4), 309–336. doi:10.1016/0030-5073(69)90013-0

Malik, M. E., & Naeem, B. (2011). Role of spirituality in job satisfaction and organizational commitment among faculty of institutes of higher learning in Pakistan. *African Journal of Business Management*, *5*(4), 1236–1244.

Manetje, O., & Martins, N. (2009). The Relation between Organizational Culture and Organizational Commitment. *Southern African Business Review*, *13*(1), 120–142.

Meyer, J. P., & Allen, N. J. (1991). A three-component conceptualization of organizational commitment. *Human Resource Management Review*, *1*(1), 61–89. doi:10.1016/1053-4822(91)90011-Z

Meyer, J. P., & Herscovitch, L. (2001). Commitment in the Workplace: Toward A General Model. *Human Resource Management Review*, *11*(3), 70–83. doi:10.1016/S1053-4822(00)00053-X

Mitroff, I. A., & Denton, E. A. (1999). A Study of Spirituality in the Workplace. *Journal Sloan Management Review*, 83-92.

Mottaz, C. J. (1988). Work satisfaction among hospital nurses. *Hospital & Health Services Administration*, *33*(1), 57–74. PMID:10286427

Myers, J. E. (1995). *Wellness throughout the Lifespan*. Guidepost.

Myers, J. E., & Allen, N. J. (1984). Testing The Side-bet Theory of Organizational commitment. *The Journal of Applied Psychology*, *69*, 327–378.

Nasel, D. D. (2004). *Spiritual orientation in relation to spiritual intelligence: Anew consideration of traditional Christianity and New Age/individualistic spirituality* (Doctoral Dissertation). University of South Australia.

Nodehi, H., & Nehardani, H. (2013). Relation between spiritual intelligence and job satisfaction. *Journal of Social Issues and Humanities*, *1*(5), 67–72.

Padala, S. R. (2011). Employees' Job Satisfactions and Organisational Commitment in Nagarjuna Fertilizers and Chemicals Limited, India. *Journal of Research in International Business and Management, 1*(1), 17-27.

Shiuan, C. B., Yn, I. D., & Relley, J. H. (2003). Organizational Commitment: The Chinese Super Visionary Commitment and Employee Outcomes in Context Proximal Hypothesis or Global Hypothesis. *Journal of Organizational Behavior*, *24*(3), 14–45.

Stamps, P. L., & Piedmonte, E. B. (1986). *Nurses and Work Satisfaction: An Index for Measurement*. Chicago: Health Administration Press.

Susan Tee Suan Chin, R. N., Anantharaman, & Kin Tong, D.Y. (2011). The Roles of Emotional Intelligence and Spiritual Intelligence at the Workplace. *Journal of Human Resource Management Research*.

Torabi, M., & Javadi, S. (2013). Studying the impact of spiritual intelligence on job engagement. *International Journal of Economy Management and Social Sciences*, *2*(9), 752–756.

Viljoen, J. P., & Rothmann, S. (2009). Occupational Stress, Ill Health and Organisational Commitment Of Employees At A University Of Technology. *SA Journal of Industrial Psychology*, *35*(1), 1–11. doi:10.4102ajip.v35i1.730

Yazdani, M., & Javad Parsa, M. (2014). The moderating effect of spiritual intelligence on the relationship between organizational commitment and organizational citizenship behavior in ZobAhan factory of Isfahan. *International Journal of Scientific Management and Development*, *2*(8), 399–403.

Zare, H., Pedram, A., & Shirvanian, A. (2011). The prediction of students' spiritual intelligence of their personality attributes. *Behavioral Sciences Researches, 10*(1), 59-67.

Zohar, D. (1997). *Rewiring the Corporate Brain: Using the New Science to Rethink How We Structure and Lead Organizations*. San Francisco: Berrett-Koehler Publishers, Inc.

Zohar, D., Marshall, I. N., & Marshall, I. (2000). *Connecting with our spiritual intelligence*. Bloomsbury Publishing USA.

Zohar, D. M. (2000). *Spiritual Intelligence: The Ultimate Intelligence*. London: Bloomsbury.

APPENDIX

Greetings and Regards

The following questionnaire is about the relationship between spiritual intelligence and organizational commitment. Therefore, we are requesting you to help us with access to valuable information that results from your experience and accuracy.

Sincerely thank you for your cooperation to complete the timely and accurate questionnaire.

Education: Bachelor () MSc () Phd ()
Gender: Male () Female ()

Table 7. Questionnaire about relationship between Spiritual Intelligence and Organizational commitment

Totally Agree	Agree	No Idea	Disagree	Totally Disagree	Questions	Row
					I am very happy to spend the rest of my service in this organization	1
					I would like to talk about the organization of work with people outside the organization	2
					I really feel that the problems of this organization are my own problem	3
					I think I can simply as much as I like to this organization to the organization I also get an attachment	4
					I do not feel like a family member in my work organization	5
					I'm not emotionally interested in this organization	6
					This organization has a lot of personal meaning and meaning for me	7
					I do not feel a lot of belonging to my work organization	8
					I am amazed by the creation world	9
					I am interested in searching for and asking basic questions about life and being	10
					I want to have a humane and compassionate relationship with others	11
					Always I feel God is watching over my actions	12
					I have a sense of gratitude and gratitude in life	13

continued on following page

Table 7. Continued

Totally Agree	Agree	No Idea	Disagree	Totally Disagree	Questions	Row
					I live with enthusiasm	**14**
					I believe in God's divine presence in the world	**15**
					Praise with God is pleasing to me and after worship I feel calm	**16**
					In the face of difficulties and suffering, I believe that God helps me	**17**
					I have the ability to express my mistakes with regard to my position	**18**
					In addition to trying to deal with problems, I also pray	**19**
					I feel responsible and committed to my duties	**20**
					The ability to stand against the general and non-voting with the general public in the event of opposition to the fundamental principles of life	**21**
					I enjoy serving others	**22**
					I do not forget God's despair	**23**
					I feel God's love for myself, both directly and through others	**24**
					I am not vulnerable to changes in the world because I believe the world is changing	**25**
					I know cause all my feelings	**26**
					My life is meaningful and with a sense of value and purpose	**27**
					I get a spiritual and spiritual connection with the when help someone	**28**
					I control my thoughts and actions	**29**
					Try to improve my development	**30**
					I benefit from tradition or custom	**31**
					I believe that there is peace, love, happiness and contentment within me, not in the world around me	**32**
					I feel in my relationship with God	**33**
					I feel secure on my own inner strengths, strengths and features	**34**
					I consider work as a tool for creativity and self-confidence	**35**
					I have the ability to love and forgive others, regardless of gender, race or nationality	**36**
					I know the achievement of perfection in the light of the perfections and spirituality	**37**

Chapter 2
A Medical Decision Support System Based on Ensemble of Complex-Valued Radial Basis Function Networks

Musa Peker
Muğla Sıtkı Koçman University, Turkey

Hüseyin Gürüler
Muğla Sıtkı Koçman University, Turkey

Ayhan İstanbullu
Balikesir University, Turkey

ABSTRACT

The use of machine learning techniques for medical diagnosis has become increasingly common in recent years because, most importantly, the computer-aided diagnostic systems developed for supporting the experts have provided effective results. The authors aim in this chapter to improve the performance of classification in computer-aided medical diagnosis. Within the scope of the study, experiments have been performed on three different datasets, which include heart disease, hepatitis, and BUPA liver disorders datasets. First, all features obtained from these datasets were converted into complex-valued number format using phase encoding method. After complex-valued feature set was obtained, these features were then classified by an ensemble of complex-valued radial basis function (^{E}CVRBF) method. In order to test the performance and the effectiveness of the medical diagnostic system, ROC analysis, classification accuracy, specificity, sensitivity, kappa statistic value, and f-measure were used. Experimental results show that the developed system gives better results compared to other methods described in the literature. The proposed method can then serve as a useful decision support system for medical diagnosis.

DOI: 10.4018/978-1-5225-5149-2.ch002

INTRODUCTION

In medical diagnostics, diagnosis of a disease is performed with considering patient's data. However, the increase in the data density and the excessive number of symptoms affecting the disease complicate diagnostic procedures. Amongst one of the most popular topics to emerge in recent years is the use of computers in medical diagnostic. Computer-aided medical diagnostic systems have been developed to help specialists, with such systems aiming to minimising the physician error. Computer-aided classification systems can minimise the potential errors. In addition, these systems facilitate and accelerate in-depth examination of medical data (Cheung, 2001; Das, 2010).

In order to test the effectiveness of newly developed computer-aided medical diagnostic systems, researchers are conducting experiments on datasets that are open to common use. The hybrid method proposed in this study has been tested with three datasets. Those are Statlog heart disease, BUPA liver disorders, and Hepatitis datasets, which are obtained from the UCI machine learning repository (Bache & Lichman, 2013). The common characteristic of these datasets is having a distribution which cannot be separated linearly. There is also a large amount of missing data on the Hepatitis dataset. Information about some of the earlier studies carried out on these datasets is given below.

In the literature, some studies performed on the Statlog heart disease dataset are as follows: Based on many attempts, Cheung (2001) has achieved the highest classification accuracy (81.48%) using the Naive Bayes algorithm among a number of other classification algorithms. Kahramanli and Allahverdi (2008) have achieved 86.8% accuracy rate by using a fuzzy neural network algorithm. Das et al. (2009) have developed an ensemble algorithm which includes three neural networks and an 89.01% classification accuracy has been obtained with the proposed model. Subbulakshmi et al. (2012) have achieved an 87.50% classification accuracy by using the extreme learning machine (ELM) method. Karabulut and Ibrikci (2012) have developed a method based on a rotation forest algorithm, and a 91.20% classification accuracy has been obtained with the proposed method.

In the literature, some studies that have been carried out on the Hepatitis dataset are as follows: Javad et al. (2012) have developed a hybrid method (SVM-SA) which includes SVM and simulated annealing (SA) algorithms. They have obtained a 96.25% accuracy rate. Shao et al. (2015) have proposed a weighted linear loss twin SVM for large-scale classification. They have obtained an 84.99% accuracy rate with the method. Aldape-Pérez et al. (2012) have developed a novel method referred to as an associative memory based classifier (AMBC) and an 85.16% classification accuracy has been obtained. Bashir et al. (2016) have developed an ensemble method with multi-layer classification using optimized weighting and enhanced bagging, and an 87.04% classification accuracy has been obtained with the method which is entitled HM-BagMoov.

In the literature, some studies have been carried out on the BUPA liver disorder dataset for the identification of liver disorders as follows: Goncalves et al. (2006) have developed a new neuro-fuzzy method entitled the inverted hierarchical neuro-fuzzy BSP System (HNFB). A 73.33% classification accuracy has been obtained using this method. Jin et al. (2007) have proposed a genetic fuzzy feature transformation method for SVMs. They have achieved a 70.80% accuracy rate. Lee and Mangasarian (2001) have developed smooth SVMs (SSVM) and reduced SVMs (RSVM) classifier methods. Using these methods, they have achieved 70.3% and 74.8% accuracy rates, respectively. Chen et al. (2012) have developed a hybrid method in which the 1-NN method and particle swarm optimization (PSO) are used together. A 68.99% classification accuracy has been obtained with the proposed hybrid method. Dehuri et al. (2012) have developed an enhanced PSO-based evolutionary functional link neural network (ISO-FLANN). A 76.8% classification accuracy has been achieved with the method. Shaoa and Deng (2012) have developed a coordinate descent margin based-twin SVM. They have obtained 73.67% classification accuracy with the method. Savitha et al. (2012) have developed a fully complex-valued radial basis function (FC-RBF) network. A 74.6% accuracy rate has been achieved with the proposed method. Mantas and Abellán(2014) have developed an algorithm entitled Credal-C4.5. A 64.53% classification accuracy has been achieved with the Credal-C4.5 method which involves a decision tree based on imprecise probabilities. López et al. (2014) have developed an SVM based method. In this method, a multivariate normalization algorithm was used to train the SVM algorithm. A 72.17% classification accuracy has been achieved with the method.

Recently, the use of complex-valued classifiers for real-valued classification problems is one of the most important research topics (Savitha, Suresh & Sundararajan, 2012; Amin, Islam & Murase, 2009). Complex-valued classifiers have been utilised in the classification stage of many studies, since they provide good results (Peker, 2016; Savitha, Suresh &Sundararajan, 2012; Amin & Murase, 2009; Amin, Islam & Murase, 2009; Li, Huang, Saratchandran & Sundararajan, 2006; Chen, Mclaughlin & Mulgrew, 1994). In this study, a new hybrid method, an ensemble version of a complex-valued radial basis function algorithm has been developed. Bagging and boosting methods have been used as an ensemble algorithm. We believe that the proposed method provides an important contribution to the literature relating to complex-valued classifiers.

The rest of the paper is organized as follows. In Section Materials and Methods, information is presented about the datasets and methods used in the study. The experimental results and discussion section is given in Section Experimental Results and Discussions. In addition, a comparison with the existing methods in the literature have been carried out in this section. General information about the obtained results is presented in Section Conclusion.

MATERIALS AND METHODS

Data Description

Studies have been carried out on three different datasets in order to evaluate the success of the proposed method. The datasets have been taken from the UCI Machine Learning Repository (Bache & Lichman, 2013). These datasets are related to heart, Hepatitis, and liver disorders. The Statlog heart disease dataset relates to 270 people (Bache & Lichman, 2013). The data of 120 of these relate to healthy individuals and 150 relate to patients. The features of this dataset have been presented in Table 1.

The Hepatitis disease dataset was donated by the Jozef Stefan Institute in Slovenia (Bache & Lichman, 2013). The dataset is used to estimate the existence or absence of Hepatitis, based on different medical tests carried out on a patient. The dataset is comprised of 155 samples with 19 features. Target features have been coded as 1 for survivors (123) and 0 for the patients who died (32). Approximately 48.30% of the dataset contains missing value. Features in the dataset have been presented in Table 2.

The BUPA liver disorders dataset contains 345 samples with 6 features and two classes (Bache & Lichman, 2013). Samples are all unmarried men. 200 of these

Table 1. The features of the Statlog heart dataset

ID	Feature	ID	Feature
1	Age	8	Maximum heart rate achieved
2	Sex	9	Exercise induced angina
3	Chest pain type (four values)	10	Old peak = ST depression induced by exercise relative to rest
4	Resting blood pressure	11	The slope of the peak exercise ST segment
5	Serum cholesterol in mg/dl	12	Number of major vessels (0–3) colored by fluoroscopy
6	Fasting blood sugar >120 mg/dl	13	Thal: 3 = normal; 6 = fixed defect and 7 = reversible defect
7	Resting electrocardiographic results (values 0, 1 and 2)		

Table 2. The features of the Hepatitis disease dataset

Feature Number	Feature Description	Values
1	Age	10, 20, 30, 40, 50, 60, 70, 80
2	Sex	Male, Female
3	Steroid	No, Yes
4	Antivirals	No, Yes
5	Fatigue	No, Yes
6	Malaise	No, Yes
7	Anorexia	No, Yes
8	Liver Big	No, Yes
9	Liver Firm	No, Yes
10	Spleen Palpable	No, Yes
11	Spiders	No, Yes
12	Ascites	No, Yes
13	Varices	No, Yes
14	Bilirubin	0.39, 0.80, 1.20, 2.00, 3.00, 4.00
15	Alk Phosphate	33, 80, 120, 160, 200, 250
16	Sgot	13, 100, 200, 300, 400, 500
17	Albumin	2.1, 3.0, 3.8, 4.5, 5.0, 6.0
18	Protime	10, 20, 30, 40, 50, 60, 70, 80, 90
19	Histology	No, Yes

data have been taken from healthy people with no liver disorder. The remaining 145 samples have been obtained from individuals with liver disorder. Five features are blood test results and daily alcohol consumption. Features in the dataset are presented in Table 3.

Table 3. The features of the BUPA liver disorder dataset.

Feature Number	Feature Description	Values
1	MCV (mean corpuscular volume)	Numeric value
2	Alkphos (alkaline phosphatase)	Numeric value
3	SGPT (alanine aminotransferase)	Numeric value
4	SGOT (aspartate aminotransferase)	Numeric value
5	Gamma GT (gamma-glutamyltranspeptidase)	Numeric value
6	Drinks (number of half-pint equivalents of alcoholic beverages drunk per day)	Numeric value

Complex-Valued Radial Basis Function Networks (CVRBF)

CVRBF was first proposed by Chen et al. (1994). Initially, it was applied to a non-linear signal processing, which includes complex signals. After this, it was used in different classification problems which have complex and real-valued input features (Chen et al., 2008; Babu, Suresh & Savitha, 2012; Savitha, Suresh & Sundararajan, 2012). CVRBF is the complex-valued version of the real-valued RBF neural network. It is structurally similar to the RBF neural network except that the parameters are complex-valued here. The CVRBF sample with a single hidden layer is given in Figure 1.

A complex-valued input data can be represented as shown in Equation (1). Here, the input value is composed of real and imaginary values.

$$x^C = x_R + ix_I \quad (1)$$

where i $= \sqrt{-1}$. x^C is the complex input value, x_R is the real value and x_I is the imaginary value. Real-valued feature values in the input layer are normalized between the range of [0, 1] at the initial phase. Normalisation formula has been given in Equation (2).

Figure 1. Structure of the CVRBF classifier

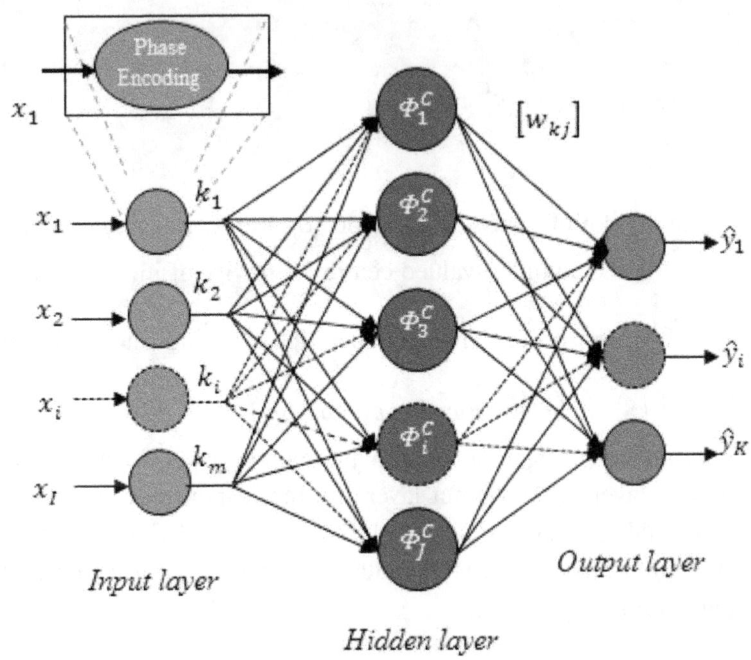

$$x_i^C = \frac{x_i - x_{(min)}}{x_{(max)} - x_{(min)}} \tag{2}$$

where x_i is the input value. $x_{(min)}$ is the minimum and $x_{(max)}$ is the maximum value. At this stage, as can be seen in the attached small picture in Figure 1, normalised values are converted to complex space with phase encoding [0, π] by using the equation '$exp\left(i\pi x\right)$'. The phase encoding method, which assures the conversion of real-valued input values to complex valued number format, has been given in Equation (3).

$$a_i^C = exp\left(i\pi x_i^C\right) \tag{3}$$

where x_i^C is the real-valued input feature normalised between the range of [0, 1]. a_i^C is the complex-valued input feature calculated based on x_i^C.

The example has been given in Figure 1 is a hidden layer with CVRBF structure. The CVRBF has 'j' hidden neurons. These hidden neurons in the hidden layer have a real radially symmetric response around the node centre. The centres of hidden nodes are some of the complex vectors in the input domain. The non-linearity of hidden node is a real function. Equation (4) is used to determine the response of each hidden node.

$$\Phi_j^C = exp\left(-\frac{1}{\sigma_j^2}\left(a_i^C - c_j^C\right)^H\left(a_i^C - c_j^C\right)\right) \tag{4}$$

where σ_j is the width of Gaussian function. a_i^C represents i th complex-valued input vector. c_j^C is the complex-valued centre of gravity of jth Gaussian CVRBF. $\left(\bullet\right)^H = \left(\left(\bullet\right)^T\right)^*$ operator is the Hermitian operation. $\left(\bullet\right)^T$ indicates vector or matrix transpose, while $\left(\bullet\right)^*$ indicates complex conjugate.

The output value of each output neuron is computed as the linear total of weights from the hidden layer to the output layer and the response of each hidden layer neuron. In the study, weights are real-valued in the CVRBF neural network. The response of output neurons is also real-valued. Equation (5) is used for the response of the output neuron.

$$y_k = \sum_{j=1}^{J} w_{kj} \Phi_j^C = \sum_{j=1}^{J} w_{kj} exp\left(-\frac{1}{\sigma_j^2}\left(a_i^C - c_j^C\right)^H \left(a_i^C - c_j^C\right)\right) \tag{5}$$

where w_{kj} is linkage value between k th output neuron and j th hidden neuron. ϕ_j^C is the radial basis function of the j th hidden node.

The error function is given in Equation (6) for CVRBF.

$$e = e_R + ie_I = y^t - \hat{y}^t \tag{6}$$

where e_R and e_I are respectively real and complex components of complex-valued error value e, $\hat{y}^t$ is the calculated output value and y^t is the real output value. In this study, the mean squared error has been used as the error function. The error function is defined as Equation (7).

$$E = \frac{1}{2}\sum_{t=1}^{N}\left(e^{t^H} e^t\right) \tag{7}$$

where H denotes the complex Hermitian operator. To minimise the deviations of the mean squared error, a gradient descent-based learning algorithm has been used. Updating rules based on this learning algorithm are as follows.

$$\Delta v_{kj} = \mu_v e_k y_h^j \,;\; k = 1,2,\ldots,n \,;\; j = 1,2,\ldots,h \tag{8}$$

$$\Delta\sigma_j = \mu_\sigma y_h^j \left[\sum_{k=1}^{n}\left(v_{kj}^R e_k^R + v_{kj}^I e_k^I\right)\right] \cdot \frac{z - c_j^{\;2}}{\sigma_j^3} \tag{9}$$

$$\Delta c_j = \mu_c y_h^j \left[\frac{\sum_{k=1}^{n}\left[v_{kj}^R e_k^R \, re\left(z - c_j\right) + iv_{kj}^I e_k^I \, im\left(z - c_j\right)\right]}{\sigma_j^2}\right] \tag{10}$$

where μ_v, μ_c and μ_σ are, respectively, the learning rate parameters for weight, centre and width of Gaussian function. v_{kj}^R and v_{kj}^I are, respectively, the real and imaginary components of v_{kj} weight value.

Ensemble of CVRBF

When ensemble learning methods are used, a single decision is made for the ensemble by gathering the results revealed by multiple classifiers. These methods put the class estimations made by the many different classifiers through voting. As a result of this voting, the best rated class is then presented as class estimation of the ensemble.

Ensemble learning methods increase the accuracy rate of predictions revealed by basic or singular learning algorithms and, for this reason, they are usually more successful than singular/individual learning methods. Bagging and Boosting are the most known and studied ensemble learning algorithms amongst them (Breiman, 1996; Freund & Schapire, 1997). In this study, these two methods are used for the ensemble version of CVRBF algorithm. The ensemble of CVRBF is named as ^{E}CVRBF.

Bagging is basically a bootstrap ensemble algorithm (Das & Sengur, 2010). The bootstrap element ensures separation during training using copies of a dataset. In other words, it means extracting and using data subsets of the dataset by relocation. Each data subset is used in the training of CVRBF. The trained CVRBFs compose an ensemble. The real result is obtained based on an absolute majority of the results of the algorithm. Bagging is simple but powerful ensemble method recommended for improving the stability and accuracy of learning algorithms (Das, Turkoglu & Sengur, 2009). The pseudo-code for the CVRBF ensemble with the Bagging algorithm is given in Figure 2.

In Boosting, as in Bagging, each CVRBF is trained on a different bootstrap sample. However, in Boosting, the existing CVRBF focuses more on previously misclassified data points. A typical application of the Boosting method is the AdaBoost method (Freund & Schapire, 1997). In the AdaBoost method, classification is usually performed by aggregating CVRBFs via weighted voting with the weight

Figure 2. The bagging algorithm for ^{E}CVRBF

Input	: Training dataset	$D = \{x_i, y_i\}_{i=1}^{N}, y_i \epsilon \{-1,1\}$;
	Base learning model	CVRBF;
	Number of iterations	T;
Process	:	
	For $t = 1,2,\dots,T$;	
	$D_t = Bootstrap(D)$; % Generate a bootstrap sample from D	
	$h_t = CVRBF(D_t)$; % Train a base learner h_t from the bootstrap sample	
	End	
	Compute $H(x) = argmax_{y \epsilon Y} \sum_{t=}^{T} 1\,(y = h_t(x))$; % Majority voting	
Output	: $H(x)$	

in the formula. The pseudo-code for the CVRBF ensemble with Boosting algorithm is given in Figure 3.

The Proposed Method

In the initial step, features were converted into a complex number format using the phase encoding method. The features obtained have been classified by the ensemble of the CVRBF algorithm. The block diagrams of the proposed method based on Bagging and Boosting ensemble learning algorithm are given in Figures 4 and 5, respectively.

EXPERIMENTAL RESULTS AND DISCUSSIONS

All experiments were performed under MATLAB environment using a computer with an Intel(R) Core™ i7-2670QM (2.2 GHz) processor and 8 GB RAM. 10-fold cross-validation method was used for training and testing data. The experiments have been repeated 5 times for the reliability of the results and the averages of obtained results have been reported.

The required parameter values to obtain high efficiency from CVRBF algorithm were found by experimentally. Accordingly, the optimal multi-layer network structures

Figure 3. The boosting algorithm for ^{E}CVRBF

Input : Training dataset $D = \{x_i, y_i\}_{i=1}^{N}, y_i \epsilon \{-1,1\}$;
Base learning model CVRBF;
Number of iterations T;

Process :

$D_1(i) = 1/N$; % Initialize the weight distribution

For $t = 1,2,\ldots,T$;

$h_t = CVRBF(D, D_t)$; % Train a base learner h_t from D using D_t

$\varepsilon_t = \Pr_{i \sim D_i}[h_t(x_i \neq y_i)]$; % Measure the error of h_t

$\sigma_t = \frac{1}{2}\ln\frac{1-\varepsilon_t}{\varepsilon_t}$; % Determine the weight of h_t

$$D_{t+1}(i) = \frac{D_t(i)}{Z_t} x \begin{cases} exp(-\sigma_t)\ if\ h_t(x_i) = y_i \\ \exp(\sigma_t)\ if\ h_t(x_i) \neq y_i \end{cases}$$ % Update the distribution, where

$$= \frac{D_t(i)exp(-\sigma_t y_i h_t(x_i))}{Z_t};$$ % Z_t is a normalization factor which enables $D_t(i)$ to % be a distribution

End

Compute $H(x) = sign(f(x)) = sign \sum_{t=1}^{T} \sigma_t h_t(x)$; % Weighted majority voting

Output : $H(x)$

Figure 4.^{E}CVRBF method with bagging

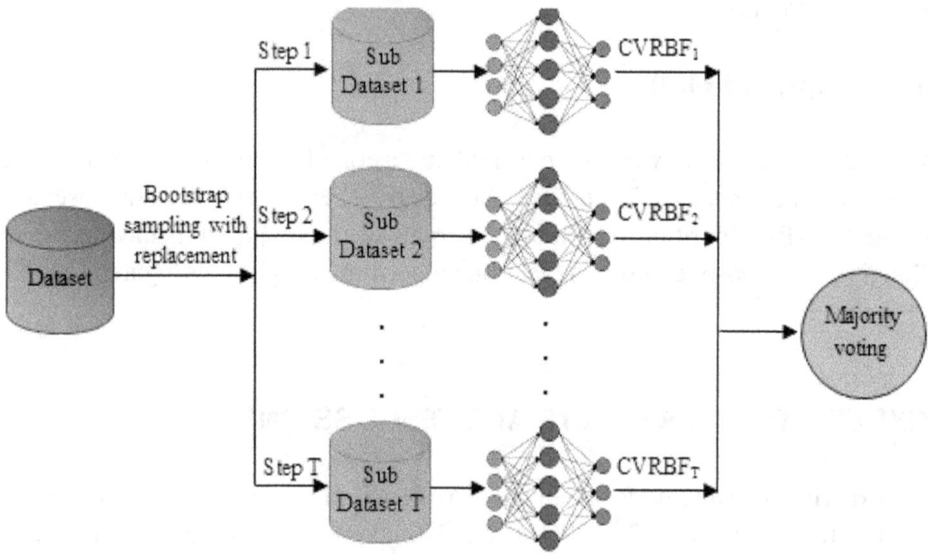

Figure 5. ^{E}CVRBF method with boosting

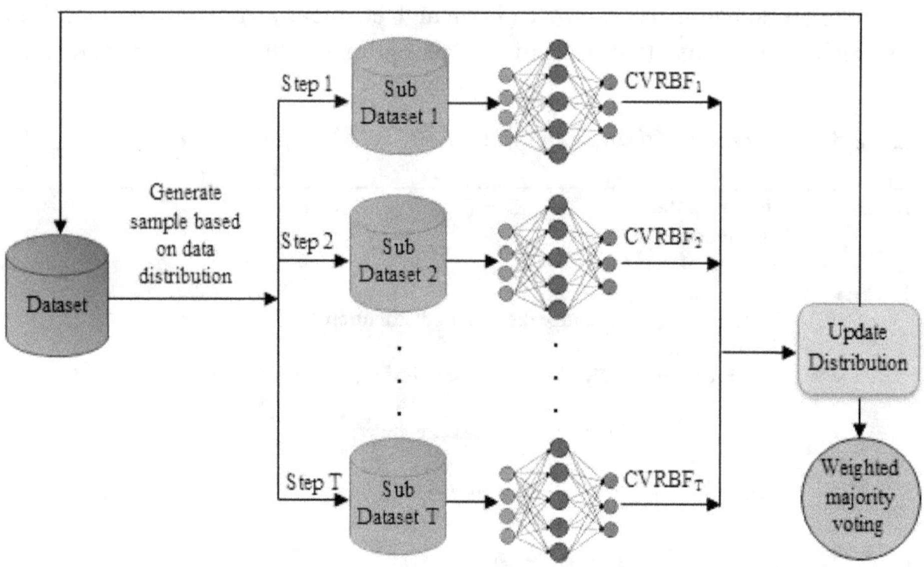

(the number of input-hidden and output neurons) have been determined as 11-10-1, 9-5-1 and 7-10-1 for heart disease, Hepatitis and BUPA liver disorder datasets, respectively. The learning rate during training process has been determined as 0.25, 0.5 and 0.15, respectively. The maximum number of iterations is set to 1000 for all datasets. The real and imaginary parts of the complex-valued weights have been initiated with the random numbers taken from a uniform distribution $\left(\mathrm{U}\left(-0.5, 0.5\right)\right)$. A gauss activation function was used. In the ensemble of CVRBF to select data subsets, a 75% random sample has been selected with a replacement of the original training dataset. That is, if a training dataset consists of 1000 parts, 750 parts will be drawn randomly with a replacement to create a subset.

The success of the ^{E}CVRBF method has been tested using six different performance evaluation criterions. These are accuracy, specificity, sensitivity, f-measure, the area under an ROC curve (AUC), and kappa statistic values. In order to see the effect of the classifiers, comparative analysis has been performed. The results obtained for each dataset are given in Table 4.

Table 4. The comparative analysis of ^{E}RBF and ^{E}CVRBF ensembles with bagging and boosting

Dataset	Performance Metrics	^{E}RBF		^{E}CVRBF	
		Bagging	Boosting	Bagging	Boosting
Heart	ACC	83.33 ± 9.56	80.37 ± 11.45	90.92 ± 4.36	91.11 ± 5.66
	Sensitivity	84.76 ± 9.10	83.44 ± 8.32	91.94 ± 5.52	90.90 ± 4.97
	Specificity	81.51 ± 10.25	89.95 ± 5.20	89.25 ± 5.85	91.37 ± 5.60
	f-measure	0.8203	0.6475	0.9163	0.9210
	Kappa	0.6622	0.6041	0.8128	0.8195
	AUC	0.8810	0.8610	0.9160	0.9670
Hepatitis	ACC	86.45 ± 7.95	87.74 ± 6.35	96.12 ± 3.85	96.77 ± 3.18
	Sensitivity	70.37 ± 12.44	74.07 ± 11.86	96.42 ± 3.25	99.88 ± 0.11
	Specificity	89.84 ± 4.87	90.62 ± 4.22	96.06 ± 3.72	96.09 ± 3.65
	f-measure	0.6440	0.6779	0.9002	0.9152
	Kappa	0.5611	0.6029	0.9364	0.9471
	AUC	0.8610	0.8440	0.9490	0.9500
BUPA liver disorder	ACC	66.08 ± 11.54	65.79 ± 9.23	87.82 ± 6.15	86.95 ± 7.98
	Sensitivity	64.28 ± 14.85	60.46 ± 13.95	88.72 ± 5.87	87.31 ± 6.95
	Specificity	66.80 ± 10.44	68.98 ± 12.76	87.26 ± 6.55	86.72 ± 7.16
	f-measure	0.5185	0.5693	0.8489	0.8387
	Kappa	0.2716	0.2873	0.7473	0.7295
	AUC	0.6790	0.6800	0.9440	0.9430

When the results in Table 4 are examined, we may observe that the ^{E}CVRBF methods give better results in terms of accuracy, sensitivity and specificity values than the ^{E}RBF methods for all three datasets. ^{E}CVRBF method also gives better results in f-measure, AUC, and kappa statistic values, as well. The superiority of the Bagging to the Boosting method can also vary in the ^{E}RBF methods. The standard deviations of ^{E}CVRBF methods are lower than the ^{E}RBF methods, demonstrating that the proposed method is more robust and reliable. In addition, the same results are given graphically in Figures 6-8.

Figures 9-11 shows ROC curves with different methods were incorporated in the evaluation for heart disease dataset, Hepatitis disease dataset and BUPA liver disorder dataset, respectively. In this phase, the number of algorithms for the comparisons are also increased. These methods are: typical CVRBF; ^{E}CVRBF with Bagging; ^{E}CVRBF with Boosting; original dataset + SVM; original dataset + RBF; and original dataset + Decision Tree. When these graphics are examined, we have seen that the best results have been obtained with ^{E}CVRBF method for three different datasets. We have also seen that, with the ^{E}CVRBF algorithm, in some cases better results were obtained with Bagging, while in some cases better results were obtained

Figure 6. The results for the heart disease dataset

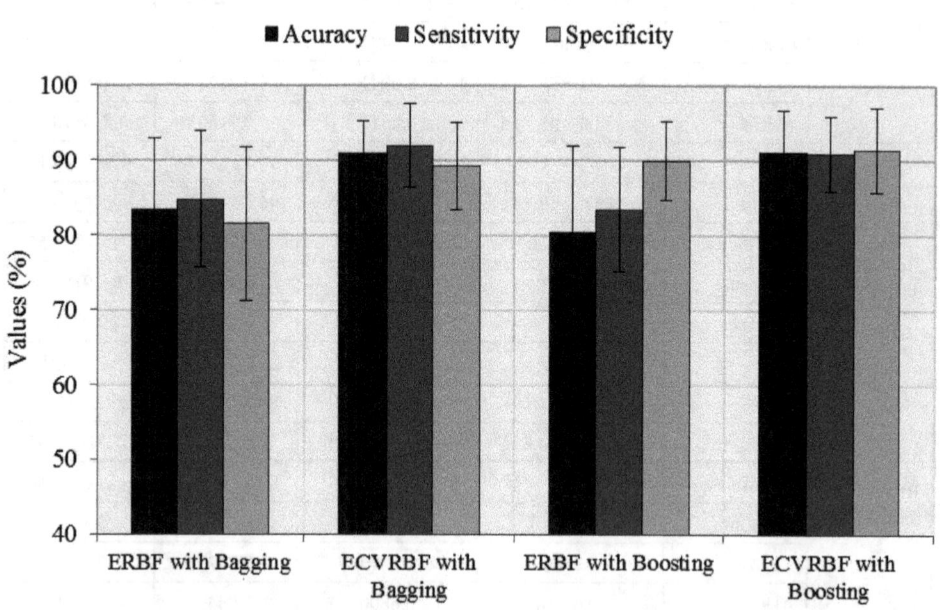

Figure 7. The results for the Hepatitis disease dataset

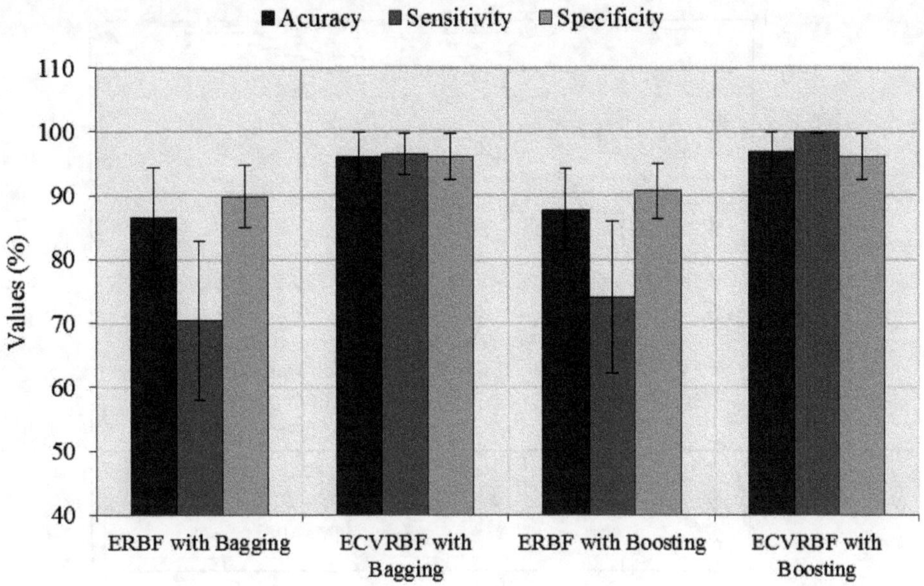

Figure 8. The results for the BUPA liver disorder dataset

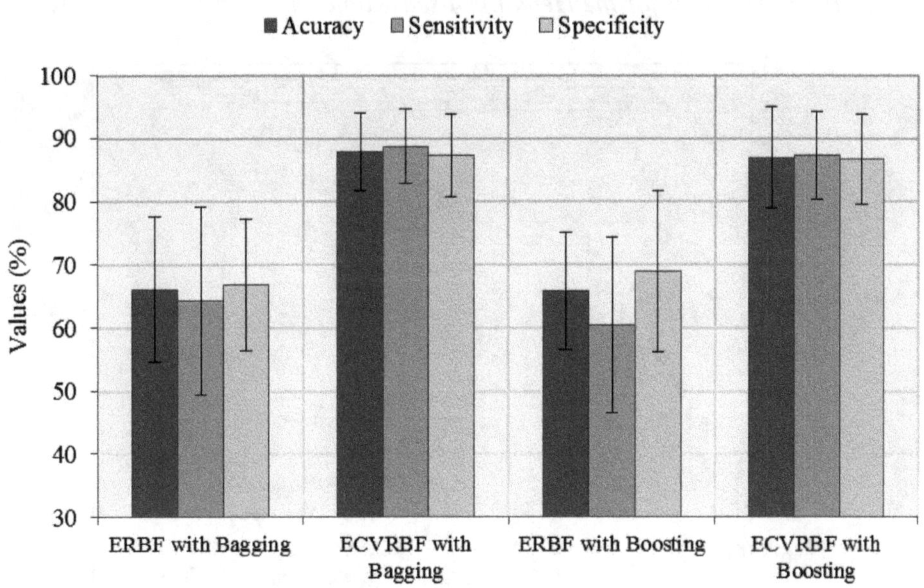

Figure 9. ROC curves for the Statlog heart disease dataset

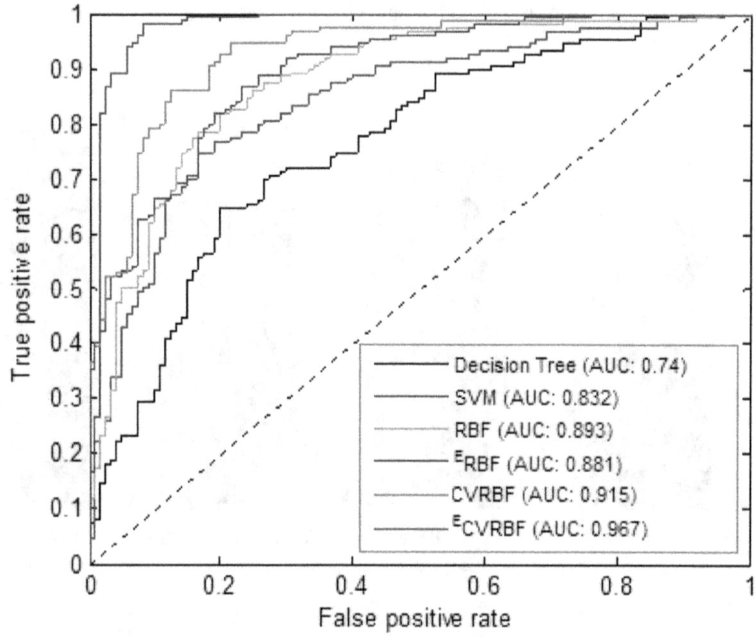

**For a more accurate representation see the electronic version.*

Figure 10. ROC curves for the Hepatitis disease dataset

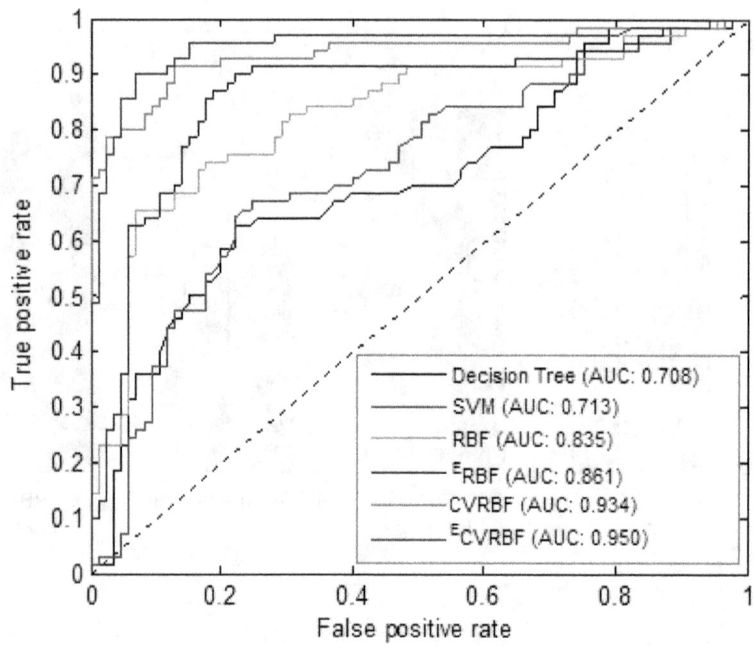

**For a more accurate representation see the electronic version.*

Figure 11. ROC curves for the BUPA liver disorder dataset

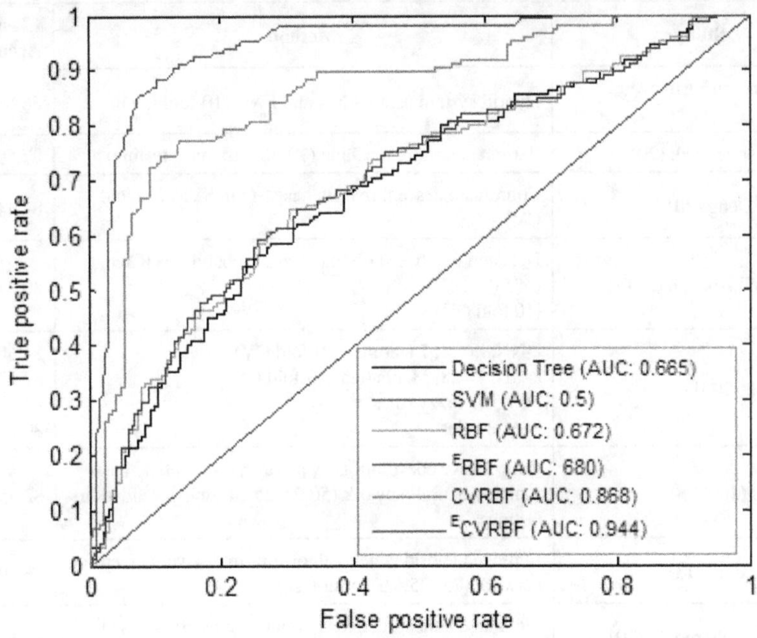

**For a more accurate representation see the electronic version.*

with Boosting. Better results have been obtained with complex valued classifiers, compared to real-valued classifiers. Considering the real-valued classifiers, we have seen that the RBF algorithm is more effective for three datasets.

The performance analysis of the proposed method was then compared with the previous studies from the literature, as listed in Tables 5 to 7. In Table 5, the analysis for the heart disease dataset is given. When the table is examined, we may observe that accuracy values in the range of 80-88% have generally been achieved by other researchers. A 91.11% accuracy rate has been obtained with the developed method for the dataset. In Table 6, the comparative analysis carried out with previous studies for the Hepatitis disease dataset is given. As seen in the table, accuracy values, generally in the range of 79-96%, have been obtained by other researchers. Compared to the other studies, the proposed method has yielded a better result with a 96.77% accuracy value. In Table 7, the comparative analysis for the BUPA liver disorder dataset is given. When we examine the table, we see that an 87.82% classification accuracy has been obtained in this study, while accuracy values in the 60-85% range have generally been obtained by other researchers. In general, the proposed method has provided better results compared to the existing methods from the literature.

Table 5. Performance comparison for the Statlog heart disease dataset

Study	Method	Classification Accuracy (%)
Kahramanli and Allahverdi (2008)	Hybrid system using ANN and FNN (10-fold CV)	86.80
Subbulakshmi et al. (2012)	Extreme learning machine (70-30% training-testing)	87.50
Shao and Deng (2015)	Coordinate descent margin based-twin SVM (10 fold CV)	84.44
Mantas and Abellán (2014)	Decision tree based on imprecise probabilities (Credal C4.5) (10 fold CV)	80.33
Duch et al. (2001)	k-NN, k=28, 7 features (10-fold CV) k-NN, k=28, Manhattan (10-fold CV) FSM, 27 fuzzy rules SSV, 3 rules	84.60–85.60 82.20–83.40 82 80.20–83.40
Tian et al. (2009)	Cooperative coevolutionary algorithm - elliptical basis function neural network (50-25-25% training-validation-testing)	82.45
Ahmad et al. (2013)	Improved hybrid genetic algorithm-multilayer perceptron network (75- 25% training-testing)	86.30
Torun and Tohumoglu (2011)	Simulated annealing and subtractive clustering based fuzzy classifier (10 fold CV)	81.11
Al-Obeidat et al. (2011)	Particle swarm optimization for PROAFT (10 fold CV)	84.27
Jaganathan and Kuppuchamy (2013)	Neural network threshold selection (10 fold CV)	85.19
Lim and Chan (2015)	Bandlerkohout-interval-valued fuzzy sets (BK-IVFS weighted) (5 fold CV)	85.56
Yang et al. (2013)	Fuzzy class – label SVM (y_i - SVM) and Fuzzy SVM (F-SVM)	85.19
Our study	**CVRBF ensemble with Bagging**	**90.92**
Our study	**CVRBF ensemble with Boosting**	**91.11**

CONCLUSION

In this study, ensembles of complex-valued radial basis function networks have been proposed. To investigate the effect of the proposed method, three benchmark medical datasets were used. The common characteristics of these datasets are having a distribution, which cannot be separated linearly and a large amount of missing data. In turn, 91.11%, 96.77% and 87.82% accuracy values were achieved respectively for Statlog heart disease, Hepatitis disease and BUPA liver disorder datasets using

Table 6. Performance comparison for the Hepatitis dataset

Study	Method	Classification Accuracy (%)
Shao et al. (2015)	Weighted linear loss twin support vector machine – 10 fold CV	84.39
Mantas and Abellán (2014)	Decision tree based on imprecise probabilities (Credal C4.5) (10 fold CV)	79.99
Yang et al. (2013)	Fuzzy class – label SVM (y_i - SVM) and Fuzzy SVM (F-SVM)	85.19
De Bock et al. (2010)	Generalized additive models (GAM) ensemble classifiers – 2 fold CV	89.20
Bascil and Oztekin (2012)	Probabilistic Neural Network – 10 fold CV	91.25
Bascil and Temurtas (2011)	Multilayer Neural Network with Levenberg Marquardt Training Algorithm - 10 fold CV	91.87
Moradi and Rostami (2015)	Integration of graph clustering with ant colony optimization (GCACO) and SVM - training set (2/3 of dataset) and test set (1/3 of dataset).	84.52
Pan et al. (2015)	K-nearest neighbor based structural twin support vector machine (KNN-STSVM) – 5 fold CV	87.54
Zhang et al. (2015)	Sparse-response backpropagation algorithm (SRBP) – 10 fold CV	84.25
Our study	**CVRBF ensemble with Bagging**	**96.12**
Our study	**CVRBF ensemble with Boosting**	**96.77**

Table 7. Performance comparison for the BUPA liver disorder dataset

Study	Method	Classification Accuracy (%)
Goncalves et al. (2006)	Inverted hierarchical neuro-fuzzy binary space partitioning system	73.33
Lee and Mangasarian (2001)	Reduced SVMs (10-fold CV)	74.90
Dehuri et al. (2012)	Improved swarm optimized functional link artificial neural network (10-fold CV)	76.80
Shao and Deng (2012)	Coordinate descent margin based-twin SVM (10-fold CV)	72.80
Savitha et al. (2012)	Fully complex valued RBF (10 fold CV)	74.60
Mantas and Abellán(2014)	Decision tree based on imprecise probabilities (Credal C4.5)	64.53
López et al. (2014)	Mahalanobis SVM	72.17
Torun and Tohumoglu (2011)	Simulated annealing and subtractive clustering based fuzzy classifier (10 fold CV)	74.13
Al-Obeidat et al. (2011)	Particle swarm optimization for PROAFT (10 fold CV)	69.31
Yang et al. (2013)	Fuzzy class – label SVM (y_i - SVM) and fuzzy SVM (F-SVM)	74.78
Van Gestel et al. (2002)	SVM with GP (10-fold CV)	69.70
Wang et al. (2014)	Spiking neural networks (SNNs)	56.60
Li et al. (2011)	A fuzzy-based nonlinear transformation method + SVM	70.85
Our study	**CVRBF ensemble with Bagging**	**87.82**
Our study	**CVRBF ensemble with Boosting**	**86.95**

the [E]CVRBF algorithm. The received results in this study are higher than the results obtained in many studies, carried out for the same data in the literature. In an important issue such as medical diagnosis, even a slight increase in classification accuracies is very important. Hence, the method proposed here will contribute significantly to the medical diagnostics. In conclusion, the system can also be used as computer-aided medical diagnosis system to help doctors.

REFERENCES

Ahmad, F., Isa, N. A. M., Hussain, Z., & Osman, M. K. (2013). Intelligent medical disease diagnosis using improved hybrid genetic algorithm-multilayer perceptron network. *Journal of Medical Systems*, *37*(2), 9934. doi:10.100710916-013-9934-7 PMID:23479268

Al-Obeidat, F., Belacel, N., Carretero, J. A., & Mahanti, P. (2011). An evolutionary framework using particle swarm optimization for classification method PROAFTN. *Applied Soft Computing*, *11*(8), 4971–4980. doi:10.1016/j.asoc.2011.06.003

Aldape-Pérez, M., Yáñez-Márquez, C., Camacho-Nieto, O., & Argüelles-Cruz, A. J. (2012). An associative memory approach to medical decision support systems. *Computer Methods and Programs in Biomedicine*, *106*(3), 287–307. doi:10.1016/j.cmpb.2011.05.002 PMID:21703713

Amin, M. F., Islam, M. M., & Murase, K. (2009). Ensemble of single-layered complex-valued neural networks for classification tasks. *Neurocomputing*, *72*(10), 2227–2234. doi:10.1016/j.neucom.2008.12.028

Amin, M. F., & Murase, K. (2009). Single-layered complex-valued neural network for real-valued classification problems. *Neurocomputing*, *72*(4), 945–955. doi:10.1016/j.neucom.2008.04.006

Asuncion, A., & Newman, D. (2007). *UCI machine learning repository*. Academic Press.

Babu, R. V., Suresh, S., & Savitha, R. (2012). Human action recognition using a fast learning fully complex-valued classifier. *Neurocomputing*, *89*, 202–212. doi:10.1016/j.neucom.2012.03.003

Bascil, M. S., & Oztekin, H. (2012). A study on Hepatitis disease diagnosis using probabilistic neural network. *Journal of Medical Systems*, *36*(3), 1603–1606. doi:10.100710916-010-9621-x PMID:21057884

Bascil, M. S., & Temurtas, F. (2011). A study on Hepatitis disease diagnosis using multilayer neural network with levenbergmarquardt training algorithm. *Journal of Medical Systems*, *35*(3), 433–436. doi:10.100710916-009-9378-2 PMID:20703548

Bashir, S., Qamar, U., & Khan, F. H. (2016). IntelliHealth: A medical decision support application using a novel weighted multi-layer classifier ensemble framework. *Journal of Biomedical Informatics*, *59*, 185–200. doi:10.1016/j.jbi.2015.12.001 PMID:26703093

Breiman, L. (1996). Bagging predictors. *Machine Learning*, *24*(2), 123–140. doi:10.1007/BF00058655

Chen, L. F., Su, C. T., Chen, K. H., & Wang, P. C. (2012). Particle swarm optimization for feature selection with application in obstructive sleep apnea diagnosis. *Neural Computing & Applications*, *21*(8), 2087–2096. doi:10.100700521-011-0632-4

Chen, S., Hong, X., Harris, C. J., & Hanzo, L. (2008). Fully complex-valued radial basis function networks: Orthogonal least squares regression and classification. *Neurocomputing*, *71*(16), 3421–3433. doi:10.1016/j.neucom.2007.12.003

Chen, S., McLaughlin, S., & Mulgrew, B. (1994). Complex-valued radial basis function network, Part II: Application to digital communications channel equalisation. *Signal Processing*, *36*(2), 175–188. doi:10.1016/0165-1684(94)90206-2

Cheung, N. (2001). *Machine learning techniques for medical analysis* (Doctoral dissertation). University of Queensland.

Das, R. (2010). A comparison of multiple classification methods for diagnosis of Parkinson disease. *Expert Systems with Applications*, *37*(2), 1568–1572. doi:10.1016/j.eswa.2009.06.040

Das, R., & Sengur, A. (2010). Evaluation of ensemble methods for diagnosing of valvular heart disease. *Expert Systems with Applications*, *37*(7), 5110–5115. doi:10.1016/j.eswa.2009.12.085

Das, R., Turkoglu, I., & Sengur, A. (2009). Diagnosis of valvular heart disease through neural networks ensembles. *Computer Methods and Programs in Biomedicine*, *93*(2), 185–191. doi:10.1016/j.cmpb.2008.09.005 PMID:18951649

De Bock, K. W., Coussement, K., & Van den Poel, D. (2010). Ensemble classification based on generalized additive models. *Computational Statistics & Data Analysis*, *54*(6), 1535–1546. doi:10.1016/j.csda.2009.12.013

Dehuri, S., Roy, R., Cho, S. B., & Ghosh, A. (2012). An improved swarm optimized functional link artificial neural network (ISO-FLANN) for classification. *Journal of Systems and Software*, *85*(6), 1333–1345. doi:10.1016/j.jss.2012.01.025

Duch, W., Adamczak, R., & Grabczewski, K. (2001). A new methodology of extraction, optimization and application of crisp and fuzzy logical rules. *IEEE Transactions on Neural Networks*, *12*(2), 277–306. doi:10.1109/72.914524 PMID:18244384

Freund, Y., & Schapire, R. E. (1995, March).A desicion-theoretic generalization of on-line learning and an application to boosting. In *European conference on computational learning theory* (pp. 23-37). Springer. 10.1007/3-540-59119-2_166

Gonçalves, L. B., Vellasco, M. M. B. R., Pacheco, M. A. C., & de Souza, F. J. (2006). Inverted hierarchical neuro-fuzzy BSP system: A novel neuro-fuzzy model for pattern classification and rule extraction in databases. *IEEE Transactions on Systems, Man and Cybernetics. Part C, Applications and Reviews*, *36*(2), 236–248. doi:10.1109/TSMCC.2004.843220

Jaganathan, P., & Kuppuchamy, R. (2013). A threshold fuzzy entropy based feature selection for medical database classification. *Computers in Biology and Medicine*, *43*(12), 2222–2229. doi:10.1016/j.compbiomed.2013.10.016 PMID:24290939

Jin, B., Tang, Y. C., & Zhang, Y. Q. (2007). Support vector machines with genetic fuzzy feature transformation for biomedical data classification. *Information Sciences*, *177*(2), 476–489. doi:10.1016/j.ins.2006.03.015

Kahramanli, H., & Allahverdi, N. (2008). Design of a hybrid system for the diabetes and heart diseases. *Expert Systems with Applications*, *35*(1), 82–89. doi:10.1016/j.eswa.2007.06.004

Karabulut, E. M., & İbrikçi, T. (2012). Effective diagnosis of coronary artery disease using the rotation forest ensemble method. *Journal of Medical Systems*, *36*(5), 3011–3018. doi:10.100710916-011-9778-y PMID:21912972

Lee, Y. J., & Mangasarian, O. L. (2001). SSVM: A smooth support vector machine for classification. *Computational Optimization and Applications*, *20*(1), 5–22. doi:10.1023/A:1011215321374

Li, D. C., Liu, C. W., & Hu, S. C. (2011). A fuzzy-based data transformation for feature extraction to increase classification performance with small medical data sets. *Artificial Intelligence in Medicine*, *52*(1), 45–52. doi:10.1016/j.artmed.2011.02.001 PMID:21493051

Li, M. B., Huang, G. B., Saratchandran, P., & Sundararajan, N. (2006). Complex-valued growing and pruning RBF neural networks for communication channel equalisation. *IEE Proceedings. Vision Image and Signal Processing*, *153*(4), 411–418. doi:10.1049/ip-vis:20050217

Lim, C. K., & Chan, C. S. (2015). A weighted inference engine based on interval-valued fuzzy relational theory. *Expert Systems with Applications*, *42*(7), 3410–3419. doi:10.1016/j.eswa.2014.12.025

López, F. M., Puertas, S. M., & Arriaza, J. T. (2014). Training of support vector machine with the use of multivariate normalization. *Applied Soft Computing*, *24*, 1105–1111. doi:10.1016/j.asoc.2014.08.020

Mantas, C. J., & Abellán, J. (2014). Credal-C4. 5: Decision tree based on imprecise probabilities to classify noisy data. *Expert Systems with Applications*, *41*(10), 4625–4637. doi:10.1016/j.eswa.2014.01.017

Moradi, P., & Rostami, M. (2015). Integration of graph clustering with ant colony optimization for feature selection. *Knowledge-Based Systems*, *84*, 144–161. doi:10.1016/j.knosys.2015.04.007

Pan, X., Luo, Y., & Xu, Y. (2015). K-nearest neighbor based structural twin support vector machine. *Knowledge-Based Systems*, *88*, 34–44. doi:10.1016/j.knosys.2015.08.009

Peker, M. (2016). An efficient sleep scoring system based on EEG signal using complex-valued machine learning algorithms. *Neurocomputing*, *207*, 165–177. doi:10.1016/j.neucom.2016.04.049

Sartakhti, J. S., Zangooei, M. H., & Mozafari, K. (2012). Hepatitis disease diagnosis using a novel hybrid method based on support vector machine and simulated annealing (SVM-SA). *Computer Methods and Programs in Biomedicine*, *108*(2), 570–579. doi:10.1016/j.cmpb.2011.08.003 PMID:21968203

Savitha, R., Suresh, S., Sundararajan, N., & Kim, H. J. (2012). A fully complex-valued radial basis function classifier for real-valued classification problems. *Neurocomputing*, *78*(1), 104–110. doi:10.1016/j.neucom.2011.05.036

Shao, Y. H., Chen, W. J., Wang, Z., Li, C. N., & Deng, N. Y. (2015). Weighted linear loss twin support vector machine for large-scale classification. *Knowledge-Based Systems*, *73*, 276–288. doi:10.1016/j.knosys.2014.10.011

Shao, Y. H., & Deng, N. Y. (2012). A coordinate descent margin based-twin support vector machine for classification. *Neural Networks*, *25*, 114–121. doi:10.1016/j.neunet.2011.08.003 PMID:21890319

Subbulakshmi, C. V., Deepa, S. N., & Malathi, N. (2012, August).Extreme learning machine for two category data classification. In *Advanced Communication Control and Computing Technologies (ICACCCT), 2012 IEEE International Conference on* (pp. 458-461). IEEE. 10.1109/ICACCCT.2012.6320822

Tian, J., Li, M., & Chen, F. (2009). A hybrid classification algorithm based on coevolutionary EBFNN and domain covering method. *Neural Computing & Applications*, *18*(3), 293–308. doi:10.100700521-008-0182-6

Torun, Y., & Tohumoğlu, G. (2011). Designing simulated annealing and subtractive clustering based fuzzy classifier. *Applied Soft Computing*, *11*(2), 2193–2201. doi:10.1016/j.asoc.2010.07.020

Van Gestel, T., Suykens, J. A., Lanckriet, G., Lambrechts, A., De Moor, B., & Vandewalle, J. (2002). Bayesian framework for least-squares support vector machine classifiers, Gaussian processes, and kernel Fisher discriminant analysis. *Neural Computation*, *14*(5), 1115–1147. doi:10.1162/089976602753633411 PMID:11972910

Wang, J., Belatreche, A., Maguire, L., & Mcginnity, T. M. (2014). An online supervised learning method for spiking neural networks with adaptive structure. *Neurocomputing*, *144*, 526–536. doi:10.1016/j.neucom.2014.04.017

Yang, C. Y., Chou, J. J., & Lian, F. L. (2013). Robust classifier learning with fuzzy class labels for large-margin support vector machines. *Neurocomputing*, *99*, 1–14. doi:10.1016/j.neucom.2012.04.009

Zhang, J., Ji, N., Liu, J., Pan, J., & Meng, D. (2015). Enhancing performance of the backpropagation algorithm via sparse response regularization. *Neurocomputing*, *153*, 20–40. doi:10.1016/j.neucom.2014.11.055

KEY TERMS AND DEFINITIONS

Classification: It is a kind of supervised machine learning in which an algorithm "learns" to classify novel observations from samples of labeled data.

Complex-Valued Neural Network: It is a variety of neural network and its parameters such as input, output, weight, and bias values consist of complex numbers.

Decision Support System: It is a computer-based information system that supports organizational or business decision-making activities.

Ensemble Methods: It is a set of classifiers whose individual decisions are integrated in some way to classify novel examples.

Machine Learning: It is the notion that a computer program can learn and adapt to novel data without human interference.

Medical Diagnosis: It is a classification operation including the decision-making process based on available medical data.

ROC Curve: It is a graphical method which assess the success of a binary classifier system.

Chapter 3
A Novel Kernel-Based Fuzzy Clustering Approach to Identify Masses in Mammograms

Arnab Chattaraj
University of Calcutta, India

Arpita Das
University of Calcutta, India

ABSTRACT

Detection of breast cancer in form of masses at initial stage becomes difficult because of obscured nature of mammograms by surrounding tissues. This poor visibility of masses addresses to the necessity of accurate contrast enhancement method. This study introduces a novel kernel-based fuzzy clustering approach to enhance the contrast of masses. Novelty of the proposed technique is incorporation of two important features of mammograms that convey the properties of masses. Local entropy and intensity mean of each kernel position play the key role to enhance masses. A kernel is moved across the mammograms to collect all possible values of those features, and hence, they are exploited as the input data of fuzzy clustering technique. Performance of the proposed approach is compared with two other conventional contrast enhancement techniques. Both subjective and objective evaluations of the proposed technique show an evidence of improvement in compare to other methods. Moreover, unwanted enhancement of obscured tissues is also suppressed in the proposed approach.

DOI: 10.4018/978-1-5225-5149-2.ch003

INTRODUCTION

Cancer is considered to be a major public health problem in the world, specifically in the developed countries. It refers to the uncontrolled multiplication of a group of cells in a particular location of the body (Schulz, 2007). For years, it has become one of the large threats to human life and it is expected to become the leading cause of death over the next few years also (WHO, 2009). According to the data from the World Health Organization (WHO), cancer accounts for 13% of all deaths in the world in recent time and deaths due to this disease are expected to increase in the future—with an estimation of 12 million people dying from cancer in 2030 (Sampat et al., 2003). Cancer is potentially fatal disease caused by different environmental factors which mutate genes encoding critical cell proteins (Malcolm, 2001). A group of these rapidly dividing cells may form a lump, micro-calcifications or architectural distortions which are usually referred to as tumors. In cancer cells the normal control systems that prevent cell overgrowth and the invasion of other tissues, are disabled. These things change normal cell division and growth procedure. Physical changes occur due to the effect of cancer and its treatment may include-

- Loss of body parts, physical stamina, hair, weight.
- Swelling of the face, arms, or other parts of body.
- Skin change, including rashes and burns.
- Decrease of physical skills, including athletic abilities, balance, and agility etc (Cueva, 2006).

Among different types of cancers, Breast Cancer is a major concern among women even men also. It is a form of benign/malignant tumor which develops from breast cells (Akay, 2009) and now it is becoming a leading cancer-related death among the women. Primary prevention of this cancer seems to be impossible since the actual causes of this disease still remain unknown. However, treatment of breast cancer in early stages is more successful; so early detection is an essential step to improve breast cancer prognosis and also to significantly reduce the mortality rate. In recent days, though a lot of advanced imaging techniques exist: including MRI, Ultrasound imaging, Positron Emission Tomography (PET) imaging, Computerized Tomography (CT) imaging, Optical Tomography/ Spectroscopy etc. Among them, Mammography is considered to be one of the best radiological screening methods for early detection of Breast Cancer (Haus et al., 1993).

Basically most important symptoms of this disease are masses and microcalcifications – which are generally different types of tumors. Spatial resolution obtained from mammography is capable of indicating any architectural distortion of the breast as well as early stage presence of masses or microcalcifications in the breast.

However, visibility of mammographic features is very poor in the mammograms. In the fatty breast, contrast of masses is very poor due to low absorption of x-ray. Sometimes presence of masses is obscured by the surrounding glandular tissues and fatty breast cells which may mislead the radiologists to detect breast cancer in early stage (Pal et al., 1981). Moreover, ambiguous nature of mass shape, size, margin, location and orientation in the mammograms also provide wrong interpretation to the radiologists (Thangavel, 1998). Hence, it is obvious that the computer assisted enhancement of mammograms produces immense importance to the radiologists and is a crucial step for automatic mammographic image analysis.

The principal objective of any image contrast enhancement technique is to improve image quality for either an automated CAD (Computer Aided Diagnosis) framework (such as- to improve subsequent image segmentation and feature extraction processes) or for manual reading (Suckling et al., 1994). Moreover, enhancement of mammographic features is a bottle neck of CAD system design which analyzes the mammograms using specific algorithms and provides a second reviewing option (Sahiner, 2001). Though CAD based analysis of mammograms has been studied over the last few years, accurate detection of suspected area or stage of the disease still remains difficult. The major reasons for this problem are mainly variable shape, size and distribution of masses which lead to potential misidentification (Jain, 2013). Presence of dense tissues in the breast, especially in younger women also reduces the contrast of suspicious regions and their surrounding tissues and hence yields a high false-positive (FP) rate in detection. Therefor to improve the visual quality of mammographic features, image enhancement is a major step for CAD based analysis of mammograms (Cheng, 1998). It may be performed by emphasizing the required image features and suppressing the noises so that the processed mammograms become more useful for detecting the masses accurately.

Much research has been done yet to discover different kind of contrast enhancement techniques to identify the suspicious regions of affected mammograms. But it has been proved in different application areas that no single image enhancement technique is the dominant/permanent solution for all types of mammographic images. However, there are also some shortcomings in these different techniques for which these techniques are unable to resolve the slight differences between normal and affected regions of mammograms. So development of a new image enhancement approach for improving the contrast of affected mammograms is of course a real challenging work.

In our proposed approach, main objective is to explore a novel Kernel based Fuzzy Clustering approach for image enhancement purpose, where this method is able to dissolve the uncertainties and vagueness present in mammograms. The slim differences between normal and suspicious regions are well captured by the proposed kernel based fuzzy c-mean clustering technique in which *entropy* and *intensity mean* of the kernels are exploited as the inputs of fcm technique. Since these two parameters are able to carry the significant differences between normal breast tissues and obscured mass regions, proposed enhancement technique is able to resolve the above-mentioned problems and achieve a result up to the mark even for analysis of difficult to diagnose masses. Moreover, it is possible to identify the accurate position, shape, size and margins of the obscured masses very clearly by using the proposed enhancement approach. In this study to describe the novelty of the proposed kernel based fcm technique, mammograms are taken as the only inputs, no other prior information or land marking is required. This computer assisted advanced procedure of contrast enhancement for difficult to diagnose mammograms has also received great attention because of its speed, consistency and robustness.

The rest of the paper is arranged as follows. Section 2 describes background of previous enhancement methods. Motivation of the proposed enhancement method is described in section 3. Section 4 describes each step of the proposed enhancement method. In section 5 different enhancement performance evaluating parameters are described thoroughly. Experimental results are given in section 6 and we have drawn some conclusions in section 7. Future direction of research and acknowledgement are included in section 8 and section 9 respectively.

BACKGROUND

A large number of researchers have already used a variety of contrast enhancement techniques to identify the suspicious regions and achieved great breakthroughs. But, due to different shortcomings in all those approaches, none of them become the ideal method for mammographic image enhancement. Conventional methods based on histogram equalization, is a commonly used contrast enhancement technique. In this method, every pixel of image is replaced by the integral of the histogram of the image in that pixel (Baert et al., 2010). This method makes the density distribution of the resultant image flat and thereby enhances the contrast of the image. Histogram equalization has an effect of stretching the dynamic range of the image. But this method has few drawbacks - it changes the original brightness of the input image which effects on deterioration of visual quality and introduction of annoying artifacts of input image.

Adaptive neighborhood contrast enhancement (ANCE) is another conventional image enhancement method to improve the medical image quality (Thangavel et al., 2005). This is an automatic method, which starts its operation with each image pixel to be processed, considering as a seed. This method adapts the size of the pixel neighborhood to the local properties. The nearest neighbors are usually 4-connected or 8-connected. These are checked to verify whether the gray values of those neighbor pixels are within a specified range from the seed gray level value or not. A local region - called the foreground, is thus generated around the seed pixel. Another region - called the background - consists of those neighborhood pixels that are outside the range of a specified gray-level deviation is also generated. The background, which surrounds the foreground, contains nearly the same number of pixels as the foreground. Only regions with low contrast are enhanced, while the high-contrast regions remain unchanged. However, this method has also drawback. The performance of the ANCE method largely depends on how to determine the parameters used in the processing steps. However, this method may enhance noise and digitization effect, for a small neighborhood, and may lose the details, for a large neighborhood. For this, this method cannot be used for all difficult type mammograms. However, the choice of the neighborhoods is not trivial, and often varies from one area of the image to another.

Morphology based mammographic image enhancement is an earlier choice, where this enhancement is done using different combinations of mathematical morphological operators- Erosion, Dilation, Opening & Closing (Gonzalez et al., 2002). These operators enhance the image by different operations like:

1. Deceasing or increasing the size of objects in binary format,
2. Smoothing the object edges,
3. Joining narrow breaks,
4. Filling small holes with the help of structuring element (SE).

But this method does not work properly in difficult type mammograms. For this, it is not a better choice. Adaptive gray level stretching (Peng et al., 2008) is an image enhancement process where it improves an image contrast, by stretching the range of intensity values uniformly. It expands the full intensity range of the recording medium. This is one type of global contrast enhancement process. For digital image processing local contrast enhancement is more suitable to detect slight abnormal changes in mammographic images – so recently this method is not widely used in digital mammography. Apart from intensity based traditional methods, wavelet-based techniques have also been used for enhancement of mammograms (Yang, 2006; Laine et al., 1995; Tang et al., 2009). Recently some advancements in wavelet theory make it able to produce satisfactory results. Tang et al (2009) have proposed an image enhancement algorithm in multi-scale wavelet domain, which improves the features of masses and calcifications in mammograms with acceptable accuracy.

Though in last few decades many new and challenging methods of image enhancement are introduced, all these enhancement processes are unable to highlight the little changes between normal and affected regions of mammograms which are basically difficult to study. Another major challenge of mammographic image enhancement is the removal of unwanted enhancement of irrelevant breast tissues. In this view, we have proposed a new kernel based fuzzy clustering approach of enhancement to overcome those shortcomings with a level of satisfaction.

MOTIVATION OF THE WORK

Like other domains of image processing, contrast enhancement is a relevant prior step for mammographic image analysis. It has been previously mentioned that mammographic images have some degree of fuzziness like - inhomogeneous background, low contrast, indistinct borders, small and irregular shapes, varying intensities of the suspicious regions etc. However, due to such fuzziness of mammographic images, when previous mentioned approaches of image enhancement are applied to various difficult to diagnose mammograms, either result in under-enhancement or over-enhancement which may lead false-negatives (FNs) or false-positives (FPs) cases respectively (Cheng et al., 2002). For this reason, our objective is to explore a new and advanced fuzzy clustering based enhancement approach which is able to capture the little uncertainties and vagueness remaining in mammograms. We have compared this new method with two other conventional methods also:

1. Histogram Equalization (HE) method and
2. Conventional Fuzzy intensity based enhancement approach.

In Histogram Equalization (HE) method, intensity value of each image pixel is changed to its integral of the histogram of that pixel and it makes the intensity distribution of the output image flat – by this it enhances the contrast of the image (Shivaramakrishna et al., 2000). Due to some drawbacks - it fades the actual contrast of the input mammogram for which output image has deterioration in visual quality. For this cause, this method is not a better one to enhance such difficult types of mammographic image. For the last few years, many researchers have investigated fuzzy logic methods for enhancing and detecting the suspected regions of mammograms. A novel fuzzy logic based contrast enhancement method was reported in Das et al., (2011) to overcome the false positive rates in detection procedure. Due to the presence of mass-like dense glandular tissues and variable shapes, sizes of masses, uncertainties are introduced to identify the accurate gradation of masses. Hence it is a good way to use fuzzy approaches to resolve those uncertainties in mammograms. Das et al (2008) also developed a fuzzy logic based contrast enhancement method to enhance mammograms using entropy as an image feature. In another study, Chuang et al. (2006) enhanced mammograms using image contrast feature as the input one of the fuzzy logic method. However, in dense mammograms, especially in younger women, this simple fuzzy logic based enhancement method is unable to resolve the problem of uncertainties. Also there are some possibilities of enhancement of irrelevant breast tissues.

PROPOSED TECHNIQUE

To achieve better response from difficult to diagnose mammograms, we have introduced a novel enhancement technique based on advanced fuzzy clustering approach. A typical overview of the proposed enhancement technique is given in Figure 1.

Each block of the above diagram is discussed in the following section —

Input Image

We have applied our proposed methodology to a variety of difficult mammographic images taken from *BIRADS* (Breast Imaging-Reporting & Data System) and *MIAS* databases (Mammographic Image Analysis Society). BI-RADS are a quality assurance tool mainly designed for study, research and use with Mammography. The system is a collaborative effort of many health groups but this is published and trademarked only by the American College of Radiology (2003). The system is mainly used by medical professionals to communicate a patient's risk for developing Breast Cancer. Similarly the Mammographic Image Analysis Society (MIAS) is an organization of UK research groups interested only in the understanding of mammograms and it has produced a large database of digital mammograms (Houssam et al., 2009).

Figure 1. Overview of the proposed approach

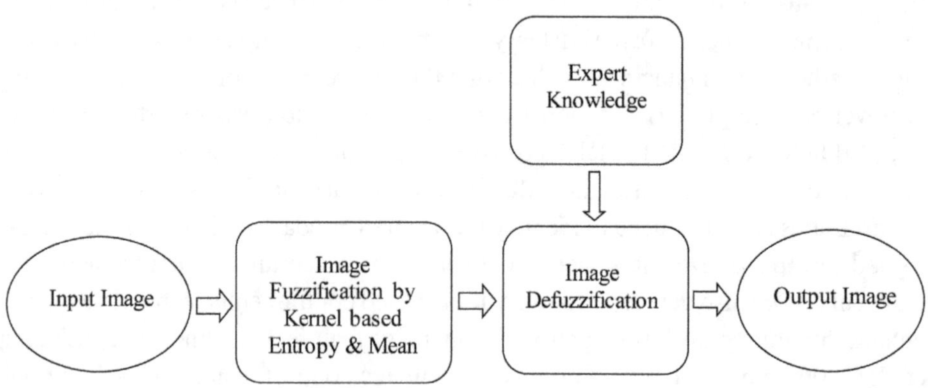

Image Fuzzification by Kernel Based Local Entropy and Mean

Fuzzy Logic Approach

Fuzzy logic is a form of many-valued logic or probabilistic logic which deals with approximate (rather than fixed and exact) reasoning. It has been extended to handle the concept of partial truth, where the truth value may range between completely true and completely false (Kumar et al., 2008). It is basically a control system where the main idea is to associate a number with each object indicating the degree to which it belongs into a special class of objects. A fuzzy logic system works on the principle of assigning a particular output depending on the probability of the state of the input. Recently this Fuzzy logic has become a better option for various control system applications since it minimizes human control. It does not require precise inputs, is inherently robust, and can process any reasonable number of inputs (Tizhoosh et al., 2000). The concept of fuzzy logic was first brought forward in 1965 in the proposal of Fuzzy Set Theory by Lotfi A. Zadeh (1965), where the concept of Fuzzy Set is given as, Let X is a space of points, where the generic elements of X are denoted by x. That is $X = \{x\}$.Fuzzy set, $\tilde{A}$ in X is generally defined by Membership Function, $\mu(x)$. This Membership Function maps each point in X in the interval [0, 1]. Now the value of this Membership Function, $\mu(x)$ at x, represents the "Degree of Membership" of x in the fuzzy set $\tilde{A}$. Here large value of Membership Function, $\mu(x)$ represents the high degree of the membership.

Conventional Fuzzy-C- Mean (FCM) Clustering Algorithm

Fuzzy C-means (FCM) clustering algorithm is one type of fuzzy clustering method which is based on the minimization of a quadratic criterion. Here clusters are represented by their respective centers. Main work of this algorithm is grouping the objects into different clusters. FCM algorithm was first proposed by Dunn in 1973 and improved by Bezdek (1981). According to the above working principle, FCM partitions a collection of n data, $X= \{x_1,\ldots,x_j,\ldots x_n\}$ into c number of fuzzy groups, and finds a cluster center in each group such that an objective function of dissimilarity measure is minimized. This objective function is minimized when large membership values are assigned to the input data patterns which are closer to their nearest cluster centers and low membership values are assigned when they are far from the centers of cluster. Objects within a given cluster have a high degree of similarity and objects within different clusters have a high degree of dissimilarity - based on these criteria FCM employs fuzzy partitioning, where a given data point can belong to different groups with the degree of belongingness specified by membership grads between [0, 1]. To suit this, membership matrix U (U is a real $c \times n$ matrix, $U = [u_{ij}]$, $i = 1$,

2…..c; j = 1, 2…..n) is allowed to have elements with values in the range [0, 1]. By giving normalization condition that the summation of degrees of belongingness for a given data set should be equal to one (Bezdek et al., 1984), given as

$$\sum_{i=1}^{c} u_{ij} = 1 \forall_j = 1, \ldots\ldots, n \tag{1}$$

where c = number of clusters [$2 \leq c < n$]

The objective function for FCM is defined in terms of the cluster centers (c_i) by the formula

$$J(U,c) = \sum_{i=1}^{c} J_i = \sum_{i=1}^{c} \sum_{j=1}^{n} u_{ij}^{m} d_{ij}^{2} \tag{2}$$

where, u_{ij} has the value in between 0 to 1, $c = (c1, c2\ldots\ldots, ci\ldots.cc)$ = vector of centers, c_i is the cluster center of fuzzy group i,$d_{ij} = \| c_i - x_j \|$ is the Euclidean distance, which determines the distance between i-th cluster center and j-th data point. It is a weighting exponent, this controls the relative weights placed on each of the squared errors d_{ij}^{2}. At $m = 1$, fuzzy c-means partitions act as hard c-means partitions. Conversely, the objective function, J approaches to inverse of cluster number (1/c) as $m \rightarrow \alpha$. Consequently increasing m tends to degrade membership towards the fuzziest state. However, no theoretical or computational evidence determines an optimal value. It has been investigated that for most data $1.5 < m < 3.0$ gives better result. In this connection we have chosen $m = 2$. Optimal fuzzy clustering of X is defined as pairs that locally minimize the objective function J. For $m > 1$, if for all j and k, may be locally optimal for J only if

$$\hat{c}_i = \frac{\sum_{j=1}^{n} \hat{u}_{ij}^{m} x_j}{\sum_{j=1}^{n} \hat{u}_{ij}^{m}} \tag{3}$$

$$\hat{u}_{ij} = \frac{1}{\sum_{k=1}^{c} \left(\frac{\hat{d}_{ij}}{\hat{d}_{kj}} \right)^{2/(m-1)}} \tag{4}$$

where, $\| \hat{c}_i - x_j \|$

Conditions expressed in equations (3) and (4) are necessary, but not sufficient; they provide important image features for improving J via simple Picard iteration, by looping back and forth from equation (3) to (4) until the iterative sequence shows small changes in successive entries.

We may explain the generalized procedure of FCM technique as follows —

1. The membership matrix $U = [u_{ij}]$ is initialized with random values in between 0 and 1 so that the constraints of eq^n-(1) are satisfied.
2. Next fuzzy cluster centers c_i (i =1, 2,…, c) are calculated using eq^n (3).
3. The objective function is computed according to eq^n (2). Computation is stopped whether improvement of this objective function over previous iteration is below a given threshold value.
4. Next a new membership matrix $\hat{U} = [\hat{u}_{ij}]$ is calculated using equation (4) and again step-2 is repeated.

Proposed Kernel Based Fuzzy Clustering Technique for Image Enhancement

It is already well known to all that fuzzy logic approach is a gradual, smooth transition characterized by membership functions. These functions model the uncertainties and impreciseness present in the nature. In this view, fuzzy logic based clustering approach is well suited in mammographic image enhancement where randomness of image features are captured and resolved accurately. Proposed Fuzzy clustering technique is a novel and advanced enhancement approach which incorporates two significant features of mammograms and used them for generation of membership functions. This image enhancement procedure is based on gray level intensity and entropy mapping of original image into a fuzzy plane, using one or more membership functions (MFs). The aim is to generate a processed image of higher contrast than the original image. In this image enhancement technique, a fixed 3×3 kernel is moved along the entire mammograms and the entropy and intensity mean of each kernel location are examined carefully. Masses in the mammograms containing specific entropy and intensity values must occupy a particular gradation of membership function which will be identified and captured as a target value. This is the novelty of proposed kernel based FCM clustering technique.

Since the presence of masses in mammograms is generally obscured by the surrounding tissues, the vague boundary between the masses and normal region can be expressed by the degree of membership functions. Proposed kernel based local entropy and intensity mean are capable to resolve those haziness of masses.

In this study simultaneous choice of two significant features of mammograms with a proper mixing ratio, improves the contrast of masses even in difficult to diagnose mammograms with a level of satisfaction. Moreover, considering local entropy and intensity mean of each kernel location reduces the unwanted enhancement of irrelevant breast tissues. During fuzzification step, we have found experimentally that there are some deviations in normal breast region and affected mass region of mammograms, which may be accurately enhanced and evaluated by using kernel based local entropy and intensity mean values simultaneously. Experimental study also shows that choice of any one of these two features is unable to enhance the mammograms accurately. Figure 2 describes this notion more clearly —

From the Figure 2 (b) we have found that kernel based local entropy feature prescribes some of the normal breast tissues as affected regions, Figure 2(c) also exhibits some over-enhancement during intensity mean based fuzzification. However,

Figure 2. (a) Original mammogram, (b) Enhanced image by using local 'entropy' based fuzzification, (c) Enhanced image by using local 'intensity mean' based fuzzification, (d) Enhanced image by the proposed method

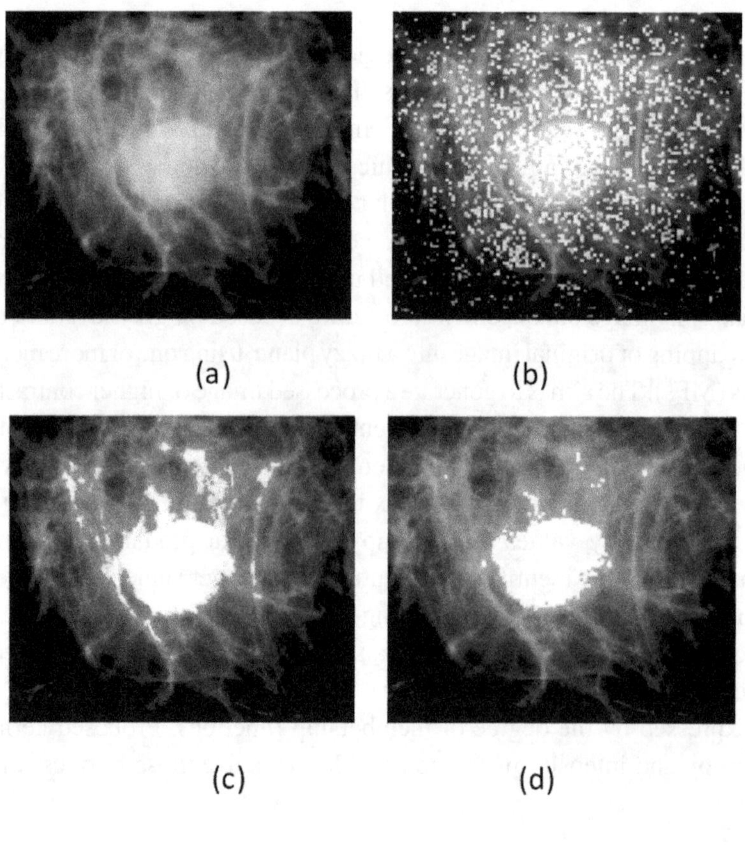

when the proposed enhancement approach (Figure 2(d)) incorporates both features with a proper ratio, affected mass is enhanced with better accuracy.

Image Defuzzification

Image Defuzzification is decoding of resulting enhanced image after image fuzzification, to obtain the output image for clear human perception. This is a process, where membership values are mapped from fuzzy plane to image pixel plane to identify the selected 'ROI's.

Expert Knowledge

We have described that two important feature values of mammograms are taken locally for fuzzification step. These two local features are collected by placing the appropriate size of kernel in the mammograms. The shape, size of the kernel is determined by exploiting the expert knowledge. Beside this, the number of required clusters during fuzzification step and proper combination ratio of two features of the kernel are also determined by the expert knowledge to achieve the best experimental results for the present dataset.

Performance Analysis and Evaluation of the Proposed Enhancement Approach

Performance of the proposed methodology is evaluated subjectively by the expert radiologists and objective evaluation is made by some quantitative measuring parameters used in image enhancement techniques. However, image quality measure has become crucial for most of the image processing techniques. The most difficult situation in image enhancement is to measure the evaluation criteria for enhancement (Li et al., 1997). Basically, it is really a tough work to determine the level of enhancement by only depending upon human visual perception. If the enhanced image can make the suspected region of interest (ROI) better for understand by the expert radiologists, then only we may say that the original image has been improved - this judgment is subjective. However, when some crucial decision is to be taken from the enhanced image, some quantitative measurement must be required to quantify the degree of enhancement. In the present study, we have used contrast improvement index, average signal to noise ratio, peak signal to noise ratio, distribution separation measure and target to background contrast enhancement as quantitative measurement parameters. The significance of these objective parameters in enhancement evaluation is described below.

Contrast Improvement Index (CII)

Contrast improvement index (*CII*) is known as the quantitative measure of a contrast enhancement algorithm. This is defined as the ratio of the contrast of processed image to the contrast of original image. This can be written by following equation no (5) —

$$CII = \frac{C_{processed}}{C_{original}} \tag{5}$$

where $C_{processed}$ is the contrast of suspected ROI in the processed image, $C_{original}$ is the contrast of suspected ROI in the original image. Now the contrast *C* of any region can be defined by the equation no (6) —

$$C = \frac{f - b}{f + b} \tag{6}$$

where *f* is mean gray-level value of the foreground region of the image, *b* is mean gray-level value of surrounding region, called background of the image. A higher value of *CII* indicates a better image enhancement performance, because in that case contrast of the processed image is higher than the contrast of the original image, which can be mathematically expressed as - $C_{processed} > C_{original}$, and this is our main aim.

Average Signal to Noise Ratio (ASNR)

ASNR is an important quantitative measuring parameter for evaluation of image enhancement performance. This *ASNR* can be defined as the ratio of difference of mean gray level value of foreground portion and background portion of the image to the standard deviation of the background portion of image. This can be written by the following equation no (7) —

$$ASNR = \frac{f - b}{\sigma} \tag{7}$$

where *f* is mean gray-level value of the foreground region of the image, *b* is mean gray-level value of surrounding region, called background of the image, σ is the standard deviation of the background portion of image.

Peak Signal to Noise Ratio (PSNR)

Similarly *PSNR* is another important quantitative measuring parameter for evaluation of image enhancement performance. *PSNR* is defined as the ratio of difference of maximum gray-level value of foreground portion and mean gray-level value of background portion of the image to the standard deviation of the background portion of image which can be written by the following equation no (8) —

$$PSNR = \frac{p - b}{\sigma} \tag{8}$$

Here p is the maximum gray-level value of the foreground and σ is standard deviation of the background portion of image. The standard deviation can be described as by the following equation no (9) —

$$\sigma = \sqrt{\frac{1}{N}\sum_{i=1}^{N}(b_i - b)^2} \tag{9}$$

where b_i is gray-level value of the surrounding background region, and N is total number of pixels in the surrounding background region. Basically the values of these two parameters, *ASNR* & *PSNR* get larger; the enhancement performance becomes much better.

Distribution Separation Measure (DSM)

Distribution Separation Measure (DSM) is a quantitative measure, based on the probability density function (PDF) of the target and the background regions of mammogram, before and after enhancement respectively [i, j]. It is a measure of quality of the enhancement process. The expression of DSM is defined as by the equation no (10) —

$$DSM = \left(|\mu_T^E - \mu_B^E| \right) - \left(|\mu_T^O - \mu_B^O| \right) \tag{10}$$

where, μ_T^O, μ_B^O are mean value of target region and background region of original mammographic image respectively. Similarly, μ_T^E, μ_B^E are mean value of target region and background region of enhanced mammographic image. A good enhancement technique must provide a positive *DSM* value. Higher value of *DSM* provides better separation between the distributions of target and background regions of mammograms and for this the performance of the enhancement technique becomes much better.

Target to Background Contrast Enhancement Based on Standard Deviation (TBC_s)

Objective of any image enhancement process is to enhance the intensity difference between background and target region of mammogram and also to ensure that the homogeneity of the target mass is increased aiding the visualization of its boundaries and location.

TBC_s is such type of measuring parameter which can measure this improvement of enhancement technique with the help of the ratio of standard deviation of the target region before and after the enhancement respectively.

The expression of TBC_s is given as by following equation no (11) —

$$TBC_S = \frac{\left(\mu_T^E / \mu_B^E\right) - \left(\mu_T^O / \mu_B^O\right)}{\sigma_T^E / \sigma_T^O} \tag{11}$$

where σ_T^O is the standard deviation of target region of original image, σ_T^E is the standard deviation of target region of enhanced image respectively. For a better enhancement technique, TBC_s must give a positive value.

EXPERIMENTAL RESULTS

In this section, we have presented *eight-sets of difficult to diagnose mammograms* to demonstrate the performance of the proposed method. In this method, we have chosen two significant image features 'entropy' and 'intensity mean' of mammograms using appropriate size of kernel and combined them with a ratio of 3:7 respectively. The kernel is moved over the entire mammograms to collect all possible values of those two features and then they are used as the data of FCM clustering technique. The mixing ratio of two image features is performed to achieve the best experimental results.

To evaluate the performance of the proposed technique, we have chosen two other conventional image enhancement techniques, like – a) histogram equalization method and b) conventional intensity based fuzzy clustering approach for comparison.

Visual interpretation shows that in most of the cases, conventional fuzzy clustering approach and histogram equalization method may provide over-enhancement. Moreover, histogram equalization method also incorporates some additional hesitancy in the suspected region of enhanced image which fade the main region of interests (ROIs).

However, the proposed method is able to highlight the suspected region of interests in the mammograms correctly with better level of accuracy. Objective evaluation parameters also exhibit this kind of impression.

- **Subjective Evaluation:** Visual interpretation by the radiologist prescribes that enhancement by histogram equalization suffers from some additional enhancement of surrounding regions which mislead the identification of actual region of interests. Enhancement by the conventional intensity based fuzzy clustering approach also suffers form over-enhancement in most of the cases and hence leads to misinterpretation to the degree of the disease. However, the proposed method is able to enhance the ROIs with better level of accuracy.
- **Objective Evaluation:** Beside the visual interpretation, to evaluate the proposed enhancement method with two other conventional methods, we have presented five quantitative evaluation parameters for each set of experimental images. This is given in tabular form below:

From the analysis of tabular data, we have found that in most of the cases, conventional intensity based FCM approach produces improved results over histogram equalization method because of its ability to model the uncertainties present in the mammograms. However, since the proposed enhancement technique has better ability to capture those uncertainties, it provides superior performances over all the methods mentioned here.

Hence, we may express that the proposed enhancement approach improves much better than other conventional methods of image enhancement. This approach is able to provide high quality results even in case of mammograms containing dense glandular breast tissues; especially present in younger women.

Apart from the quantitative assessment of given eight sets of mammograms, some graphical representations of those five evaluating parameters for other dataset is shown in Figure 4 –Figure 8. In this graphical analysis, we have also found the superior performance of the proposed approach against two existing enhancement techniques.

Figure 3. (a) Original mammogram, (b) Enhanced image by Histogram Equalization method, (c) Enhanced image by conventional intensity based FCM technique, (d) Enhanced image by the proposed method

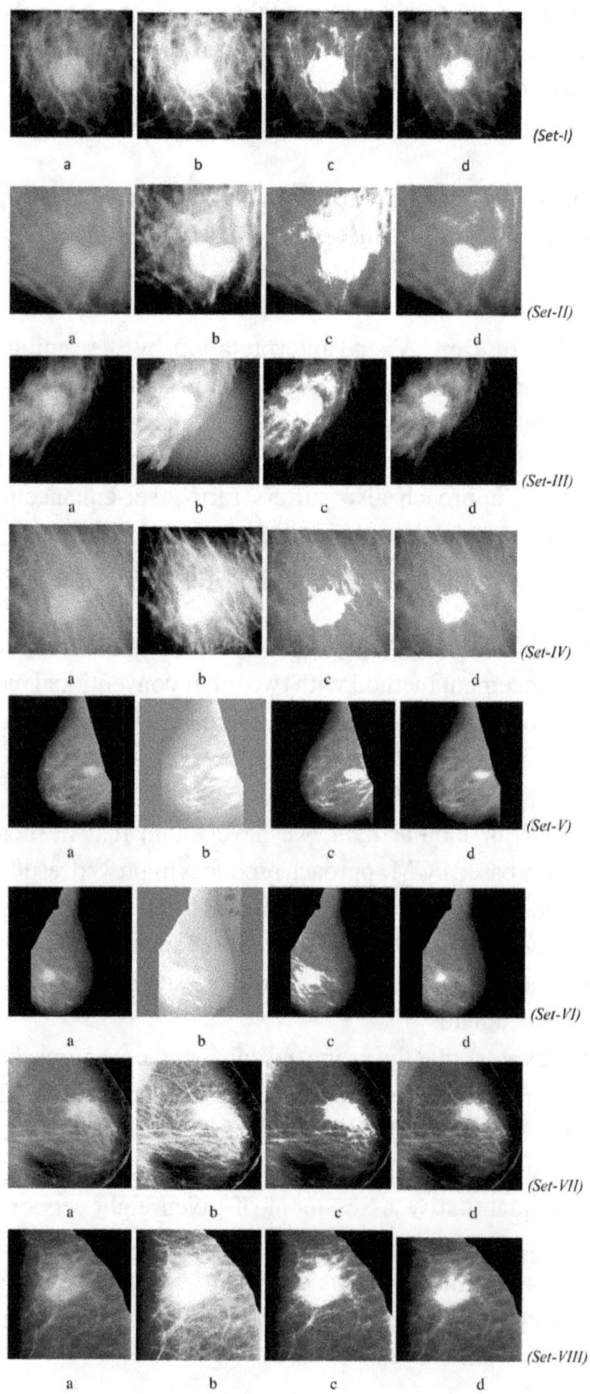

Table 1. Objective evaluation of the proposed method

IMAGE NO	ENHANCEMENT METHODS	ENHANCEMENT MEASURING PARAMETERS				
		CII	ASNR	PSNR	DSM	TBC_s
SET I	Histogram Equalization	1.2966	1.4326	4.0503	0.0676	0.1562
	Intensity based FCM	1.5260	3.9749	5.2072	0.4409	2.6986
	Proposed Method	2.2420	4.6930	5.7046	0.5634	3.8529
SET II	Histogram Equalization	2.5352	1.9849	3.9527	0.1938	0.2190
	Intensity based FCM	2.2986	3.6975	4.4238	0.4225	0.3284
	Proposed Method	4.2081	3.8711	5.2471	0.4347	1.3026
SET III	Histogram Equalization	1.0265	2.2566	4.2359	0.0204	0.0970
	Intensity based FCM	1.2380	3.3664	4.4985	0.4207	1.0078
	Proposed Method	1.8209	4.3995	5.4575	0.6317	3.8004
SET IV	Histogram Equalization	1.8630	3.1247	5.9138	0.1454	0.1732
	Intensity based FCM	2.2047	5.6008	7.2542	0.3406	0.2603
	Proposed Method	2.8152	6.0298	7.9190	0.4202	1.0491
SET V	Histogram Equalization	1.2194	2.2109	4.0371	0.2093	1.0973
	Intensity based FCM	1.2013	4.0054	4.3228	0.4186	1.0733
	Proposed Method	1.5796	4.1459	5.0006	0.5981	3.2376
SET VI	Histogram Equalization	1.0480	2.3225	4.2363	0.2208	0.8636
	Intensity based FCM	1.1544	4.5053	4.8141	0.4471	1.1273
	Proposed Method	1.2955	5.0463	5.4664	0.5572	3.5281
SET VII	Histogram Equalization	1.8039	1.7631	4.8602	0.1903	0.3862
	Intensity based FCM	1.4801	4.3551	6.5719	0.4273	0.5878
	Proposed Method	2.4741	5.4285	7.0177	0.5878	3.9932
SET VIII	Histogram Equalization	1.4143	1.5024	4.5717	0.1005	0.1634
	Intensity based FCM	1.4578	4.3126	5.5620	0.4211	0.8455
	Proposed Method	2.4250	4.5304	5.9565	0.5298	2.4109

CONCLUSION

This study shows an advanced fuzzy logic based approach for mammographic image enhancement to detect the suspected mass regions. The key idea of the proposed method is to enhance the ROI's of mammograms and not to enhance the existing noise and surrounding unwanted breast tissues. Choice of two significant features of mammograms and their proper mixing ratio serve this purpose successfully. This is because, we have found experimentally that there are some small deviations

Figure 4. Plot of CII for 10 different mammograms

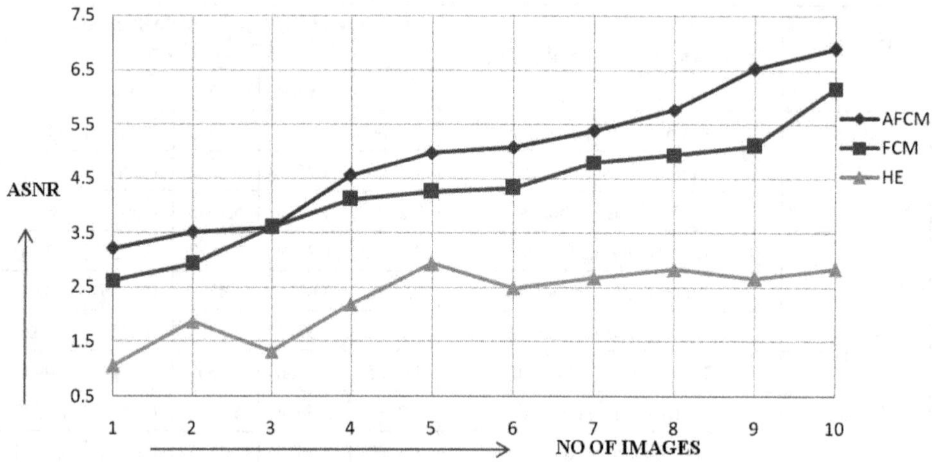

Figure 5. Plot of ASNR for 10 different mammograms

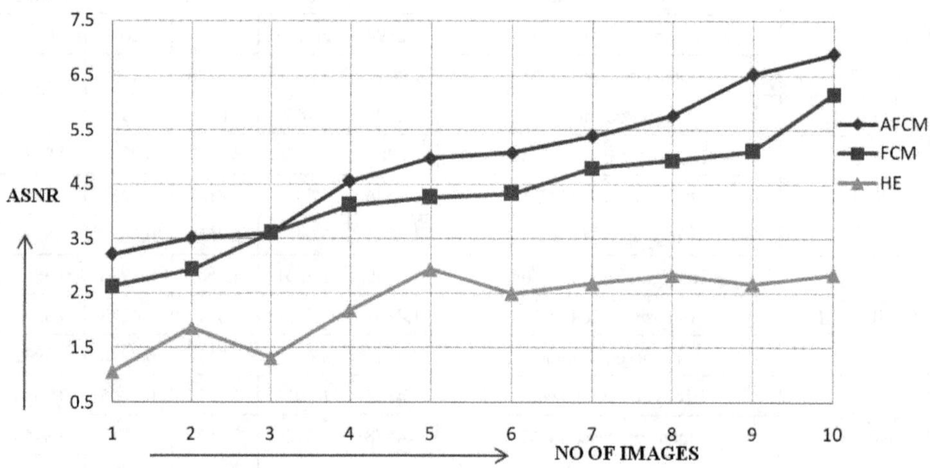

in the normal breast region and affected mass region of the mammograms which may be accurately captured and evaluated by these two important image features simultaneously. The inherent uncertainty modeling capability of fuzzy logic approach is fully exploited in this novel methodology in a more intelligent way. Both subjective and objective performance evaluations are made and verified with other conventional techniques and we have found that the proposed approach performs better for the present dataset.

The advantages and scope of the proposed approach are:

Figure 6. Plot of PSNR for 10 different mammograms

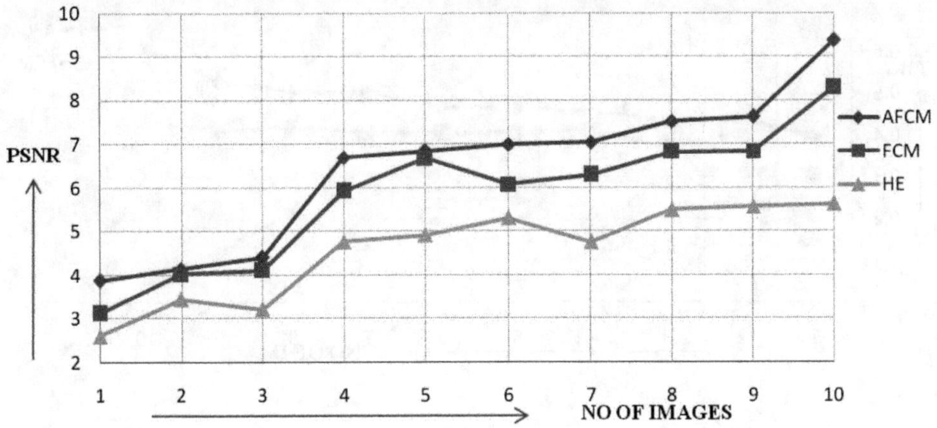

Figure 7. Plot of DSM for 10 different mammograms

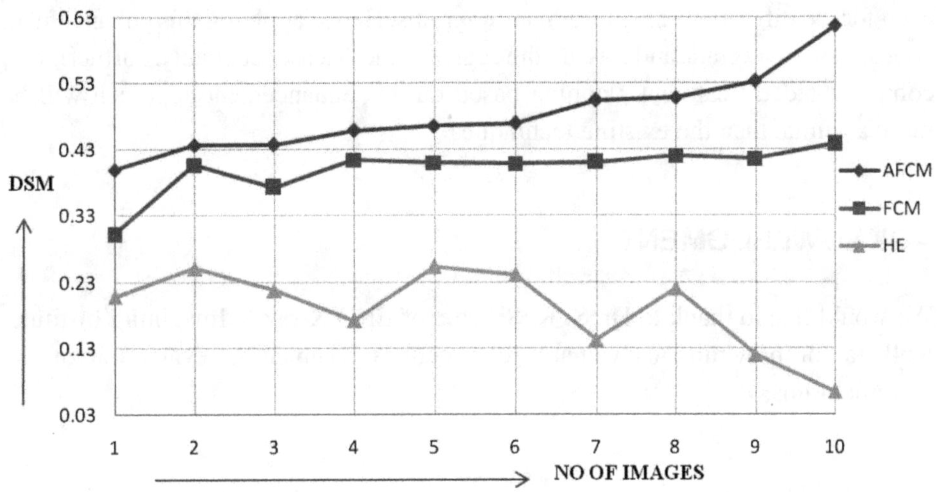

1. The effected regions causing breast cancer are accurately detected even in presence of very dense glandular tissues.
2. The irrelevant breast-structures can be easily identified and removed.
3. Some parameters can be adjusted in order to find out different levels of TP (True Positive) and FP (False Positive) rates.
4. The experimental results are encouraging for further processing such as categorizing the masses into benign and malignant stages in its early stage.

Figure 8. Plot of TBC_s for 10 different mammograms

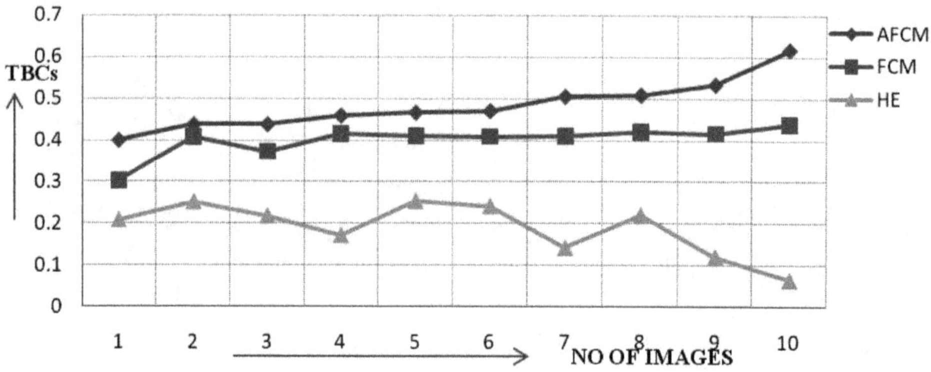

FUTURE RESEARCH DIRECTIONS

Proposed enhancement approach produces encouraging and satisfactory results even for the difficult to diagnose mammograms. Hence applying this enhancement approach we may grade and classify the degree of the disease accurately. Furthermore, computer aided treatment planning based on this enhancement approach will be more accurate than the existing techniques.

ACKNOWLEDGMENT

We would like to thank to Dr. S. K. Sharma of EKO X-ray & Imagining Institute, Kolkata for providing us valuable comments on subjective evaluation of the mammograms.

REFERENCES

Akay. (2009). Support vector machines combined with feature selection for breast cancer diagnosis. *Expert Syst. With Applicat.*, *36*(2), 3240–3247. 10.1016/j.eswa.2008.01.009

American College of Radiology (ACR) Breast Imaging Reporting and Data System Atlas. (2003). *BI-RADS Atlas*. Reston, VA: American College of Radiology.

Baert, A., Reiser, M., Hricak, H., & Kanuth, M. (2010). *Digital Mammography*. Springer.

Bezdek, J. C. (1981). *Pattern Recognition with Fuzzy Objective Function Algorithms*. Norwell, MA: Kluwer Academic Publishers. doi:10.1007/978-1-4757-0450-1

Cancer Fact SheetsW. H. O. (2009). Available: http://www.who.int/mediacentre/factsheets/fs297/en/index.html

Cheng, H. D., Wu, C. Y., & Li, J. (1998). VLSI architectures for moments and their applications to pattern recognition. In C. H. Chen, L. F. Pau, & P. S. P. Wang (Eds.), *Handbook of Pattern Recognition and Computer Vision* (2nd ed.). Singapore: World Scientific.

Cheng, H. D., & Xu, H. (2002). A novel fuzzy logic approach to mammogram contrast enhancement. *Information Sciences*, *148*(1-4), 167–184. doi:10.1016/S0020-0255(02)00293-1

Chuang, K.-S., Tzeng, H.-L., Chen, S., Wu, J., & Chen, T. J. (2006). Fuzzy c-means clustering with spatial information for image segmentation. *Computerized Medical Imaging and Graphics, Elsevier*, *30*(1), 9–15. doi:10.1016/j.compmedimag.2005.10.001 PMID:16361080

Cueva, M., Kuhnley, R., Stueckemann, C., Lanier, A. P., & McMahon, P. (2010). *Understanding Cancer*. Alaska Native Tribal Health Consortium.

Das, A., & Bhattacharya, M. (2011). Computerized Decision Support System for Mass Identification in Breast Using Digital Mammogram: A Study on GA Based Neuro Fuzzy Approaches. *Advances in Experimental Medicine and Biology*, *696*(6), 523–533. doi:10.1007/978-1-4419-7046-6_53

Das, A., & Bhattacharya, M. (2008). GA based Neuro Fuzzy Techniques for Breast Cancer Identification. *Proc. of Int. Machine Vision and Image Processing Conference (IMVIP-08)*, 136-141. 10.1109/IMVIP.2008.19

Gonzalez, R., & Woods, R. (2002). Digital Image Processing (2nd ed.). PHI.

Haus, A. G., & Yaffe, M. J. (Eds.). (1993). *A categorical course in physics, technical aspects of breast imaging*. Presented at the *79 Scientific Assembly and Annual Meeting of RSNA*.

Jain, A., Singh, S., & Bhateja, V. (2013). A Robust approach for denoising and enhancement of mammographic breast masses. *Int. J. Converg. Comput*, *1*, 38–49. doi:10.1504/IJCONVC.2013.054659

James, C. (1984). Bezdek, Robert Ehrlich, William Full, 'FCM: The Fuzzy C-Means Clustering Algorithm'. *Computers & Geosciences*, *10*(2-3), 191–203. doi:10.1016/0098-3004(84)90020-7

Laine, A., Fan, J., & Yang, W. (1995). *Wavelet For Contrast Enhancement of Digital Mammography*. IEEE Engineering in Medicine & Biology.

Li, H., Ray Liu, K. J., & Lo Shih-Chung, B. (1997). Fractal Modeling and Segmentation for the Enhancement of Microcalcifications in Digital Mammograms. *IEEE Transactions on Medical Imaging*, *16*(6), 785–798. doi:10.1109/42.650875 PMID:9533579

Malcolm, R. (2001). *Cancer*. London, UK: Imperial College School of Medicine.

Milind Kumar, Sarode, Ladhake, & Deshmukh. (2008). Fuzzy system for color image enhancement. *Proceedings of World Academy Of science, Engineering and Technology, 36*.

Nassif, H., Woods, R., Burnside, E., Ayvaci, M., Shavlik, J., & Page, D. (2009). *Information Extraction for Clinical Data Mining: A Mammography Case Study*. IEEE International Conference on Data Mining (ICDM'09) Workshops, Miami, FL.

Pal & Kin. (1981). Image Enhancement Using Smoothing with Fuzzy Sets. *IEEE Trans. Systems, Man, And Cybernetics, 11*(7), 494-501.

Peng, R., Varshney, P. K., Chen, H., & Michels, J. H. (2008). Digital mammogram enhancement based on ROI enhancement and background suppression. In *Medical Imaging 2008: Image Processing*. San Diego, CA: SPIE. doi:10.1117/12.770649

Sahiner, B., Chan, H. P., Petrick, N., Helvie, M. A., & Hadjiiski, L. M. (2001). Improvement of mammographic mass characterization using speculation measures and morphological features. *Medical Physics*, *28*(7), 1455–1465. doi:10.1118/1.1381548 PMID:11488579

Sampat, Markey, & Bovik. (2003). Computer-Aided Detection and Diagnosis in Mammography. In *Handbook of Image and Video Processing*. London, UK: Elsevier.

Schulz, W. (2007). *Molecular Biology of Human Cancers*. New York: Springer.

Shivaramakrishna, R., Obuchowski, N., & Cardenosa, W. (2000). Comparing the performance of Mammographic Enhancement Algorithms. *AJR*, *175*(1), 45–51. doi:10.2214/ajr.175.1.1750045 PMID:10882244

Suckling, J., Parker, J., Dance, D. R., Astley, S., Hutt, I., Boggis, C. R. M., ... Savage, J. (1994). The mammographic image analysis society mammogram database. *Proc. 2nd Int. Workshop Digital Mammography*, 375–378.

Tang, J., Liu, X., & Sun, Q. (2009). A Direct Image Contrast Enhancement Algorithm in the Wavelet Domain for Screening Mammograms. *IEEE Journal of Selected Topics in Signal Processing*, *3*(1), 74–80. doi:10.1109/JSTSP.2008.2011108

Thangavel, K., Karnan, M., & Sivakumar, R. (2005). *Automatic Detection of Microcalcification in Mammogram - A Review*. ICGST.

Thangavel, K., Karnan, M., Sivakumar, R., & Kaja Mohideen, A. (1998). Automatic detection of microcalcification in mammograms - a review. *Journal on Graphics Vision and Image Processing*, *5*(5), 31–61.

Tizhoosh, H. R. (2000). Fuzzy Image Enhancement: An Overview. In Fuzzy Techniques in Image Processing. Springer.

Yang, C. (2006). Image enhancement by modified contrast-stretching manipulation. *Optic & Laser Technology (Elmsford, N.Y.)*, *38*, 196–201.

Zadeh, L. A. (1965). Fuzzy sets. *Information and Control*, *8*(3), 338–353. doi:10.1016/S0019-9958(65)90241-X

Chapter 4
Design and Development of Capacitance Sensor Array for Analyzing the Non-Homogeneity in Biological Materials:
A Smart Sensing Approach

Sahana Apparsamy
Madras Institute of Technology, India

Kamalanand Krishnamurthy
Madras Institute of Technology, India

ABSTRACT

Soft tissues are non-homogeneous deformable structures having varied structural arrangements, constituents, and composition. This chapter explains the design of a capacitance sensor array for analyzing and imaging the non-homogeneity in biological materials. Further, tissue mimicking phantoms are developed using Agar-Agar and Polyacrylamide gels for testing the developed sensor. Also, the sensor employs an unsupervised learning algorithm for automated analysis of non-homogeneity. The reconstructed capacitance image can also be sensitive to topographical and morphological variations in the sample. The proposed method is further validated using a fiberoptic-based laser imaging system and the Jaccard index. In this chapter, the design of the sensor array for smart analysis of non-homogeneity along with significant results are presented in detail.

DOI: 10.4018/978-1-5225-5149-2.ch004

INTRODUCTION

The group of tissue that bind, support and protect our human body and organs are known as soft tissues. These soft tissues are present all over the body. The various soft tissues in the human body are fat, muscle, fibrous tissue, synovial tissue, blood vessels, lymph vessels and peripheral nerves. Every soft tissue has its own specific set of functions. They give shape to our body and support the structures of the body. These soft tissues also protect other tissues and hold them together (Marieb, 2000). Human soft tissues are deformable, viscoelastic and are complex, fiber-reinforced composite structures. Their mechanical properties vary significantly from one tissue to another tissue. Their electrical and mechanical behaviors are strongly influenced by the concentration and structural arrangements of their tissue constituents. So, soft tissues are generally non-homogeneous in composition (Holzapfel, 2001).

A biological material can be made of a single substance or combination of two or more substances. Each substance retains their own identity (Ji & Gao, 2004). A material, in general, is broadly classified as homogeneous material and non-homogeneous material. The homogeneous materials are uniform in composition and character. The particles are uniformly distributed and have the same properties at every point, without irregularities (Nasser & Hori, 2013).

Non-homogeneous materials are non-uniform in composition or character. The particles in these materials are not uniformly distributed and they also have localized regions with different properties. They have different concentration at some areas (Nasser & Hori, 2013). Few examples of non-homogeneous materials are tumor cells, sea water, blood, etc. The non-homogeneity in biological materials is mostly due to abnormal growth of malignant cells, tumor formation or the presence of foreign particles. Presence of these factors may change the regular structural arrangements or composition of the biological material, thus showing non-homogeneity in the biological tissue material (Nymeyer & Zhou, 2008). Figure 1 (a) and 1 (b) shows a pictorial representation of homogeneous arrangement and non-homogeneous arrangement in a material, respectively.

In recent years, capacitance sensors have been employed, for measuring many physical and electrical quantities for biomedical analysis. The two most important characteristics of capacitance sensors are low energy consumption and simple construction (Jong & Meijer, 1997). The capacitance (*C*) of a capacitor is determined by the following well known equation.

$$C = \frac{\varepsilon_0 \varepsilon_r A}{d}$$

Figure 1. A representation of (a) Homogeneous arrangement in a material (b) Non-homogeneous arrangement in a material

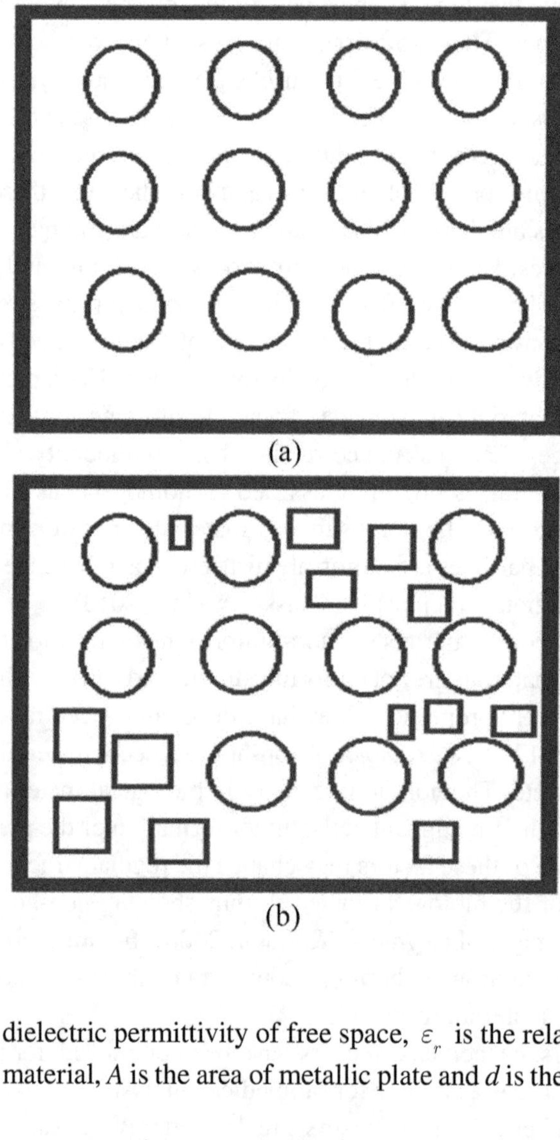

where, ε_0 is the dielectric permittivity of free space, ε_r is the relative permittivity of the dielectric material, *A* is the area of metallic plate and *d* is the plate separation distance.

The capacitance output of the capacitance sensor can be varied by changing ε_r, *A* and *d*. In the process of measuring the capacitance, there are several sources of measurement uncertainties. One of the uncertainties may be due to dielectric properties varying in the test item. The dielectric parameters generally vary based on the geometric characters like configuration, chemical composition, size and structure and surface profile (Assender, Bliznyuk & Porfyrakis, 2002). The distribution of the electric field intensity in the test surface is referred to as field topography.

The surface profile variation also called topography is one of the major characteristics of biological tissue material which affects the dielectric properties. The size and structure of the biological material accounts to their morphological properties. Also, the variations in the chemical composition of biological materials also affect their dielectric characteristics (Kim & Economou, 2002).

Tissue mimicking phantoms are often used as physical models to simulate the properties of biological soft tissues (Madsen, Zagzebski, & Frank, 1982). Phantoms are used in medical research to substitute for real tissue in studies where in vivo models are inappropriate. Phantoms are generally used to reproduce the properties of the actual biological materials that are unavailable for testing in the laboratory. These phantoms are similar to real mammalian soft tissues. Several tissue mimicking phantoms play major roles in research areas of biomedical fields and several other applications like testing and investigation in laboratories (Krishnamurthy, Sridhar, Rajeshwari, & Swaminathan, 2009; Kamalanand, Sridhar, Rajeshwari & Ramakrishnan, 2010). Phantoms can be modelled for mimicking anatomical features, such as vessels and vascular trees, including structures such as white and grey matter and lesions, or mechanical and electrical properties (Surry, Austin, Fenster, & Peters, 2004). Since the properties of phantom materials closely resemble the properties of real tissues, these phantoms are of great importance in testing and clinical validation of new technologies (Erkamp, Skovoroda, Emelianov, & O'Donnell, 2004; Takegami, Kaneko, Watanabe, Maruyama, Matsumoto, & Nagawa, 2004). A variety of tissue mimicking materials such as agar, urethanes, epoxies and other natural materials are used to simulate the geometry and mechanics of the human tissue (Rowan, & Pedersen, 2006). They are used in the development and calibration of medical systems and for validation of various algorithms. Tissue mimicking phantoms provide a more clinically realistic testing environment for studying the properties of biological tissues (Cook, Bouchard & Emelianov, 2011).

Grouping of data points into different groups on the basis of similarity between data points is called clustering. These groups are called clusters. K-mean clustering method is one of the simplest algorithms for pure numeric datasets because of its low time-complexity (Ahmad & Hashmi 2016). K-mean is an unsupervised and iterative method of clustering. In k-mean, each cluster is represented by the mean value of objects in the cluster. In this algorithm, a set of n object is partitioned into k clusters. Similarity is calculated from the mean value of objects in a cluster (Yadav & Sharma 2013; Manickavasagam, Sutha & Kamalanand, 2014).

This chapter describes a method to design a capacitance sensor array for analyzing the non-homogeneous biological materials and also to develop non-homogeneous tissue mimicking phantoms. Further to automate the identification of non-homogeneity, K-Mean algorithm has been applied. Also, using the intensity profile measurements and Jaccard index, the developed system has been validated.

BACKGROUND

Capacitive Sensing

Capacitive sensors have the capacity to analyze non-homogeneity in several medical and engineering applications (Zhu & Spronck, 1991; Robert Puers, 1993; Xin Zhou, An Huang & Qin, 2005; Chu Chiang, Lin & Shuang Ju, 2007; Sepúlveda, Fachin, Villoria, Wardle, Viana, Pontes & Rocha, 2011). Arunachalam *et al.* (2014) have developed a capacitance sensor for minimally invasive diagnosis of normal, cirrhotic, and malignant liver. The authors have used finite element methods to design and simulate the sensor for minimally invasive assessment of liver disorders. Further, in their study, the authors have designed capacitive sensors using four different biocompatible metals namely, Gold, Silver, Palladium and Platinum. Nymeyer *et al.* (2008) have developed a new method for determining the dielectric profile in a complex non-homogenous system. Further, the authors have found that the disadvantage of this method is that it requires multiple stimulations for the sample placement of the test material. Further, the authors have reported that the test particle radius can be chosen by the usage of multiple test charges. Further, the authors have reported that the developed method has its own uncertainty. The proposed method is useful for the understanding and explanation of complex dielectric profiles. Assender *et al.* (2002) have presented a paper on how surface topography relates to material properties. The authors state that the topography of a surface is due to the nature of the material. The authors have analyzed the topography of the sample taken using atomic force microscopy techniques. The authors have also concluded that topographical changes are due to the number of properties like optical finishing and interactions of a surface with some secondary material surface.

Matiss (2014) has utilized the multi parameter capacitance technique by scanning the test item using an electric field of different topography. The author has designed a simple capacitance testing hardware for measuring the thickness of various profiles. Further, the author has designed a sensor consisting of an array of coplanar electrodes adapted to the surface profile of the test item. Also, the author has discussed the uses of such sensors with which two parameters can be measured, namely the thickness and the dielectric permittivity. Further, the author has concluded that the measurements obtained should be subjected to data processing and optimization in order to have more reliable values. Zhu *et al.* (1991) have developed a capacitive displacement sensor based on the application of two different techniques namely the spatial sampling technique and the Doppler measurement technique. Further, the authors have discussed that the capacitive sensor measures linear displacement with high resolution, for a small range and for large scale applications. Finally, the authors have concluded that the developed sensor has linearity over long range, high stability and low sensitivity to electromagnetic disturbance.

Puers (1993) has discussed about capacitive sensors and their applicability. The author has discussed about several capacitive sensors, their construction, performance and their applications. The author has also provided review over all the technologies used and had given complete overview of capacitive sensors. Jong and Meijer (1997) have presented an efficient retrieving algorithm for accurate capacitive position sensors. For solving the problems of mechanical origin in capacitive position sensors, multi capacitive sensing elements have been introduced. The authors have presented an overview of the capacitive position sensors and also have discussed about the design aspect of the various system parts and the related retrieving algorithm. The authors have concluded that the retrieving algorithm is efficient in providing high accuracy and low cross sensitivity. Li and Meijer (2002) have discussed on accurate interfaces for the capacitive sensors. The authors have developed a new interface with the help of a first order charge balance SC-oscillator. The developed oscillator was also shunted by parasitic conductance. The authors have also introduced two-port measurement for eliminating the effect of stray capacitances. Further, the authors have also eliminated the additive and multiplicative errors of the interface using the chopping and auto-calibration techniques.

Tissue Mimicking Phantoms

Kamalanand *et al.* (2010) have made use of poly-acrylamide based tissue mimicking phantoms to measure the dielectric permittivity and correlated them with their mechanical properties. Further, the authors have prepared the tissues mimicking phantoms as per the standard protocol and used them for the assessment of soft tissue behaviors. Also, the authors have utilized various concentrations of tissues mimicking phantoms for analysis of different behavior of soft tissues and correlated them with their mechanical properties. Kawabata *et al.* (2004) have developed a tissue mimicking phantom for analyzing the elastic properties of tissues. Further, the authors have analyzed the stability of the tissue mimicking phantoms to obtain reproducible data and found that polyacrylamide gel which is a chemical gel, shows greater stability than physical gels such as agar-agar. Also, the authors have analyzed the test results and proved that the elastic properties of both physical and chemical gels vary with the concentrations. Finally, the authors have proved that the Polyacrylamide gel used is thermally irreversible and have advantage over other phantom get material.

Cook *et al.* (2011) have discussed that an accurate tissue-mimicking phantom for photoacoustic and ultrasonic (PAUS) imaging can be constructed for most soft tissues. Also, the authors have demonstrated that the phantoms were stable over the duration of the testing and were sealed in air-tight molds in a 4°C refrigerator between tests. By further investigations, the authors have shown that gelatin phantoms maintain good stability for several months with similar recipes by preventing desiccation of the phantoms. Further, the authors have demonstrated that storing the phantom at low temperatures slows bacterial growth within the phantom and temporal stability. Further, the authors have finalized that the careful manipulation of the concentrations of each of the ingredients can be used to create an accurate tissue-mimicking phantom for the continued development of PAUS imaging of soft tissues. Madsen *et al.* (2005) have developed five 9 cm × 9 cm × 9 cm phantoms, each with a 2-cm-diameter cylindrical inclusion with various dry-weight concentrations of agar and gelatin. Also, the authors have monitored the strain ratios over a period of 7 to 10 months and finalized that the mechanical properties of the phantoms were stable. Further, they have concluded that the only dependable method for determining the storage moduli of the inclusions is to make measurements on samples excised from the phantoms.

Earle *et al.* (2016) have experimented whether agar models are superior and can produce ultrasound images superior to gelatin models. The authors have also concluded that agar models do not require refrigeration and can produce an ultrasound image similar to real tissues. The authors have also proved that agar models have multiple advantages over gelatin for ultrasound training in austere conditions. Menter (2000) has described a practical approach for the polymerization of acrylamide. The author has also explained the important parameters necessary for the polymerization. The author has further described about the substances required for polymerization, the initiator type, the concentration, the contaminants in buffer, the temperature, the amount of oxygen required, gel additives, the pH level, the cross linkers, the monomer concentration, the time for polymerization and the polymerization protocols. The authors have also showed the different types of polymerization and their corresponding result profiles of the polymerization reaction. The author has discussed about commonly occurring polymerization problems and also their probable causes and solutions.

Clustering Algorithms

Yadav and Sharma (2013) have analyzed the shortcomings and benefits of the K-mean algorithm. Also, the authors have proposed three dissimilar modified K-mean algorithms to gradually improve the speed and efficiency of the algorithm and also to remove the limitations of the existing K-mean algorithm. In the first algorithm, the authors have avoided the difficulty of proposing the K value beforehand and in the second algorithm, the authors have reduced the computational complexity. Further, the authors have increased the speed of clustering in the third algorithm.

Yedla *et al.* (2010) have proposed a study on enhancing the K-mean algorithm with an improved center taken initially. Further, the authors have analyzed the existing K-mean algorithm which mostly depends upon correcting the initially selected random centroids. Also, the authors have found that the existing K-mean algorithm converges to local minimum instead of considering global optimum. The authors have proposed a new inventive method to find the best initial centroid. Further, the authors have proposed an improved method to assign the data points to preferred clusters so that the time complexity reduces. The authors have also concluded that the proposed method has less computation time and more accuracy. Manickavasagam et al. (2014) have developed a system for automated classification of plasmodium specied in thin blood smear images using 2D empirical mode decomposition and k-means clustering algorithm.

Ahmad and Hashmi (2016) have given a brief discussion on K-harmonic measurement type clustering algorithm for mixed datasets consisting of numerical and categorical attributes which has cluster center initialization problem. The authors have used K-Harmonic means clustering for overcoming the problem of pure numeric data. The authors have carried out experiments with pure categorical and mixed datasets. The results also prove that the proposed clustering algorithm is insensitive to cluster center initialization problem and also produce better clustering results. Ortega *et al.* have presented a paper discussing the research issues on K-means algorithm with an experimental trial using Matlab. The authors have discussed the results on the K-mean algorithm to overcome the shortcomings. The authors have conducted experiments of the K-means in Matlab package and Unique Client Identifier (UCI) repository databases and also established a framework for the proposed improvement of the K-means algorithm.

Nazeer and Sebastian (2009) have presented a paper on improving the Accuracy and Efficiency of the k-means Clustering Algorithm. The authors have discussed about the emerging modern techniques for collection of scientific data. These data have also resulted in accumulation in large scale which supports diverse fields. The authors have also discussed about the conventional database querying methods. These conventional database querying methods are found to be inadequate to extract information from large data banks. Hence the authors have introduced the k-means clustering algorithm which is one of the major data analysis methods widely used for many practical applications. The authors have proposed several methods in this paper for improving the performance of the k-means clustering algorithm since the original k-means algorithm is computationally expensive and also the resulting clusters mostly depends on the selection of initial centroids. In this paper, the authors have proposed a method for making the algorithm effective and efficient for getting a better clustering with reduced complexity.

Fiber Optic Measurement Systems

Idanboylu and Efendioglu (2009) have discussed about fiber optic sensors and their applications in several fields. Further, the authors have presented a brief study about the most widely used sensor types based on intensity, phase, wavelength and polarization. Initially, the authors have given an elaborate explanation about the basics of fiber optics, their evolution history, and working principle of fiber optics. The authors have presented major sensors like micro bending sensors, evanescent wave sensors, optical fiber interferometer and polarization modulated fiber optic sensors categorized under sensor types. Finally, the authors have presented the applications of these sensors. Sherif *et al.* (2007) have presented a review on fiber optic sensors for detection of toxic and biological threats. The authors have developed a new fiber optic chemical sensor for the detection of toxic and biological materials. The authors have designed the fiber optic sensor using cladding modification approach. The authors have used total intensity and modal power distribution measurements to detect the changes in the output power through the sensing fibers. The authors have also presented results that showed drastic improvement in sensor sensitivity when the modal power distribution method was applied. Sumathi and Pratheep (2012) have described about intensity based fiber optic deflection sensor. The authors have developed a low cost intrinsic fiber optic sensor. Using that sensor, the authors were able to measure and detect angular displacement of articulated arm. The authors have also presented experimental results that showed that the sensor output is changing according to angular displacement. The authors have also concluded that this deflection sensor can be used in several applications like medical equipment.

Jaccard Index

Niwattanakul *et al.* (2013) have utilized Jaccard coefficient technique for the identification of keywords similarity. The authors have also presented their test results which demonstrated the advantages and disadvantages of the Jaccard similarity coefficient measurement. Shikalgar and Dixit (2014) have used the Jaccard Index based clustering algorithm for the purpose of mining. The authors have investigated the opinion analysis problem. In this paper, the authors have also proposed the usage of Jaccard index based clustering algorithm for supporting the mining of online reviews and also for predicting the sales performance beforehand. The authors have also recommended Jaccard index based clustering algorithm for good feature selection. Hyuk cha (2007) has prepared a comprehensive survey on distance and similarity measures between several probability density functions. Seifoddini and Djassemi (1991) have discussed the production data-based similarity coefficient and Jaccard's similarity coefficients. In their paper, the authors have compared the performance of Jaccard's similarity coefficient with the performance of production data-based simi1arity coefficient. Hyuk cha *et al.* (2009) have given a brief description on anomaly between Jaccard and Tanimoto coefficients. The authors have taken over 100 binary similarity measures for comparing two binary patterns.

DESIGN OF THE CAPACITANCE SENSOR ARRAY

Capacitive sensors are constructed from many different media, such as copper, Indium tin oxide (ITO) and printed ink. Copper capacitive sensors can be implemented on standard PCBs too. Size and spacing of the capacitive sensor are very important to the sensor's performance. A single sided copper clad board was utilized. Required design was drawn on the board using an etch-resistant marker. Ferric chloride etching solution was used for etching. The board with copper side up was put in the plastic container filled with the etching solution. The exposed copper begins to dissolve and takes 15-20 minutes for all the exposed copper to dissolve. The marker marks can be removed using thinner to expose the copper clad circuit. Thus, a 5x5 matrix array on the copper board was obtained after etching. Further, burge sticks have been soldered on the copper clad board. This sensor array can be used for analyzing the properties of biological materials. Figure 2 shows the developed capacitive sensor array.

Figure 2. The developed capacitance sensor array

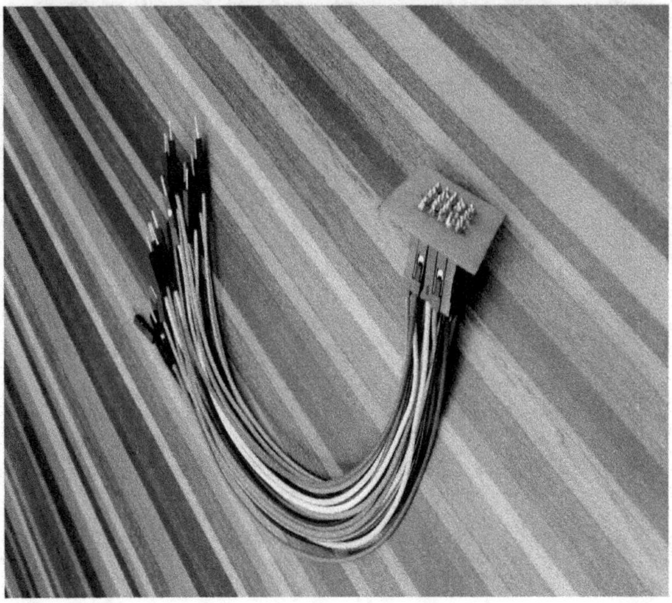

Working of the Sensor

The developed sensor array along with another metallic plate (ground plate) acts as the capacitance sensor array. When the material to be analyzed is placed in between the two plates, it acts as dielectric medium. By using this prototype, the dielectric characteristics of the given material using an LCR meter, at two selectable test frequencies of 120 Hz and 1 KHz can be analyzed. With the obtained values, the homogeneity or the non-homogeneity of the material can be analyzed.

The designed capacitance sensor array was initially analyzed by using air as the dielectric medium. The distance between the two plates can be varied and the capacitance values were measured at each point. Reduction in the distance between the plates minimizes the effect of other interference factors on the sensor. Also, a homogeneous material like rubber was analyzed for homogeneity by measuring capacitance values using the LCR meter at 120Hz. By the analysis of the rubber material, it can be understood that the error variations at all the points was very less and can be neglected. The capacitance image of the rubber material was also of a single color denoting that the material is homogeneous in nature. Figure 3 shows the obtained capacitance image of the homogeneous rubber material.

Figure 3. The capacitance image of the homogeneous rubber material

DEVELOPMENT OF TISSUE MIMICKING PHANTOMS

Tissue mimicking phantoms are materials that reproduce the properties of the natural biological materials. Biological substances have been used to create these tissue mimicking phantoms and these phantoms are utilized for investigations (Lazebnik, Madsen, Frank, & Hagness, 2005). Hydrogels are very similar to soft tissues in many properties and are often used as tissue mimicking phantoms. Hydrogels are of two types namely, the physical gels that are obtained through physical procedures such as heating and cooling (e.g. Agar and gelatin), and chemical gels are obtained through chemical reactions like polymerization (e.g. Polyacrylamide gels) (Kawabata, Waki, Matsumura & Umemura, 2004).

Preparation of Agar-Agar Phantoms

Agar-agar is a jelly-like substance obtained from polysaccharide agarose. Agar is a polysaccharide complex which has the capacity to hold water within its structure due to the presence of hydrophilic groups. Agar is mostly used in microbiology and plant biology. Agar is a promising material for preparing tissue phantoms since it doesn't require refrigeration. It resists melting and spoilage and can be reused. Agar models provide images similar to real tissue and they are one of the commonly used models (Earle, De Portu & DeVos, 2016).

Agar powder (1 gram) is taken and mixed well with 50 ml of distilled water. This forms 2% of agar solution. A magnetic stirrer is used to achieve uniform distribution. The stir cycles are repeated until all the agar dissolves and liquid becomes light brown but clear. After complete mixing, the mixture is heated at a temperature of about 60-70 degree Celsius. Then, the liquid is poured separately in different molds and is set to cool. After 5 - 10 minutes, the mixture cools at room temperature and forms a gel material. This gel material can be used as a tissue mimicking phantom to study various properties of biological materials, in a laboratory. Figure 4 shows the prepared agar-agar gel phantom.

The Agar gel concentrations used in this study provided a solid medium and helped in its easy manipulation. The 2% concentration produced a rigid gel and was less brittle and less prone to fracture during its evaluation. The prepared homogeneous agar-agar phantom material has been analyzed and capacitance values were obtained for 1 kHz. Figure 5 shows the capacitance image of the homogeneous agar-agar phantom. The difference in the capacitance values between various leads may be due to the topographical variations in the developed Agar-Agar phantom material. Since the capacitance values obtained were homogeneous, it showed a blue colour image with only slight variations. These variations are due to the topography of the tissue mimicking agar-agar phantom.

Figure 4. The prepared Agar-Agar gel

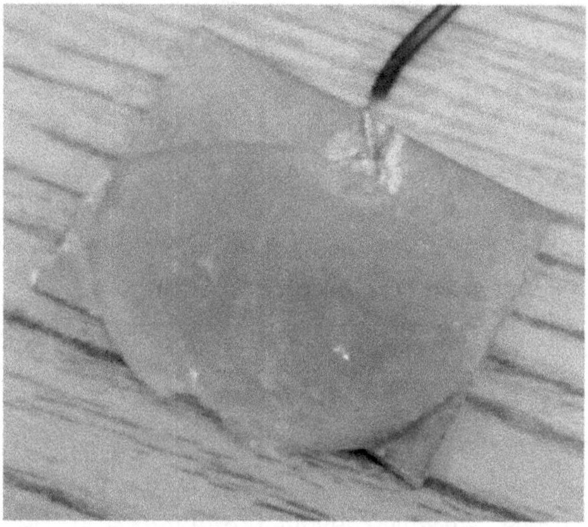

Figure 5. The capacitance image of the homogeneous agar-agar phantom

Preparation of Polyacrylamide Phantoms

Chemical gels when compared to physical gels are more stable and are thus easier to handle once prepared. Polyacrylamide gel is a typical chemical gel used in many biomedical applications as tissue mimicking phantoms. It is obtained through the polymerization of acrylamide, which is driven by appropriate initiators and catalysts of radical chain reactions (Kawabata, Waki, Matsumura & Umemura, 2004). To prepare Polyacrylamide gel, following materials are required.

- Acrylamide (extra pure)
- Bis-acrylamide (extra pure)
- Ammonium per-sulphate
- TEMED (N.N.N'.N' tetrametylethylenediamine)

Polyacrylamide gels are formed by copolymerization of acrylamide and bis-acrylamide ("bis", N, N'-methylene-bis-acrylamide). Polymerization is initiated by ammonium per-sulphate and TEMED. TEMED accelerates the rate of formation of free radicals from per-sulphate and these in turn catalyze polymerization. The per-sulphate free radicals convert acrylamide monomers to free radicals which react with un-activated monomers to begin the polymerization chain reaction. The elongating polymer chains are randomly cross-linked by bis-acrylamide resulting in a gel with a characteristic porosity which depends on the polymerization conditions and monomer concentrations (Menter, 2000).

A 20% Polyacrylamide gel required a mixture of 19g of acrylamide (extra pure) and 1g bis-acrylamide (extra pure) in 100 ml of deionized water. APS (ammonium per-sulphate) and TEMED (N.N.N'.N'-tetrametylethylenediamine) were added to initiate and catalyze the polymerization reaction. The solution was poured into a suitable mold and left undisturbed for about 10 min for the polymerization of acrylamide. The preparation of Polyacrylamide gels of higher or lower concentrations involves the proportional increase or decrease of the quantity of Acrylamide and Bis-acrylamide (Kamalanand, Sridhar, Rajeshwari, & Ramakrishnan, 2010). Figure 6 shows the prepared polyacrylamide tissue mimicking phantom, used in this study.

The prepared homogeneous Polyacrylamide phantom material has been analyzed and capacitance values were obtained at 1 KHz. Figure 7 shows the capacitance image of the homogeneous polyacrylamide phantom. Since the capacitance values obtained were homogeneous, it showed a blue colour image with only little variations. These variations were due to the topography variations in the tissue mimicking polyacrylamide phantom.

Capacitive Imaging of Non-Homogeneous Phantoms

A 10% polyacrylamide gel was made from the mixture of 0.9g of acrylamide (extra pure) and 0.1g Bis-acrylamide (extra pure) in 10 ml of deionized water along with APS (ammonium per- sulphate) and TEMED (N.N.N'.N'-tetrametylethylenediamine) to initiate and catalyze the polymerization reaction.The solution was poured into a

Figure 6. The prepared polyacrylamide tissue mimicking phantom

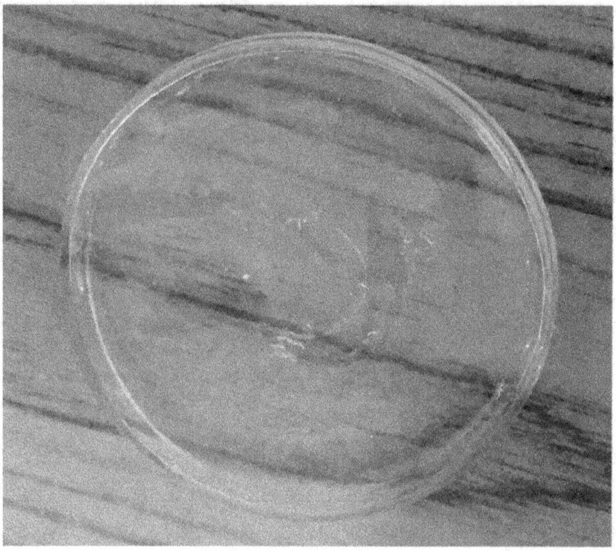

suitable mold and left undisturbed for about 10 minutes for the polymerization of acrylamide. To create non-homogeneity, a small portion of the prepared phantom was removed after the polymerization reaction. A 20% concentration of agar-agar gel was prepared by mixing 8gms of Agar-Agar powder in 40 ml of distilled water and set to boil. When the gel attained the boiling temperature after 10 minutes, they were poured into the empty portion between the prepared polyacrylamide phantom and set to cool. This non-homogeneous biological phantom was then taken for analysis of non-homogeneity using the developed capacitance sensor array and capacitance values were obtained at 1 KHz. Figure 8 (a) shows the photograph of the nonhomogeneous phantom prepared using both agar-agar and polyacrylamide material. Figure 8 (b) shows the corresponding capacitance image of the non-homogeneous phantom shown in Figure 8 (a). The agar and polyacrylamide regions are clearly differentiable in the capacitance image obtained.

Automation Using K-Means Clustering Algorithm

K-mean algorithm is an unsupervised learning algorithm which solves clustering problems. K-means clustering aims to partition n observations into k clusters in which each observation belongs to the cluster with the nearest mean. Given a set of

Figure 7. The capacitance image of the homogeneous polyacrylamide phantom

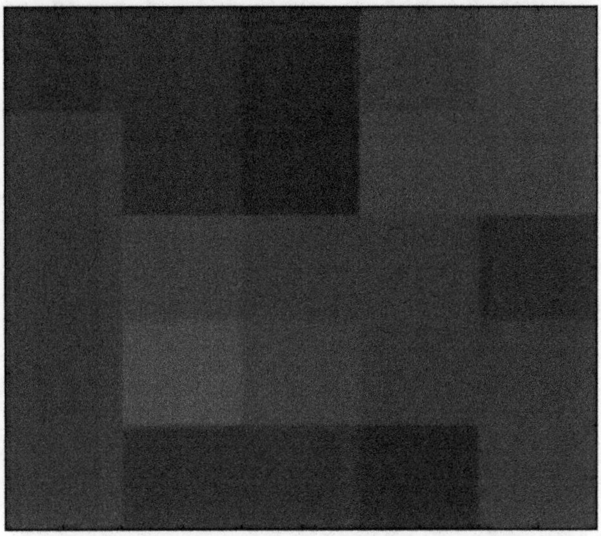

n observations $X=[x_1, x_2, x_3, x_4, \ldots.., x_n]$, where each observation is a d-dimensional real vector, k-means clustering aims to partition the n observations into K sets ($k \leq n$) $S=\{S_1, S_2, S_3, S_4 \ldots\ldots.., S_k\}$ so as to minimize the within-cluster sum of squares given by (Manickavasagam, Sutha & Kamalanand, 2014; Cheung, 2003):

$$\arg\min_{S} \sum_{i=1}^{k} \sum_{x_j \in S_i} \| x_j - \mu_i \|^2$$

where, μ_i is the mean of points in S_i. The algorithm follows a simple method to classify the given data set through a certain number of clusters using the following steps (Yadav & Sharma, 2013):

Step 1: Arbitrarily choose k data items from dataset X, as initial cluster centroid.
Step 2: After choosing a cluster centroid, assign each data item x_i to the cluster to which object is most similar, based on the mean value of the object in cluster.
Step 3: Calculate the new mean value of the data items for each cluster and update the mean until no change is found.

Figure 8(a) The prepared non-homogeneous phantom of agar-agar and polyacrylamide and (b) the capacitance image of the non-homogeneous phantom

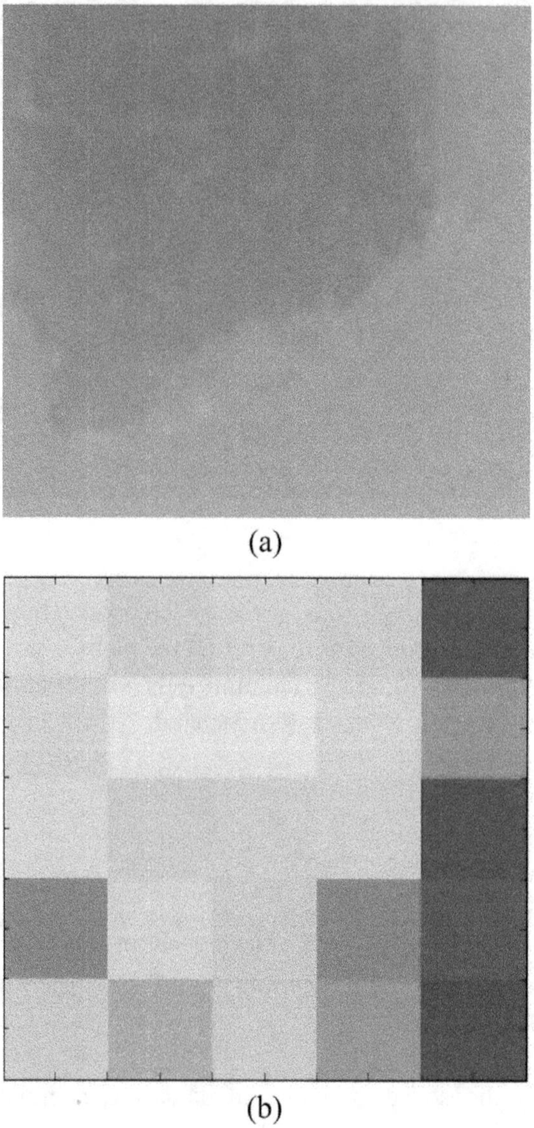

K- Mean algorithm was applied to the capacitance image data obtained from the non-homogeneous phantom prepared using agar-agar and polyacrylamide. The algorithm partitioned the points into two clusters, one cluster corresponding to agar and the other cluster corresponding to polyacrylamide. The k-means algorithm partitions the capacitance data into values 1 and 2, in the following way:

$$\begin{pmatrix} 2 & 2 & 2 & 2 & 1 \\ 2 & 2 & 2 & 2 & 1 \\ 2 & 2 & 2 & 2 & 1 \\ 1 & 2 & 2 & 1 & 1 \\ 1 & 1 & 1 & 1 & 1 \end{pmatrix}$$

which can then be imaged to view the non-homogeneity in the test sample. The capacitance image of the non-homogeneous phantom after applying K-means algorithm, is showed in Figure 9 which proved that the Agar-Agar and Polyacrylamide phantom is non-homogeneous in nature.

VALIDATION OF THE DEVELOPED SENSOR

In this work, the intensity profile of the adopted phantom of the biological material is obtained from a fiber optic sensor. An optical fiber sensor system consists of an optical laser source, optical fibers, and optical detector and processing electronics (Fidanboylu & Efendioglu, 2009). When laser light is passed through any material, due to absorption properties, topography and morphological properties, the intensity of transmitted light varies accordingly. This intensity profile of the developed non-

Figure 9. The image of the non-homogeneous phantom after applying k-mean algorithm

homogeneous phantom was analyzed for validating the capacitive images produced by the developed capacitive sensor array. The diode laser was turned on and the beam was directed through the 10x microscope objective onto the optical fiber which passed through the developed phantom. At the output end of the detecting fiber, the intensity of the light coming out of the phantom was measured. Figure 10 shows the fiber optic measurement system (available at Department of Instrumentation Engineering, MIT campus, Anna University) which was used to for intensity profile measurements.

The Jaccard Index also known as the Jaccard similarity coefficient is a statistic method also used for comparing the similarity and diversity of sample sets. The Jaccard index measures similarity between finite sample sets and the Jaccard distance measures dissimilarity between sample sets. The Jaccard coefficient is defined as the size of the intersection divided by the size of the union of the sample sets. (Real & Vargas, 1996). Jaccard index approach was applied to the data obtained from the non-homogeneous phantom of agar-agar and polyacrylamide to obtain the similarity between the sample sets (capacitance image and intensity image). The Jaccard coefficient which measures similarity between finite sample sets and the Jaccard distance which measures dissimilarity between sample sets was obtained as:

Figure 10. The Fiber optic measurement system used for intensity profile measurement

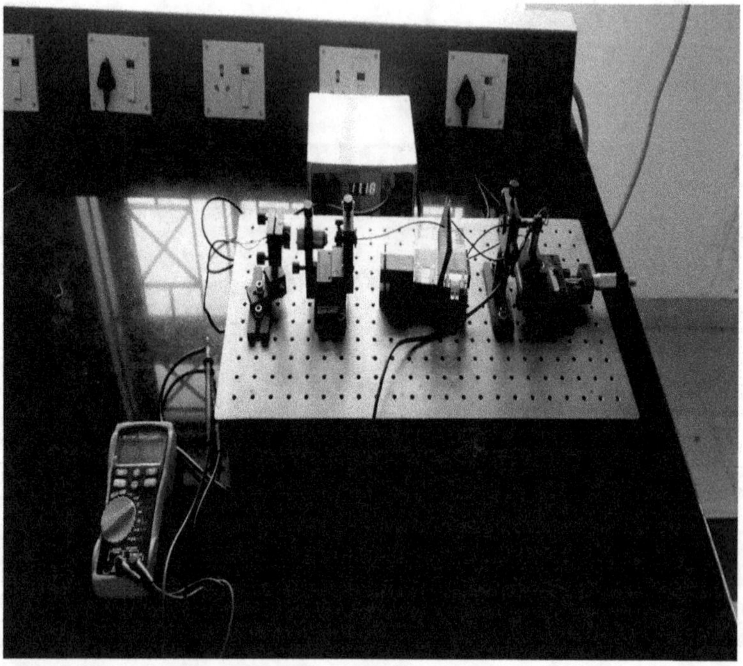

- Jaccard Index = 1
- Jaccard Distance = 0

CONCLUSION

Soft tissues that are found all over our body are complex and highly deformable structures. These soft tissues have varied structural arrangements, constituents, and composition. Hence, soft tissues are generally non-homogeneous in nature. Since soft tissues are not easy to handle, tissue mimicking phantoms have been developed that mimic the properties of biological tissues. These tissue mimicking phantoms can be used instead of soft tissues to study their properties and behavior.

Non-homogeneity in biological tissue may be due to abnormal growth of malignant cells, tumor formation or the presence of foreign particles. Presence of these factors may change the regular structural arrangements or composition of the biological material, thus showing non-homogeneity in the biological tissue material. In this work, an attempt has been made to develop a suitable capacitance sensor array for analyzing the non-homogeneity in biological materials. The sensor array consists 5x5 matrix of conductive points with burge sticks soldered on to it. The array size and spacing can be increased according to imaging requirements. Using this designed sensor array, capacitance values can be obtained from the biological materials to analyze the non-homogeneity in them.

For testing the developed sensor, tissue mimicking phantoms such as agar-agar and polyacrylamide gels have been utilized. Results demonstrate that the sensor is efficient in analyzing the non-homogeneity of biological phantoms. K-mean algorithm has been applied to automatically detect the non-homogeneity in biological materials. The intensity profile of these prepared biological phantoms was obtained to validate the proposed method using Jaccard index. This work appears to be of high significance since the developed capacitance sensor may further be used for diagnostic purposes.

REFERENCES

Ahmad, A., & Hashmi, S. (2016). K-Harmonic means type clustering algorithm for mixed datasets. *Applied Soft Computing*, *48*, 39–49. doi:10.1016/j.asoc.2016.06.019

Arunachalam, K., Jacob, L. V., & Kamalanand, K. (2014). Design and analysis of finite element based sensors for diagnosis of liver disorders using biocompatible metals. *Technology and Health Care*, *22*(6), 867–875. PMID:25391529

Assender, H., Bliznyuk, V., & Porfyrakis, K. (2002). How surface topography relates to materials' properties. *Science*, *297*(5583), 973–976. doi:10.1126cience.1074955 PMID:12169724

Bude, R. O., & Adler, R. S. (1995). An easily made, low-cost, tissue-like ultrasound phantom material. *Journal of Clinical Ultrasound*, *23*(4), 271–273. doi:10.1002/jcu.1870230413 PMID:7797668

Cha, S. H. (2007). Comprehensive survey on distance/similarity measures between probability density functions. *City*, *1*(2), 1.

Cha, S. H., Choi, S., & Tappert, C. C. (2009). Anomaly between jaccard and tanimoto coefficients. *Proceedings of Student-Faculty Research Day, CSIS*. Pace University.

Cheng-Yu, H., Yi-Fan, Z., Guo-Wei, L., Meng-Xi, Z., & Zi-Xiong, L. (2017). Recent progress of using Brillouin distributed fiber sensors for geotechnical health monitoring. *Sensors and Actuators. A, Physical*.

Cheung, Y. M. (2003). k*-Means: A new generalized k-means clustering algorithm. *Pattern Recognition Letters*, *24*(15), 2883–2893. doi:10.1016/S0167-8655(03)00146-6

Chévez, P., Barbero, D., Martini, I., & Discoli, C. (2017). *Application of the k-means clustering method for the detection and analysis of areas of homogeneous residential electricity consumption at the Great La Plata region*. Buenos Aires, Argentina: Sustainable Cities and Society.

Chiang, C. C., Lin, C. C. K., & Ju, M. S. (2007). An implantable capacitive pressure sensor for biomedical applications. *Sensors and Actuators. A, Physical*, *134*(2), 382–388. doi:10.1016/j.sna.2006.06.007

Cook, J. R., Bouchard, R. R., & Emelianov, S. Y. (2011). Tissue-mimicking phantoms for photoacoustic and ultrasonic imaging. *Biomedical Optics Express*, *2*(11), 3193–3206. doi:10.1364/BOE.2.003193 PMID:22076278

Datla, N. V., Konh, B., Koo, J. J., Choi, D. J., Yu, Y., Dicker, A. P., ... Hutapea, P. (2014). Polyacrylamide phantom for self-actuating needle–tissue interaction studies. *Medical Engineering & Physics*, *36*(1), 140–145. doi:10.1016/j.medengphy.2013.07.004 PMID:23932314

De Jong, G. W., & Meijer, G. C. (1997). An efficient retrieving algorithm for accurate capacitive position sensors. *Sensors and Actuators. A, Physical*, *58*(1), 75–84. doi:10.1016/S0924-4247(97)80227-0

Earle, M., De Portu, G., & DeVos, E. (2016). Agar ultrasound phantoms for low-cost training without refrigeration. *African Journal of Emergency Medicine*, *6*(1), 18–23. doi:10.1016/j.afjem.2015.09.003

El-Sherif, M., Bansal, L., & Yuan, J. (2007). Fiber optic sensors for detection of toxic and biological threats. *Sensors (Basel)*, *7*(12), 3100–3118. doi:10.33907123100 PMID:28903282

Erkamp, R. Q., Skovoroda, A. R., Emelianov, S. Y., & O'Donnell, M. (2004). Measuring the nonlinear elastic properties of tissue-like phantoms. *IEEE Transactions on Ultrasonics, Ferroelectrics, and Frequency Control*, *51*(4), 410–419. doi:10.1109/TUFFC.2004.1295426 PMID:15139542

Farrer, A. I., Odéen, H., de Bever, J., Coats, B., Parker, D. L., Payne, A., & Christensen, D. A. (2015). Characterization and evaluation of tissue-mimicking gelatin phantoms for use with MRgFUS. *Journal of Therapeutic Ultrasound*, *3*(1), 9. doi:10.118640349-015-0030-y PMID:26146557

Fidanboylu, K. A., & Efendioglu, H. S. (2009, May). Fiber optic sensors and their applications. *5th International Advanced Technologies Symposium (IATS'09)*, 6.

Goodall, D. W. (1966). A new similarity index based on probability. *Biometrics*, *22*(4), 882–907. doi:10.2307/2528080

Guha, S., Rastogi, R., & Shim, K. (2000). ROCK: A robust clustering algorithm for categorical attributes. *Information Systems*, *25*(5), 345–366. doi:10.1016/S0306-4379(00)00022-3

Holzapfel, G. A. (2001). Biomechanics of soft tissue. The handbook of materials behavior models, 3, 1049-1063.

Ji, B., & Gao, H. (2004). Mechanical properties of nanostructure of biological materials. *Journal of the Mechanics and Physics of Solids*, *52*(9), 1963–1990. doi:10.1016/j.jmps.2004.03.006

Johnston, J. W. (1976). *Similarity Indices I: What Do They Measure?* Academic Press.

Kamalanand, K., Sridhar, B. T. N., Rajeshwari, P. M., & Ramakrishnan, S. (2010). Correlation of Dielectric Permittivity with Mechanical Properties in Soft Tissue-Mimicking Polyacrylamide Phantoms. *Journal of Mechanics in Medicine and Biology*, *10*(02), 353–360. doi:10.1142/S0219519410003411

Kawabata, K. I., Waki, Y., Matsumura, T., & Umemura, S. I. (2004, August). Tissue mimicking phantom for ultrasonic elastography with finely adjustable elastic and echographic properties. In *Ultrasonics Symposium*, 2004 *IEEE* (*Vol. 2*, pp. 1502-1505). IEEE. 10.1109/ULTSYM.2004.1418087

Kersey, A. D., Davis, M. A., Patrick, H. J., LeBlanc, M., Koo, K. P., Askins, C. G., & Friebele, E. J. (1997). Fiber grating sensors. *Journal of Lightwave Technology*, *15*(8), 1442–1463. doi:10.1109/50.618377

Kim, D., & Economou, D. J. (2002). Plasma molding over surface topography: Simulation of ion flow, and energy and angular distributions over steps in RF high-density plasmas. *IEEE Transactions on Plasma Science*, *30*(5), 2048–2058. doi:10.1109/TPS.2002.805326

Koerdel, M., Alatas, F., Schick, A., Rupitsch, S. J., & Lerch, R. (2011). Contactless inspection of planar electronic devices by capacitive coupling: Development of a model describing the sensor signal and its impact on signal post-processing. *Sensors and Actuators. A, Physical*, *172*(1), 88–97. doi:10.1016/j.sna.2011.02.040

Krishnamurthy, K., Sridhar, B. T. N., Rajeshwari, P. M., & Swaminathan, D. R. (2009). Correlation of Electrical Impedance with Mechanical Properties in Models of Tissue Mimicking Phantoms. In *13th International Conference on Biomedical Engineering* (pp. 1708-1711). Springer Berlin Heidelberg. 10.1007/978-3-540-92841-6_424

Kuru, E. A., Orakdogen, N., & Okay, O. (2007). Preparation of homogeneous polyacrylamide hydrogels by free-radical crosslinking copolymerization. *European Polymer Journal*, *43*(7), 2913–2921. doi:10.1016/j.eurpolymj.2007.04.019

Lafon, C., Kaczkowski, P. J., Vaezy, S., Noble, M., & Sapozhnikov, O. A. (2001). Development and characterization of an innovative synthetic tissue-mimicking material for high intensity focused ultrasound (HIFU) exposures. In *Ultrasonics Symposium*, 2001 *IEEE* (*Vol. 2*, pp. 1295-1298). IEEE. 10.1109/ULTSYM.2001.991957

Lazebnik, M., Madsen, E. L., Frank, G. R., & Hagness, S. C. (2005). Tissue-mimicking phantom materials for narrowband and ultrawideband microwave applications. *Physics in Medicine and Biology*, *50*(18), 4245–4258. doi:10.1088/0031-9155/50/18/001 PMID:16148391

Lee, T. (2003). *Design, fabrication and characterization of fiber optic sensors for physical and chemical applications* (Doctoral dissertation). Cochin University.

Li, X., & Meijer, G. C. (2002). An accurate interface for capacitive sensors. *IEEE Transactions on Instrumentation and Measurement*, *51*(5), 935–939. doi:10.1109/TIM.2002.807793

Madsen, E. L., Hobson, M. A., Shi, H., Varghese, T., & Frank, G. R. (2005). Tissue-mimicking agar/gelatin materials for use in heterogeneous elastography phantoms. *Physics in Medicine and Biology*, *50*(23), 5597–5618. doi:10.1088/0031-9155/50/23/013 PMID:16306655

Madsen, E. L., Zagzebski, J. A., & Frank, G. R. (1982). Oil-in-gelatin dispersions for use as ultrasonically tissue-mimicking materials. *Ultrasound in Medicine & Biology*, *8*(3), 277–287. doi:10.1016/0301-5629(82)90034-5 PMID:7101576

Manickavasagam, K., Sutha, S., & Kamalanand, K. (2014). An automated system based on 2 d empirical mode decomposition and k-means clustering for classification of Plasmodium species in thin blood smear images. *BMC Infectious Diseases*, *14*(S3), 13. doi:10.1186/1471-2334-14-S3-P13 PMID:24405683

Manickavasagam, K., Sutha, S., & Kamalanand, K. (2014). Development of systems for classification of different plasmodium species in thin blood smear microscopic images. *Journal of Advanced Microscopy Research*, *9*(2), 86–92. doi:10.1166/jamr.2014.1194

Marieb, E. N. (2000). *Essentials of human anatomy & physiology*. Benjamin Cummings.

Matiss, I. (2014). Multi-element capacitive sensor for non-destructive measurement of the dielectric permittivity and thickness of dielectric plates and shells. *NDT & E International*, *66*, 99–105. doi:10.1016/j.ndteint.2014.05.003

Menter, P. (2000). Acrylamide Polymerization— A Practical Approach. *Bio-Rad Tech Note, 1156*.

Mordacq, J. C., & Ellington, R. W. (1994). Polyacrylamide gel electrophoresis (PAGE) of blood proteins. *Tested Studies for Laboratory Teaching, 15*, 15-44.

Nayakam, G. N. (2013). Study of Similarity Coefficients Using MapReduce Programming Model. *Circulation*, *701*, 8888.

Nazeer, K. A., & Sebastian, M. P. (2009, July). Improving the Accuracy and Efficiency of the k-means Clustering Algorithm. In *Proceedings of the World Congress on Engineering* (*Vol. 1*, pp. 1-3). Academic Press.

Nemat-Nasser, S., & Hori, M. (2013). *Micromechanics: overall properties of heterogeneous materials* (Vol. 37). Elsevier.

Niwattanakul, S., Singthongchai, J., Naenudorn, E., & Wanapu, S. (2013, March). Using of Jaccard coefficient for keywords similarity. *Proceedings of the International MultiConference of Engineers and Computer Scientists*, *1*, 6.

Nymeyer, H., & Zhou, H. X. (2008). A method to determine dielectric constants in nonhomogeneous systems: Application to biological membranes. *Biophysical Journal*, *94*(4), 1185–1193. doi:10.1529/biophysj.107.117770 PMID:17951302

Ortega, J. P., Del, M., Rojas, R. B., & Somodevilla, M. J. Research issues on k-means algorithm: An experimental trial using matlab. *CEUR Workshop Proceedings: Semantic Web and New Technologies*.

Podolak, E., Kinn, J. B., & Westura, E. E. (1969). Biomedical applications of a commercial capacitance transducer. *IEEE Transactions on Biomedical Engineering*, *BME-16*(1), 40–44. doi:10.1109/TBME.1969.4502601 PMID:5775604

Puers, R. (1993). Capacitive sensors: When and how to use them. *Sensors and Actuators. A, Physical*, *37*, 93–105. doi:10.1016/0924-4247(93)80019-D

Real, R., & Vargas, J. M. (1996). The probabilistic basis of Jaccard's index of similarity. *Systematic Biology*, *45*(3), 380–385. doi:10.1093ysbio/45.3.380

Rowan, M., & Pedersen, P. (2006, October). P2C-3 an injury mimicking ultrasound phantom as a training tool for diagnosis of internal trauma. In *Ultrasonics Symposium, 2006. IEEE* (pp. 1612-1617). IEEE.

Seifoddini, H., & Djassemi, M. (1991). The production data-based similarity coefficient versus Jaccard's similarity coefficient. *Computers & Industrial Engineering*, *21*(1-4), 263–266. doi:10.1016/0360-8352(91)90099-R

Sepulveda, A. T., Fachin, F., de Villoria, R. G., Wardle, B. L., Viana, J. C., Pontes, A. J., & Rocha, L. A. (2011). Nanocomposite flexible pressure sensor for biomedical applications. *Procedia Engineering*, *25*, 140–143. doi:10.1016/j.proeng.2011.12.035

Shikalgar, N. R., & Dixit, A. M. (2014). JIBCA: Jaccard Index based Clustering Algorithm for Mining Online Review. *International Journal of Computers and Applications*, *105*(15).

Sumathi, M., & Pratheep, R. (2012, October). *Intensity Based Fiber Optic Deflection Sensor*. ICOP-2009-International Conference on Optics and Photonics, CSIO, Chandigarh.

Surry, K. J. M., Austin, H. J. B., Fenster, A., & Peters, T. M. (2004). Poly (vinyl alcohol) cryogel phantoms for use in ultrasound and MR imaging. *Physics in Medicine and Biology*, *49*(24), 5529–5546. doi:10.1088/0031-9155/49/24/009 PMID:15724540

Takegami, K., Kaneko, Y., Watanabe, T., Maruyama, T., Matsumoto, Y., & Nagawa, H. (2004). Polyacrylamide gel containing egg white as new model for irradiation experiments using focused ultrasound. *Ultrasound in Medicine & Biology*, *30*(10), 1419–1422. doi:10.1016/j.ultrasmedbio.2004.07.016 PMID:15582242

Thada, V., & Jaglan, V. (2013). Comparison of jaccard, dice and cosine similarity coefficient to find best fitness value for web retrieved documents using genetic algorithm. *International Journal of Innovations in Engineering and Technology*, *2*(4), 202–205.

Tsang, K. M., & Chan, W. L. (2011). Dual capacitive sensors for non-contact AC voltage measurement. *Sensors and Actuators. A, Physical*, *167*(2), 261–266. doi:10.1016/j.sna.2011.02.019

Wang, B., Lv, Z., Zhao, J., Wang, X., & Zhang, T. (2016, December). An Adaptively Disperse Centroids K-Means Algorithm Based on MapReduce Model. In *Computational Intelligence and Security (CIS), 2016 12th International Conference on* (pp. 142-146). IEEE. 10.1109/CIS.2016.0041

Yadav, J., & Sharma, M. (2013). A Review of K-mean Algorithm. *International Journal of Engineering Trends and Technology*, *4*(7), 2972–2975.

Yedla, M., Pathakota, S. R., & Srinivasa, T. M. (2010). Enhancing K-means clustering algorithm with improved initial center. *International Journal of Computer Science and Information Technologies, 1*(2), 121-125.

Yuan, Y., Wyatt, C., Maccarini, P., Stauffer, P., Craciunescu, O., MacFall, J., & Das, S. K. (2012). A heterogeneous human tissue mimicking phantom for RF heating and MRI thermal monitoring verification. *Physics in Medicine and Biology*, *57*(7), 2021–2037. doi:10.1088/0031-9155/57/7/2021 PMID:22430012

Zhou, M. X., Huang, Q. A., & Qin, M. (2005). Modeling, design and fabrication of a triple-layered capacitive pressure sensor. *Sensors and Actuators. A, Physical*, *117*(1), 71–81. doi:10.1016/j.sna.2004.05.036

Zhu, F., Spronck, J. W., & Heerens, W. C. (1991). A simple capacitive displacement sensor. *Sensors and Actuators. A, Physical*, *26*(1-3), 265–269. doi:10.1016/0924-4247(91)87003-L

Zurek, S., & Meydan, T. (2006). A novel capacitive flux density sensor. *Sensors and Actuators. A, Physical*, *129*(1), 121–125. doi:10.1016/j.sna.2005.11.027

KEY TERMS AND DEFINITIONS

Agar-Agar: A substance obtained from polysaccharide agarose.

APS: Ammonium Per-Sulphate.

Fiber Optic Sensor: A sensor that uses optical fiber either as the sensing element or as a means of relaying signals from a remote sensor to the electronics.

ITO: Indium Tin Oxide.

Jaccard Similarity Coefficient: A statistic used for comparing the similarity and diversity of different sample sets.

K-Mean Algorithm: An unsupervised and iterative method for clustering of data points.

Morphology: Form, shape, or structure of a material.

PAUS Imaging: Photoacoustic and ultrasonic imaging.

PCB: Printed circuit board.

Polyacrylamide: A polymer formed from acrylamide subunits.

TEMED: Tetramethylethylenediamine.

Tissue Mimicking Phantoms: Artificial materials that reproduces the properties of the natural biological tissues.

Topography: The distribution of parts or features on the surface of a material.

UCI: Unique client identifier.

Chapter 5
Development of an Automated Decision Support System for Diagnosis of Digestive Disorders Using Electrogastrograms:
An Approach Based on Empirical Mode Decomposition and K-Means Algorithm

Arivarasu Rajagopal
Madras Institute of Technology, India

Paramasivam Alagumariappan
Madras Institute of Technology, India

Kamalanand Krishnamurthy
Madras Institute of Technology, India

ABSTRACT

The disorders of the digestive tract lead to various problems such as bleeding, bloating, nausea, etc. In order to diagnose various digestive abnormalities, the electrogastrograms (EGG) can serve as an efficient tool. In an EGG, several electrodes are placed onto the abdomen over the stomach and the electrical signals originating from the stomach muscles are recorded. By analyzing these electrical patterns, the abnormalities in digestive system can be analyzed. This chapter describes the developed system for measuring EGG signals along with the decision support

DOI: 10.4018/978-1-5225-5149-2.ch005

system developed for automated classification of digestive disorders. The normal and abnormal EGG signals were acquired at Balaji Medical Hospital, Chennai. Further, the features were extracted using descriptive statistics and empirical mode decomposition (EMD) algorithm. Finally, an automated classification system was developed using k-means algorithm. This chapter explains the recording of electrogastrograms and a method for classification of normal and abnormal EGG signals.

INTRODUCTION

The digestive system consists of the digestive tract, a tube extending from the mouth to the anus, and its associated accessory organs, primarily glands, which secrete fluids into digestive tract (Tortora & Derrickson, 2008). The function of digestive system includes: Ingestion, mastication, propulsion, mixing, secretion, digestion, absorption and elimination. Digestion is a multistage process in which food is broken down and nutrients are absorbed (Paramasivam, Rajagopal, & Krishnamurthy, 2016). Digestive system is highly interconnected since disorder in digestive system affects other systems.

Digestive diseases are disorders of the digestive tract and problems in the digestive tract include several symptoms like heartburn, nausea, vomiting, bleeding, bloating, diarrhea, constipation etc (Alagumariappan, Krishnamurthy, Kandiah, & Ponnuswamy, 2017). The clinical pattern of digestive diseases differ in different parts of the world and even vary from area to area in the same country. Racial, hereditary factors, climatic conditions, dietetic habits etc. are some of the important factors involved in the genesis of these variations (Vakil, 1960; Inoue, Iwamura, & Yoshida, 2001). Digestive diseases significantly affect millions of humans worldwide resulting in decreased quality of life. Several diagnostic techniques such as biopsy, endoscopy, ultrasound scanning, Electrogastrography etc. are used to investigate the digestive system disorders. Nowadays Endoscopy procedure is followed to investigate the problems in the digestive system disorders, which is a tedious, expensive and invasive method (Gopu, Neelaveni, & Porkumaran, 2008).

One of the primary disadvantages of ultrasound is that it is operator dependent and the accuracy of the examination is limited by the comfort level of patient and skill of the examiner. Although ultrasound can provide exquisitely detailed pictures, it is not intended to evaluate diffuse pain. Limitations of abdominal ultrasound generally are related to factors which limit transmission of the ultrasound beam. These limitations include obesity, excessive bowel gas, and barium in the intestines from recent fluoroscopic procedure. Obese patients are more difficult to image by ultrasound because greater amounts of tissue attenuate (weaken) the sound waves as they pass deeper into the body.

Electrogastrography is an efficient and noninvasive alternative for diagnosis of digestive disorders. EGG signals are electrical activity generated by the stomach (Alagumariappan, Krishnamurthy, Kandiah, & Ponnuswamy, 2017; Yin & Chen, 2013; Ding, Qin, Miao, Xi, Li, & Wang, 2010). The EGG signals are measured by placing cutaneous electrodes onto the abdomen over the stomach (Alagumariappan, Krishnamurthy, Kandiah, & Ponnuswamy, 2017). The features of the EGG signals of normal individuals differ when compared to the features of the signals obtained from human subjects with digestive abnormalities (Gopu, Neelaveni, & Porkumaran, 2008; Paramasivam, Rajagopal, & Krishnamurthy, 2016). By analyzing such features, various digestive diseases such as Gastroesophageal Reflux Disease (GERD), Diabetic Neuropathy, Anorexia Nervosa, Idiopathic Gastroparesis, Motion Sickness, Pan Gastro Neoplastic Syndrome, Bradygastria, Tachygastria, Functional Dyspepsia, Epigastric Pain Syndrome etc can be diagnosed. Electrogastrogram is a low cost, painless method and is an initial mode of investigation for gastric disorders before encouraging the Endoscope procedure for uncomplicated gastric disease and benign tumors.

Several electrodes such as wet electrodes, gelled electrodes, dry electrodes etc. are commonly used for acquisition of biological signals (Neuman, 1998). The silver/silver chloride (Ag/Agcl) electrodes are most commonly used cutaneous electrodes since it provides stable recordings for various physiological measurements even at low voltage and low frequency signals (Alagumariappan, Krishnamurthy, Kandiah, & Ponnuswamy, 2017). The Ag/Agcl electrodes are disposable and the recordings are highly optimal.

For normal individuals, the gastric electrical activity occurs at a frequency of 3 cycles per minute (cpm) in the stomach. The intestinal cells of Cajal (ICC) is responsible for rhythmic depolarization's of the gastric slow wave. Depolarizations occur at frequencies lower than normal frequency leads to Bradygastria and depolarization occur at frequencies higher than normal frequency leads to Tachygastria (Parkman, Hasler, Barnett, & Eaker, 2003). Several components are essential for the performance of EGG such as cutaneous Ag/AgCl electrodes, Amplifiers and filters. The Ag/AgCl electrodes are employed to facilitate reliable acquisition of EGG signals. Amplifiers are required since the EGG signals ranges 100uV to 400uV and filters are used to eliminate respiration and motion artifacts (Komorowski, & Tkacz, 2015). The electrical signals recorded from the stomach contains not only the desired EGG signal but also other physiological interferences such as electrical activity of the abdominal muscles, respiration artifacts and some non-physiological interferences such as powerline interference and motion artifacts (Taralunga, Ungureanu, Hurezeanu, Gussi, & Strungaru, 2015; Komorowski, & Tkacz, 2015). Thus, more complex signal processing is required to remove physiological and non-physiological interferences from raw EGG signal. One of the most promising techniques for denoising biological signal is the Empirical Mode Decomposition (EMD) method. The EMD method is fully data-driven and no prior knowledge about the signal of interest is required. The EMD decomposes non-stationary complicated data in a finite and small number of oscillations named intrinsic mode functions (IMFs). The process is based on the local characteristics of data on the time scale, thus, it is fully data driven and adaptive, making it suitable for decomposing non-stationary data (Taralunga, Ungureanu, Hurezeanu, Gussi, & Strungaru, 2015).

The most widely used clustering formulations based on minimizing a formal objective function is K-means clustering. Clustering based on K-means is closely related to a number of other clustering and location problems (Kanungo, Mount, Netanyathu, Piatko, Silverman, & Wu, 2002). These include the Euclidean k-medians, in which the objective is to minimize the sum of distances to the nearest center and the geometric sum of distances to the nearest center and the geometric K-center problem in which the objective is to minimize the maximum distance from every point to its closest center. K-means algorithm is one of the most popular heuristics for solving the K-means problem which is based on a simple iterative scheme for finding a locally minimal solution. In this chapter, the development of an automated decision support system for diagnosis of digestive disorders using Electrogastrograms has been described in detail.

BACKGROUND

In recent years, EGG has become an attractive tool for several researchers to investigate the electrophysiology of the stomach and pathophysiology of gastric motility disorders. Yin et al. (2013) have discussed the methodology, validation and applications of EGG. Firstly, the authors have stated the correlation between the gastric slow wave and gastric motility. Also, the authors have discussed briefly about the recording method for electrogastrogram and its pitfalls in the recording. The authors have concluded that the EGG is an accurate measure of gastric slow wave when it is recorded appropriately and provides clinically, physiologically or pathophysiologically meaningful information when it is properly analyzed and interpreted. Calder et al. (2014) have developed a boundary element model to investigate the relationship between the gastric electrical activity and the electrogastrogram. Further, the authors have calculated a dipole to represent the equivalent net activity of gastric slow waves. Also, the authors have analyzed the simulated EGG results using the Fast Fourier Transforms (FFT), spatial distribution of EGG potential and a resultant EGG based on a three-lead configuration. Liang and Chen (1997) have investigated the detectability of the propagation of the gastric slow wave from the cutaneous electrogastrogram (EGG). Further, the authors have developed a mathematical model based on the volume conductor theory to simulate the transfer of serosal gastric slow wave from the stomach to the abdominal surface and conducted number of computer simulations on the developed model. Further, the authors have concluded that the propagation of gastric slow wave is detectable from the multichannel EGG signals.

Li and Ren (2008) from Chongqing University of Posts and Telecommunications have developed a signal processing device to investigate the complex course of the electrical and mechanical processes of functional dyspepsia (FD). Further, the authors have separated impedance gastric motility and EGG signals impedance signals due to breathing and blood flow using wavelet transform. Zhao et al. (2012) have proposed a new method by combining EGG and impedance gastric motility for noninvasive measurement of gastric motility. Obioha et al. (2013) have analyzed the effects of body mass index (BMI) on the sensitivity of Magnetogastrogram (MGG) and Elecrogastrogram. Further, the authors have concluded that the Second Order Blind Identification (SOBI) has increased sensitivity of EGG and MGG recordings irrespective to BMI or waist circumference. Riezzo et al. (2013) have reviewed the state of the art about the pathophysiological background of the gastric electrical activity, the recording and processing methology of the EGG with particular attention to multichannel recording, and the possible clinical application of the EGG in adult and children.

Haddab and Laghrouche (2009) have designed a device to monitor the EGG signals of a patient outside the hospital environment and the signal acquisition is achieved by means of an ambulatory system carried by the patient which is connected through surface electrodes. The signal acquired by the proposed device is transmitted via the Bluetooth to a mobile phone where the data are stored to the memory and then transferred via the GSM network to the processing and diagnostic unit in the hospital. Further, the authors have proposed a neural network method for removal of motion artefacts and biological signal separation.

Li et al. (2008) have proposed a new noninvasive method using Bio-Impedance and synchronous electrogastrogram to assess gastric motility. Further, the authors have employed wavelet transform to separate Electrical impedance signals (EIP) breath and heart activity signals. Also, the authors have discussed the temporal-domain and frequency-domain parameters for EIP and heart activity signals to evaluate gastric motility. Finally, the authors have concluded that there is a significant difference in the temporal-domain and frequency-domain properties between two groups, such as slow waves of EGG and EIP, signal power spectrum etc. Contreras et al. (2010) have developed a system for acquisition and analysis of three electrogastrogram (EGG) signals and two monitor signals such as respiration, muscle movement and its route along the stomach wall. The proposed system records the signals using three pairs of electrodes affixed to the external abdominal wall and filtered with a low pass filter with cut-off frequency of 1 Hz. Further, the authors have concluded that the proposed system is capable of computing parameters associated with the pacemaker frequency such as percentages of bradygastria, tachygastria, arrhythmia and typical range during recording time.

Barroso et al. (2011) have discussed the visual analysis of the EGG, denoised processes, filtering, wavelet analysis of the signals from EGG database. Familoni et al. (1995) have developed a model for gastric electrical activity which is applicable both in health and disease. Further, the authors have investigated the correlation between the amplitude of the simulated cutaneous EGG and the velocity of propagation of the myogenic activity. Also, the authors have compared a similar investigation of the oscillations in the amplitude of the cutaneous EGG with the velocity of propagation of the serosal activity measured in humans. Finally, the authors have concluded that the amplitude of the electrogastrogram increases with the propagation velocity of GEA.

Komorowski et al. (2015) have examined a noninvasive method for an investigation of stomach slow wave propagation. Further, the authors have proposed an adaptive filtering method and concluded that the proposed method has a possibility to obtain simultaneously recorded signals such as non-standard derivation of ECG, heart rate variability signal, respiratory signal and EGG signal that allow investigating mutual interferences among internal human systems.

Gharibans et al. (2016) have developed a high resolution (EGG) for estimation of direction and speed of gastric slow-waves using array of electrodes. Kolev (1999) has proposed a method with simple compressed presentation of long term EGG recordings, without losing information such as amplitude and frequency. Leahy et al. (1999) have discussed about the assessment of the specificity of electrogastrography as well as the prevalence and pattern of abnormalities in functional dyspepsia and irritable bowel syndrome. Gopu et al. (2008) have proposed a method to find the digestive system's disorders using Virtual Instrumentation (VI) based EGG. Further, the authors have concluded that the digestive system's disorder dissimilarity is found in its frequency, amplitude, power spectrum analysis and the statistical analysis compared with its normal individual.

In the past two decades, several biomedical researchers have adopted various feature extraction techniques for extraction of normal and abnormal EGG signal features. Al-Subari et al. (2015) have introduced a new toolbox called EMDLAB provides an alternative decomposition technique. Further, the authors have concluded that the proposed toolbox is more convenient to analyze non-stationary time series data sets, mainly EEG data, with heuristic signal decomposition techniques. Liang et al. (2000) have proposed Empirical Mode Decomposition (EMD) method to remove a variety of artifacts from EGG recordings. Further, the authors have concluded that the proposed EMD method effectively separates, identify and remove variety of artifacts in EGG recordings. Taralunga et al. (2015) have proposed the empirical mode decomposition method for Electrohysterographic (EHG) signals denoising. Further, the authors have reported that the proposed method is very simple and more suitable for non-stationary data like EHG.

Kanungo et al. (2002) have proposed a simple and efficient implementation of Lloyd's K-means clustering algorithm (filtering algorithm). Further, the authors have concluded that the proposed algorithm is easy to implement and requires a kd-tree as the only major data structure. Xia et al. (2015) have proposed a method for quick detection of QRS complexes and R-waves using a wavelet transform and K-means clustering. Further, the authors have concluded that the proposed method has an average R-peak detection sensitivity of 99.72% and a positive predictive value of 99.80%.

Khanmohammedi et al., (2016) have proposed a hybrid method that combines k-harmonic means and overlapping K-means algorithm (KHM-OKM) to overcome limitation such as low sensitivity to initial cluster centroids. Further, the authors have tested the proposed algorithm using FBcubed metric, which is shown to be the most effective measure to evaluate overlapping clustering algorithms regarding homogeneity, completeness, rag bag, and cluster size-quantity tradeoff. Also, the authors have concluded that the proposed algorithm is very efficient for clustering medical datasets.

Orhan et al. (2011) have proposed a multilayer perceptron neural network (MLPNN) based classification model as a diagnostic decision support mechanism for epilepsy treatment. Further, the authors have decomposed EEG signals into sub-bands using discrete wavelet transform (DWT) and clustered wavelet coefficients using the K-means algorithm. Ning et al. (2015) have developed a new method by combining the K-mean clustering method (KMC) and a modified convolution kernel compensation method (CKC) for decomposition of multichannel surface electromyogram (EMG). Further, the authors have evaluated the performance of K-means clustering and modified convolution kernel compensation approach by reconstructing innervations pulse train from simulated and experimental surface EMG signals.

Merino et al. (2015) have proposed an offline version and a real-time implementation of a new algorithm to determine QRS localization in the ECG signals using Envelopment filter and K-means clustering algorithm. Further, the authors have reported that the proposed algorithm has low computational load with accuracy of 99.7%. Liang (2005) has proposed two-stage combined method (independent component analysis and adaptive signal enhancement) for extraction of gastric slow waves in each of the multichannel EGGs. Tokmakci (2007) has analyzed the EGG using discrete wavelet transform and statistical methods to detect Gastric Dysrhythmia.

In recent years, computational methods have been utilized for development of diagnostic assistance tools for biomedical analysis (Wojewnik, & Zmigrodzki, 2013; Manickavasagam, Sutha, & Kamalanand, 2014; Rajinikanth, & Couceiro, 2014; Kamalanand, & Jawahar, 2012, 2013, 2015, 2016; Berradja & Boughanmi, 2016; Ben Hassen, Ben Zakour, & Taleb, 2016; Khanmohammadi, Adibeig, & Shanehbandy, 2017; Lakshmi, Tebby, Shriranjani, & Rajinikanth, 2016; Rajinikanth, Satapathy, Fernandes, & Nachippan, 2017). Alagumariappan et al., (2016) have proposed a method to analyze complexity on normal and abnormal electrogastrograms using Tsallis entropy. Further, the authors have concluded that the complexity of normal EGG signals is high when compared to the complexity of abnormal EGG signals.

EXPERIMENTAL SETUP

The two lead EGG measurement system using Instrumentation Amplifier (INA) designed by three op-amp is used. The amplitude of EGG signal for normal individual ranges from 100 uV to 400 uV (Koch & Stern, 2004; Komorowski, & Tkacz, 2015). The INA is used to amplify the microvolt EGG signal into the range of volts so as to be within the range of Data acquisition (DAQ). DAQ is the process of measuring an electrical phenomenon such as voltage, current, temperature etc., with a computer. In the proposed system, the DAQ system consists of DAQ measurement hardware, and a computer with NI-LabVIEW (V 14.0.1) software. Figure 1 shows a circuit diagram of two lead EGG measurement system.

The opamps labeled U1 and U2 are the input buffers and the gains of these buffers are not unity because of R1 and Rg. The op-amp labeled U3 is a standard differential amplifier. Two cutaneous electrodes are employed, one as reference electrode and the other as measurand electrode which are connected to non-inverting pins of op-amps U1 and U2 respectively. The voltage gain of the instrumentation amplifier can be expressed as

$$Voltage\ gain(A_v) = V_0 / (V_2 - V_1) = (1 + 2R_1 / R_g).R_3 / R_2 \tag{1}$$

Figure 1. Circuit diagram of two lead EGG measurement system

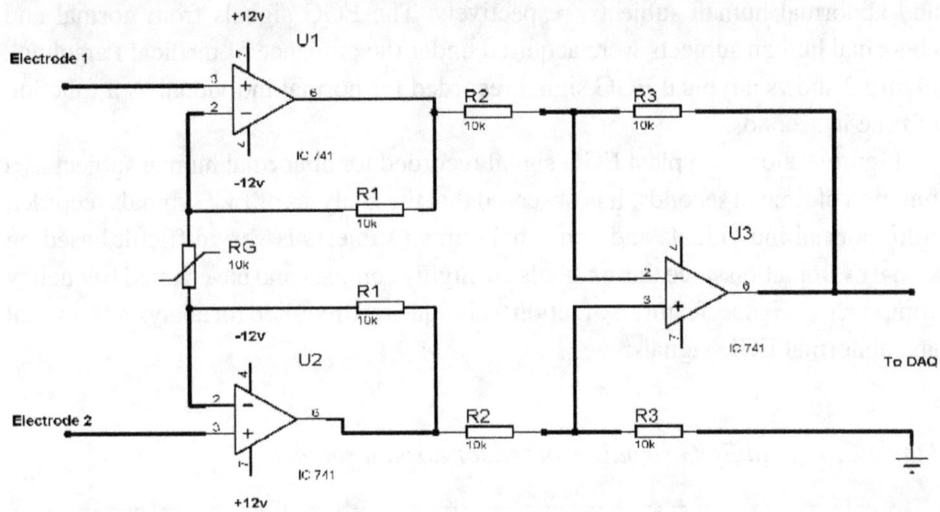

For variable gain, the Rg can be replaced with a suitable potentiometer. According to standard electrode placement protocol, the measurand electrode is placed between the umbilicus and the xyphoid process, and the reference electrode is placed on the left side of the abdomen, one-third of the distance from the ventral mid-line to the left axial mid-line, 1 cm below the lowest rib (Patterson, Rintala, Lloyd, Abernethy, Houghton, & Williams, 2001). LabVIEW is a platform and development environment for a visual programming language from National Instruments. A new VI page consists of Front Panel window and the Block Diagram window. The block diagram contains the graphical source code and the Front Panel objects appear as terminals on the block diagram window. Once a DAQ is interfaced with PC, a popup menu appears, in which the signal acquisition type whether to acquire or generate is selected. Then channel and signal mode is selected in the next window. The amplified EGG signal output of the instrumentation amplifier is fed to PC by interfacing USB DAQ6008 along with NI-LabVIEW software (Alagumariappan, Krishnamurthy, Kandiah & Ponnuswamy, 2017). Thus, the EGG signals acquired from normal individuals and abnormal subjects can be monitored and logged using the NI-LabVIEW software.

MEASUREMENT AND ANALYSIS OF NORMAL AND ABNORMAL EGG SIGNALS

The EGG signals originating from the stomach were measured using the proposed system. The permission was granted by the superintendent of medicine at local

Medical Hospital, Chennai and EGG signals were acquired from normal individuals and abnormal human subjects, respectively. The EGG signals from normal and abnormal human subjects were acquired under the guidance of medical Personnel. Figure 2 shows a typical EGG signal recorded for normal individual as a function of time in seconds.

Figure 3 shows a typical EGG signal recorded for abnormal human subject as a function of time in seconds. It is observed that the analyses of EGG signals recorded from normal individuals and abnormal human subjects is very difficult based on visual examination since these signals are highly complex and have varied frequency components. Hence, feature extraction techniques are required for analysis of normal and abnormal EGG signals.

Figure 2. Typical EGG signal recorded for normal subject

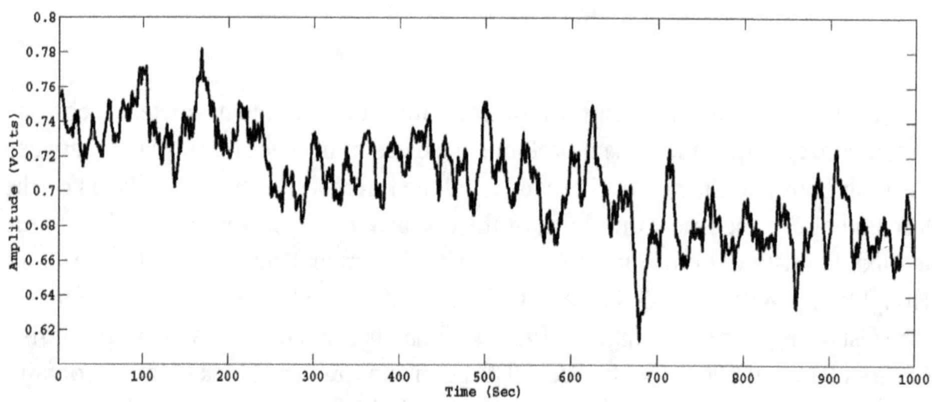

Figure 3. Typical EGG signal recorded for abnormal subject

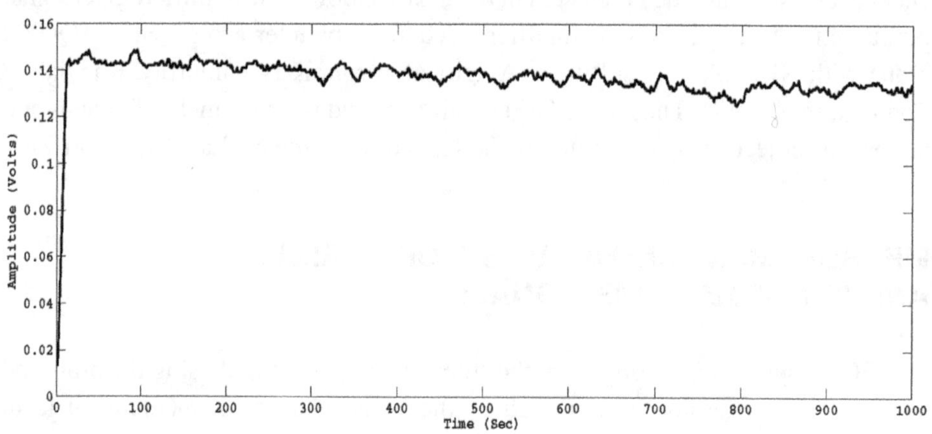

The Descriptive statistics such as mean, mode, median, standard deviation, kurtosis, standard deviation, skewness and the statistical features of intrinsic mode functions obtained from Empirical mode decomposition (EMD) were calculated for EGG signals recorded from normal individuals and abnormal human subjects.

Table 1 represents descriptive statistics such as Variance, Mode, Median, Mean, Standard Deviation, Kurtosis and Skewness of normal EGG signals. Table 2 represents descriptive statistics such as Variance, Mode, Median, Mean, Standard Deviation, Kurtosis and Skewness of abnormal EGG signals. The variations in the descriptive statistics such as the Mean, Mode, Standard Deviation, Variance, Kurtosis and Skewness of the signals were observed between normal and abnormal cases. It is seen that the Variance, Kurtosis and Skewness of EGG signals acquired from normal individuals is higher than the Variance, Kurtosis and Skewness of EGG signals acquired from abnormal subjects. Further, it is observed that the Mode,

Table 1. Descriptive statistics of normal EGG signals

Significant	Normal Subject									
Cases	1	2	3	4	5	6	7	8	9	10
Variance	0.0068	0.0103	0.0226	0.0216	0.0183	0.0284	2.2752	0.0347	2.8605	1.3224
Mode	0.6409	0.8699	1.1546	1.6470	0.1819	0.6798	0.1012	2.4853	0.1012	0.5757
Median	0.6084	0.8199	1.2413	1.6118	0.1986	0.1012	0.1012	2.4867	0.1021	0.5717
Mean	0.5799	0.8005	1.2392	1.5455	0.1582	0.6989	0.1008	2.4651	0.1016	0.5717
Standard Deviation	0.0827	0.1016	0.1504	0.1468	0.1351	0.1686	0.0051	0.1863	0.0053	0.0115
Kurtosis	5.5779	5.5106	3.4343	15.719	3.2340	10.926	14.665	5.8335	12.415	2.7947
Skewness	-1.416	-0.915	-0.215	-2.726	-1.138	-2.432	-10.76	-7.244	-9.694	-0.021

Table 2. Descriptive statistics of abnormal EGG signals

Significant	Abnormal Subject									
Cases	1	2	3	4	5	6	7	8	9	10
Variance	7.7844	0.0140	0.0145	0.0347	3.3779	4.6946	4.6946	4.9111	4.7008	0.0015
Mode	0.1420	2.4111	2.444	2.4853	0.0743	0.6409	0.6404	1.7407	0.6409	0.7188
Median	0.1374	2.4167	2.4371	2.4867	0.0729	0.6353	0.6350	1.7416	0.6353	0.7276
Mean	0.1369	2.0486	2.4261	2.4657	0.0715	0.6334	0.6334	1.7406	0.6334	0.7367
Standard Deviation	0.0088	0.1182	0.1207	0.1863	0.0194	0.0217	0.0220	0.0222	0.0217	0.0381
Kurtosis	9.5461	1.726	165.91	58.333	2.6283	2.3192	2.3189	2.4809	2.3143	3.8157
Skewness	-8.025	-1.235	-12.02	-7.244	-0.091	-0.114	-0.113	-0.277	-0.116	-1.219

Median, Mean and Standard Deviation values of normal EGG signals is lesser when compared to the Mode, Median, Mean and Standard Deviation values of abnormal EGG signals. Significant variations were observed in the Kurtosis and mean values of normal and abnormal EGG signals.

EMPIRICAL MODE DECOMPOSITION

The EMD is locally adaptive and suitable for analysis of nonlinear or non-stationary processes (Manickavasagam, Sutha, & Kamalanand, 2014). EMD is an adaptive and data driven multi-resolution technique, in which a multi-component waveform is resolved into several components. These components, referred to as intrinsic mode functions (IMF), are expected to be mono-component in nature. Application of Hilbert transform yields their analytic forms, from which their instantaneous amplitudes and frequencies can be extracted. However, the original EMD technique fails to separate participating modes whose instantaneous frequencies simultaneously lie within an octave. The use of a masking signal based EMD was initially proposed to improve the filtering characteristics of the EMD (Deering & Kaiser, 2005)

The steps involved in the EMD method are as follows:

Step 1: Identify local maxima and minima of input signal, $x(t)$
Step 2: Perform cubic spline interpolation between the maxima and the minima to obtain the envelopes $U_1(t)$ and $L_1(t)$, respectively.
Step 3: Compute mean of the envelopes, $m(t) = \left(U_1(t) + L_1(t)\right) / 2$
Step 4: Extract $h_1(t) = x(t) - m(t)$,
Step 5: $h_1(t)$ is an IMF if the number of local extrema of $h_1(t)$, is equal to or differs from the number of zero crossings by one, and the average of $h_1(t)$ reasonably zero. If $h_1(t)$ is not an IMF, then repeat steps 1-4 on $h_1(t)$ instead of $x(t)$, until the obtained new $h_1(t)$ satisfies the conditions of an IMF,
Step 6: Compute the residue, $r_1(t) = x(t) - h_1(t)$,
Step 7: If the residue, $r_1(t)$ is above a threshold value of error tolerance, then repeat steps 1-6 on $r_1(t)$, to obtain the next IMF and a new residue.

An appropriate stopping criterion, in step A5, avoids 'over-improving' $c_1(t)$ as that can lead to significant loss of information (Rilling, Flandrin, & Goncalves, 2003). If n orthogonal IMFs are obtained in this iterative manner, the original signal can be reconstructed from its IMFs as,

$$x(t) = \sum_{k=1}^{n} a_k(t)_{\varphi_k}(t) \quad (2)$$

The first IMF obtained, consists of the highest frequency components present in the original signal. The subsequent IMFs obtained, contain progressively lower frequency components of the signal.

K-MEANS CLASSIFIER

K-means clustering is a method of vector quantization which is popular for cluster analysis in data mining, originated from signal processing (Manickavasagam, Sutha, & Kamalanand, 2014). *K-means* clustering aims to partition *n* observations into *k* clusters in which each observation belongs to the cluster with the nearest mean, serving as a prototype of the cluster. The problem is computationally difficult, however, there are efficient heuristic algorithms that are commonly employed and converge quickly to a local optimum. These are usually similar to the expectation – maximization algorithm for mixtures of Gaussian distributions via an iterative refinement approach employed by both algorithms. Additionally, they both use cluster centers to model the data; however, *k*-means clustering tends to find clusters of comparable spatial extent, while the expectation-maximization mechanism allows clusters to have different shapes.

The most common algorithm uses an iterative refinement technique. Due to its ubiquity it is often called the *k*-means algorithm. Assign each observation to the cluster whose mean yields the least within-cluster sum of squares (WCSS). Since the sum of squares is the squared Euclidean distance, this is intuitively the "nearest" mean.

$$S_i^{(t)} = \{x_p : \| x_p - m_i^{(t)} \|^2 \le \| x_p - m_j^{(t)} \|^2 \ \forall j, 1 \le j \le k\}, \quad (3)$$

where each x_p is assigned to exactly one $S^{(t)}$, even if it could be assigned to two or more of them. Calculate the new means to be the centroids of the observations in the new clusters.

$$m_i^{(t+1)} = \frac{1}{|S_i^{(t)}|} \sum_{x_j \in S_i^{(t)}} x_j \quad (4)$$

Since the arithmetic mean is a least-squares estimator, this also minimizes the within-cluster sum of squares (WCSS) objective.

In a more specific form, the four algorithm steps can be identified (Ortega, Rojas, & Somodevilla, 1999):

Step 1 - (Initialization): A set of objects to be partitioned, the number of groups and a centroid for each group are defined.

Step 2 - (Classification): For each database object its distance to each of the centroids is calculated, the closest centroid is determined, and the object is incorporated to the group related to this centroid.

Step 3 - (Centroid Calculation): For each group generated in the step 2, its centroid is recalculated.

Step 4 - (Convergence Condition): Several convergence conditions are utilized: stopping when reaching a given number of iterations, stopping when there is no exchange of objects among groups, or stopping when the difference among centroids at two consecutive iterations is smaller than a given threshold. If the convergence condition is not satisfied, steps 2, 3 and 4 of the algorithm are repeated.

There are four outcomes from the classifier. If the outcome is normal for the input corresponding to a normal subject then it is called a True Negative (TN). However if the outcomes refers to abnormal subject then it is called False positive (FN). True Positive (TP) and False Negative (FN) are the case where the abnormal is classified as abnormal and normal respectively. The performance of the developed classifiers was assessed using standard performance measures. The accuracy, sensitivity, specificity, positive predictive value and negative predictive value were calculated using the followings relations.

- Accuracy = (TP+TN)/ (TP+FP+TN+FN)
- Sensitivity = TP/ (TP+FN)
- Specificity=TN/ (TN=FP)
- Positive predictive value=TP/ (TP+FP)
- Negative predictive value=TN/ (TN+FN)
- TN=True Negative
- FP=False positive
- TP=True positive
- FN=False Negative

PERFORMANCE OF THE DEVELOPED K-MEANS CLASSIFIER

The variation of accuracy, sensitivity, specificity, positive predictive values and negative predictive values, when different features such as the descriptive statistics and also the features obtained from IMF components are given as inputs to the classifier. It is found that the developed classifier was able to classify the normal and abnormal EGG signals with a high degree of accuracy and sensitivity. Also, significant classification performance was achieved in terms of PPV and NPV values.

Further, two different feature sets consisting of:

- Feature set 1 = [statistics of IMF components of EGG signals]
- Feature set 2 = [statistics of EGG signals]

was given as individual inputs to the classifier and the performance of the classifier was analyzed for each case.

Table 3 represents the results of the classification performance for two different feature sets such as Feature set 1 and Feature set 2. Figure 4 shows variation of accuracy, sensitivity, specificity, positive predictive value and negative predictive value for Feature set 1 and Feature set 2. Results demonstrate that high degree of accuracy is obtained when Feature set 1 is used as the input to the classifier. Further, the sensitivity value of 90% is observed when Feature set 1 is adopted. No significant variations in the specificity values were observed when feature set 1 is compared to the specificity values of feature set 2. Also, the PPV and NPV values of feature set 1 is higher when compared to the PPV and NPV values of feature set 2. The overall performance of the classifier was found to the high when feature set 1 is used, when compared to the use of feature set 2.

Table 3. Performance of classifier for different feature sets

PERFORMANCE OF CLASSIFIER	FEATURE SET (1)	FEATURE SET(2)
Accuracy	85	50
Sensitivity	90	70
Specificity	80	80
Positive Predictive Value	81	77
Negative Predictive value	88	72

Figure 4. Variation of accuracy, sensitivity, specificity, positive predictive value and negative predictive value for feature set 1 & feature set 2

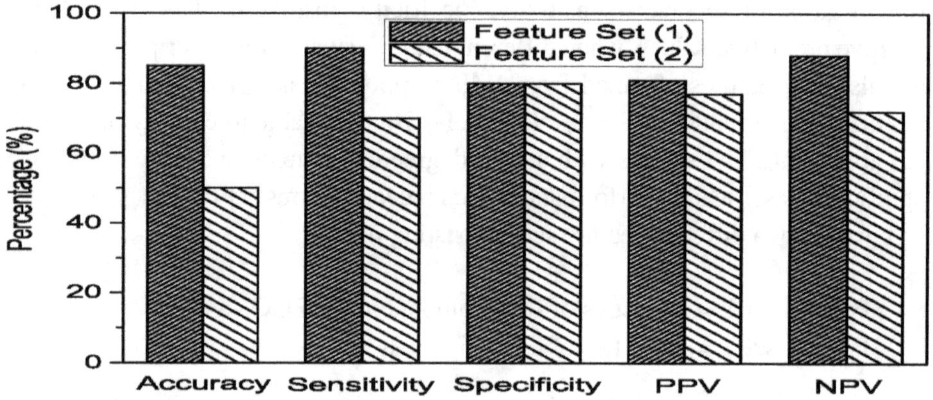

CONCLUSION

EGG is a non-invasive method for measurement of gastric myoelectrical activity that controls gastric motility. In this technique, the electrical signals originating from the stomach muscles are recorded using cutaneous electrodes placed on the abdominal skin (Alagumariappan, Krishnamurthy, Kandiah, & Ponnuswamy, 2017). The features of the obtained EGG signals from normal individuals differ when compared to the features of the EGG signals obtained from abnormal human subjects. By analyzing such features, several digestive disorders can be diagnosed. The permission were granted by superintendent of medicine at local Hospital, Chennai and EGG signals were acquired from normal and abnormal human subjects. In this chapter, the development of an automated decision support system for diagnosis of digestive disorders using electrogastrograms has been explained in detail. The features extracted from the EGG signals are the descriptive statistics and statistics of IMF components obtained using Empirical Mode Decomposition algorithm from normal and abnormal EGG signals. Further, the variation in such statistics was analyzed. Also, an automated classification system was developed using k-means Classifier. Results demonstrate that a high degree of accuracy was obtained using the K-Means classifier. The developed classifier is efficient for classification of normal and abnormal EGG signals. Further, a classification accuracy of 85% and classification sensitivity of 90% were observed. This work appears to be of high clinical relevance, since the features of EGG signal is highly useful for non-invasive analysis of various pathological and physiological states of the digestive system.

REFERENCES

Al-Subari, K., Al-Baddai, S., Tome, A. M., Goldhacker, M., Faltermeier, R., & Lang, E. W. (2015). EMDLAB: A toolbox for analysis of single-trial EEG dynamics using empirical mode decomposition. *Journal of Neuroscience Methods*, *253*, 193–205. doi:10.1016/j.jneumeth.2015.06.020 PMID:26162614

Alagumariappan, P., Krishnamurthy, K., Kandiah, S., & Ponnuswamy, M. J. (2017). Effect of electrode contact area on the information content of the recorded electrogastrograms: An analysis based on Renyi entropy and Teager-Kaiser Energy. *Polish Journal of Medical Physics and Engineering*, *23*(2), 37–42. doi:10.1515/pjmpe-2017-0007

Alagumariappan, P., Rajagopal, A., & Krishnamurthy, K. (2016). Complexity Analysis on Normal and Abnormal Electrogastrograms Using Tsallis Entropy. In *3rd International Electronic and Flipped Conference on Entropy and Its Applications*. Multidisciplinary Digital Publishing Institute. 10.3390/ecea-3-A003

Barroso-Alvarado, A. J., Tovar-Corona, B., Contreras-Uribe, T. J., Santiago-Godoy, R., González-Navarro, Y. E., Solís-Villela, J. G., . . . Garay-Jiménez, L. I. (2011, October). Wavelet analysis of an electrogastrogram database. In *Electrical Engineering Computing Science and Automatic Control (CCE), 2011 8th International Conference on* (pp. 1-5). IEEE. 10.1109/ICEEE.2011.6106644

Ben Hassen, D., Ben Zakour, S., & Taleb, H. (2016). A Hybrid Fuzzy-SVM classifier for automated lung diseases diagnosis. *Polish Journal of Medical Physics and Engineering*, *22*(4), 97–103. doi:10.1515/pjmpe-2016-0017

Berradja, K., & Boughanmi, N. (2016). Assessment of myocardial metabolic rate of glucose by means of Bayesian ICA and Markov Chain Monte Carlo methods in small animal PET imaging. *Polish Journal of Medical Physics and Engineering*, *22*(3), 69–75. doi:10.1515/pjmpe-2016-0012

Bradshaw, L. A., Cheng, L. K., Chung, E., Obioha, C. B., Erickson, J. C., Gorman, B. L., ... Richards, W. O. (2016). Diabetic gastroparesis alters the biomagnetic signature of the gastric slow wave. *Neurogastroenterology and Motility*, *28*(6), 837–848. doi:10.1111/nmo.12780 PMID:26839980

Calder, S., Cheng, L. K., & Du, P. (2014, August). A theoretical analysis of the electrogastrogram (EGG). In *Engineering in Medicine and Biology Society (EMBC), 2014 36th Annual International Conference of the IEEE* (pp. 4330-4333). IEEE.

Contreras, T. J., Mayen, M. A., Servin, A., & Garay, L. I. (2010, September). System for acquisition and analysis of multichannel electrogastrogram. In *Electrical Engineering Computing Science and Automatic Control (CCE), 2010 7th International Conference on* (pp. 220-224). IEEE. 10.1109/ICEEE.2010.5608577

Deering, R., & Kaiser, J. F. (2005). The use of masking signal to improve empirical mode decomposition. *IEEE Int. Conf. Acoustics, Speech Signal Processing (ICASSP '05)*, 4, 485-488. 10.1109/ICASSP.2005.1416051

Ding, W., Qin, S., Miao, L., Xi, N., Li, H., & Wang, Y. (2010, December). Processing and analysis of bio-signals from human stomach. In *Robotics and Biomimetics (ROBIO), 2010 IEEE International Conference on* (pp. 769-772). IEEE. 10.1109/ROBIO.2010.5723423

Familoni, B. O., Abell, T. L., & Bowes, K. L. (1995). A model of gastric electrical activity in health and disease. *IEEE Transactions on Biomedical Engineering*, *42*(7), 647–657. doi:10.1109/10.391163 PMID:7622148

Gharibans, A. A., Kim, S., Kunkel, D. C., & Coleman, T. P. (2017). High-Resolution Electrogastrogram: A Novel, Noninvasive Method for Determining Gastric Slow-Wave Direction and Speed. *IEEE Transactions on Biomedical Engineering*, *64*(4), 807–815. doi:10.1109/TBME.2016.2579310 PMID:27305668

Gopu, G., Neelaveni, R., & Porkumaran, K. (2008). Acquisition and analysis of electrogastrogram for digestive system disorders using a novel approach. *Proceedings of International Conference on Electrical and Computer Engineering*, 65–69. 10.1109/ICECE.2008.4769174

Gopu, G., Neelaveni, R., & Porkumaran, K. (2008). Investigation of digestive system disorders using Electrogastrogram. In *Computer and Communication Engineering, 2008. ICCCE 2008. International Conference on* (pp. 201-205). IEEE. 10.1109/ICCCE.2008.4580596

Haddab, S., & Laghrouche, M. (2009). Microcontroller-based system for electrogastrography monitoring through wireless transmission. *Measurement Science Review*, *9*(5), 122–126. doi:10.2478/v10048-009-0022-6

Inoue, M., Iwamura, S., & Yoshida, M. (2001). EGG measurement under various situations. In *Engineering in Medicine and Biology Society, 2001. Proceedings of the 23rd Annual International Conference of the IEEE* (*Vol. 4*, pp. 3356-3358). IEEE.

Jin, X., Katsuura, T., Iwanaga, K., Shimomura, Y., & Inoie, M. (2007). The influence of taste stimuli and illumination on electrogastrogram measurements. *Journal of Physiological Anthropology*, *26*(2), 191–195. doi:10.2114/jpa2.26.191 PMID:17435364

Jonderko, K., Kasicka-jonderko, A., Krusiec-świdergoł, B., Dzielicki, M., Strój, L., Doliński, M., ... Błońska-fajfrowska, B. (2005). How reproducible is cutaneous electrogastrography? An in-depth evidence-based study1. *Neurogastroenterology and Motility*, *17*(6), 800–809. doi:10.1111/j.1365-2982.2005.00707.x PMID:16336495

Kamalanand, K., & Jawahar, P. M. (2012). Coupled jumping frogs/particle swarm optimization for estimating the parameters of three dimensional HIV model. *BMC Infectious Diseases*, *12*(1Suppl 1), 82. doi:10.1186/1471-2334-12-S1-P82 PMID:22471518

Kamalanand, K., & Jawahar, P. M. (2013). Particle swarm optimization based estimation of HIV-1 viral load in resource limited settings. *African Journal of Microbiological Research*, *7*(20), 2297–2304. doi:10.5897/AJMR12.1924

Kamalanand, K., & Jawahar, P. M. (2015). Prediction of Human Immunodeficiency Virus-1 Viral Load from CD4 Cell Count Using Artificial Neural Networks. *Journal of Medical Imaging and Health Informatics*, *5*(3), 641–646. doi:10.1166/jmihi.2015.1430

Kamalanand, K., & Mannar Jawahar, P. (2016). Comparison of particle swarm and bacterial foraging optimization algorithms for therapy planning in HIV/AIDS patients. *International Journal of Biomathematics*, *9*(02), 1650024. doi:10.1142/S1793524516500248

Kanungo, T., Mount, D. M., Netanyahu, N. S., Piatko, C. D., Silverman, R., & Wu, A. Y. (2002). An efficient k-means clustering algorithm: Analysis and implementation. *IEEE Transactions on Pattern Analysis and Machine Intelligence*, *24*(7), 881–892. doi:10.1109/TPAMI.2002.1017616

Khanmohammadi, S., Adibeig, N., & Shanehbandy, S. (2017). An improved overlapping k-means clustering method for medical applications. *Expert Systems with Applications*, *67*, 12–18. doi:10.1016/j.eswa.2016.09.025

Koch, K. L., & Stern, R. M. (2004). *Handbook of electrogastrography*. Oxford University Press.

Kolev, V. (2000). Compressed time and frequency recording of the electrogastrogram by individual wave detection. *Physiological Measurement*, *21*(1), N1–N10. doi:10.1088/0967-3334/21/1/401 PMID:10720016

Komorowski, D., Pietraszek, S., Tkacz, E., & Provaznik, I. (2015). The extraction of the new components from electrogastrogram (EGG), using both adaptive filtering and electrocardiographic (ECG) derived respiration signal. *Biomedical Engineering Online*, *14*(1), 60. doi:10.118612938-015-0054-0 PMID:26099312

Komorowski, D., & Tkacz, E. (2015, August). A new method for attenuation of respiration artifacts in electrogastrographic (EGG) signals. In *Engineering in Medicine and Biology Society (EMBC), 2015 37th Annual International Conference of the IEEE* (pp. 6006-6009). IEEE.

Lakshmi, V. S., Tebby, S. G., Shriranjani, D., & Rajinikanth, V. (2016). Chaotic cuckoo search and Kapur/Tsallis approach in segmentation of T. cruzi from blood smear images. *International Journal of Computer Science and Information Security*, *14*, 51–56.

Leahy, A., Besherdas, K., Clayman, C., Mason, I., & Epstein, O. (1999). Abnormalities of the electrogastrogram in functional gastrointestinal disorders. *The American Journal of Gastroenterology*, *94*(4), 1023–1028. doi:10.1111/j.1572-0241.1999.01007.x PMID:10201477

Li, Z., Guan, F., Ren, C., Liu, S., Sha, H., Zhao, S., . . . Wang, Y. (2008, May). Bio-Impedance and Synchronous Electrogastrogram to Evaluate Gastric Motility. In *Bioinformatics and Biomedical Engineering, 2008. ICBBE 2008. The 2nd International Conference on* (pp. 689-692). IEEE. 10.1109/ICBBE.2008.168

Li, Z., & Ren, C. (2008). Gastric motility measurement and evaluation of functional dyspepsia by a bio-impedance method. *Physiological Measurement*, *29*(6), S373–S382. doi:10.1088/0967-3334/29/6/S31 PMID:18544817

Liang, H. (2005). Extraction of gastric slow waves from electrogastrograms: Combining independent component analysis and adaptive signal enhancement. *Medical & Biological Engineering & Computing*, *43*(2), 245–251. doi:10.1007/BF02345962 PMID:15865135

Liang, H., Lin, Z., & McCallum, R. W. (2000). Artifact reduction in electrogastrogram based on empirical mode decomposition method. *Medical & Biological Engineering & Computing*, *38*(1), 35–41. doi:10.1007/BF02344686 PMID:10829388

Liang, J. I. E., & Chen, J. D. Z. (1997). What can be measured from surface electrogastrography (computer simulations). *Digestive Diseases and Sciences*, *42*(7), 1331–1343. doi:10.1023/A:1018869300296 PMID:9246026

Lin, Z., Sarosiek, I., Forster, J., Damjanov, I., Hou, Q., & McCallum, R. W. (2010). Association of the status of interstitial cells of Cajal and electrogastrogram parameters, gastric emptying and symptoms in patients with gastroparesis. *Neurogastroenterology and Motility*, *22*(1), 56–e10. PMID:19614868

Manickavasagam, K., Sutha, S., & Kamalanand, K. (2014). An automated system based on 2 d empirical mode decomposition and k-means clustering for classification of Plasmodium species in thin blood smear images. *BMC Infectious Diseases*, *14*(S3), 13. doi:10.1186/1471-2334-14-S3-P13 PMID:24405683

Manickavasagam, K., Sutha, S., & Kamalanand, K. (2014). Development of systems for classification of different plasmodium species in thin blood smear microscopic images. *Journal of Advanced Microscopy Research*, *9*(2), 86–92. doi:10.1166/jamr.2014.1194

Merino, M., Gómez, I. M., & Molina, A. J. (2015). Envelopment filter and K-means for the detection of QRS waveforms in electrocardiogram. *Medical Engineering & Physics*, *37*(6), 605–609. doi:10.1016/j.medengphy.2015.03.019 PMID:25922210

Neuman, M. R. (1998). Biopotential amplifiers. *Medical instrumentation: Application and design*, 292-296.

Ning, Y., Zhu, X., Zhu, S., & Zhang, Y. (2015). Surface EMG decomposition based on K-means clustering and convolution kernel compensation. *IEEE Journal of Biomedical and Health Informatics*, *19*(2), 471–477. doi:10.1109/JBHI.2014.2328497 PMID:25486655

Obioha, C., Erickson, J., Suseela, S., Hajri, T., Chung, E., Richards, W., & Bradshaw, L. A. (2013). Effect of Body Mass Index on the sensitivity of Magnetogastrogram and Electrogastrogram. *Journal of Gastroenterology and Hepatology Research*, *2*(4), 513. PMID:27077053

Orhan, U., Hekim, M., & Ozer, M. (2011). EEG signals classification using the K-means clustering and a multilayer perceptron neural network model. *Expert Systems with Applications*, *38*(10), 13475–13481. doi:10.1016/j.eswa.2011.04.149

Ortega, J. P., Del, M., Rojas, R. B., & Somodevilla, M. J. (n.d.). Research issues on k-means algorithm: An experimental trial using matlab. *CEUR Workshop Proceedings: Semantic Web and New Technologies.*

Parkman, H. P., Hasler, W. L., Barnett, J. L., & Eaker, E. Y. (2003). Electrogastrography: A document prepared by the gastric section of the American Motility Society Clinical GI Motility Testing Task Force. *Neurogastroenterology and Motility*, *15*(2), 89–102. doi:10.1046/j.1365-2982.2003.00396.x PMID:12680908

Patterson, M., Rintala, R., Lloyd, D., Abernethy, L., Houghton, D., & Williams, J. (2001). Validation of electrode placement in neonatal electrogastrography. *Digestive Diseases and Sciences*, *46*(10), 2245–2249. doi:10.1023/A:1011931502985 PMID:11680604

Patterson, M., Rintala, R., Lloyd, D., Abernethy, L., Houghton, D., & Williams, J. (2001). Validation of electrode placement in neonatal electrogastrography. *Digestive Diseases and Sciences*, *46*(10), 2245–2249. doi:10.1023/A:1011931502985 PMID:11680604

Rajinikanth, V., & Couceiro, M. S. (2014, October). Multilevel Segmentation of Color Image using Lévy driven BFO Algorithm. In *Proceedings of the 2014 International Conference on Interdisciplinary Advances in Applied Computing* (p. 19). ACM. 10.1145/2660859.2660925

Rajinikanth, V., Satapathy, S. C., Fernandes, S. L., & Nachiappan, S. (2017). Entropy based Segmentation of Tumor from Brain MR Images–A study with Teaching Learning Based Optimization. *Pattern Recognition Letters*, *94*, 87–95. doi:10.1016/j.patrec.2017.05.028

Rilling, G., Flandrin, P., & Goncalves, P. (2003). On empirical decomposition and its algorithms. *IEEE-EURASIP Workshop on Nonlinear Signal Image Process Grado*.

Sarosiek, I., Song, G., Sun, Y., Sandoval, H., Sands, S., Chen, J., & McCallum, R. W. (2017). Central and Peripheral Effects of Transcutaneous Acupuncture Treatment for Nausea in Patients with Diabetic Gastroparesis. *Journal of Neurogastroenterology and Motility*, *23*(2), 245–253. doi:10.5056/jnm16097 PMID:28163260

Taralunga, D. D., Ungureanu, M., Hurezeanu, B., Gussi, I., & Strungaru, R. (2015, August). Empirical mode decomposition applied for non-invasive electrohysterograhic signals denoising. In *Engineering in Medicine and Biology Society (EMBC), 2015 37th Annual International Conference of the IEEE* (pp. 4134-4137). IEEE. 10.1109/EMBC.2015.7319304

Taralunga, D. D., Ungureanu, M., Hurezeanu, B., Gussi, I., & Strungaru, R. (2015, August). Empirical mode decomposition applied for non-invasive electrohysterograhic signals denoising. In *Engineering in Medicine and Biology Society (EMBC), 2015 37th Annual International Conference of the IEEE* (pp. 4134-4137). IEEE. 10.1109/EMBC.2015.7319304

Tokmakçi, M. (2007). Analysis of the electrogastrogram using discrete wavelet transform and statistical methods to detect gastric dysrhythmia. *Journal of Medical Systems*, *31*(4), 295–302. doi:10.100710916-007-9069-9 PMID:17685154

Tortora, G. J., & Derrickson, B. H. (2008). *Principles of anatomy and physiology*. John Wiley & Sons.

Vakil, B. J. (1960). The pattern of certain gastro-intestinal diseases in India. *Postgraduate Medical Journal*, *36*(420), 614–618. doi:10.1136/pgmj.36.420.614 PMID:13779649

Wojewnik, P., & Żmigrodzki, J. (2013). An infrared-based device for non-invasive monitoring of eyelid movement during sleep. *Polish Journal of Medical Physics And Engineering*, *19*(2), 85–91.

Xia, Y., Han, J., & Wang, K. (2015). Quick detection of QRS complexes and R-waves using a wavelet transform and K-means clustering. *Bio-Medical Materials and Engineering*, *26*(s1), S1059–S1065. doi:10.3233/BME-151402 PMID:26405862

Yin, J., & Chen, J. D. (2013). Electrogastrography: Methodology, validation and applications. *Journal of Neurogastroenterology and Motility*, *19*(1), 5–17. doi:10.5056/jnm.2013.19.1.5 PMID:23350042

Zhao, S., Sha, H., Li, Z. Y., & Ren, C. S. (2012). Electrical bioimpedance gastric motility measurement based on an electrical-mechanical composite mechanism. *World Journal of Gastroenterology*, *18*(25), 3282–3287. PMID:22783053

KEY TERMS AND DEFINITIONS

DAQ: Data acquisition (DAQ) is the process of measuring an electrical phenomenon with computer system.

Descriptive Statistics: Descriptive statistics are the basic features of a given data set, which can be either a representation of the entire population or a sample of it.

Digestive Diseases: Digestive diseases are disorders of the digestive tract.

EGG: Electrogastrography (EGG) is an efficient and noninvasive technique for diagnosis of digestive disorders.

EMD: Empirical mode decomposition (EMD) is a technique to decompose a given signal into a set of elemental signals called intrinsic mode functions.

K-Means: K-means is an unsupervised learning algorithm used to solve the well-known clustering problem based on vector quantization.

LABVIEW: Laboratory Virtual Instrumentation Engineering Workbench (LABVIEW) is a platform and development environment for a visual programming language from National Instruments.

Chapter 6
Effect of a Romantic Song on the Autonomic Nervous System and the Heart of Indian Male Volunteers

Soumanti Das
National Institute of Technology Rourkela, India

Rohit Kumar Verma
National Institute of Technology Rourkela, India

Suraj Kumar Nayak
National Institute of Technology Rourkela, India

Anilesh Dey
Kaziranga University, India

Kunal Pal
National Institute of Technology Rourkela, India

ABSTRACT

In this chapter, the effect of an old generation romantic music (stimulus) on the autonomic nervous system (ANS) activity and the cardiac electrophysiology of Indian male volunteers was investigated. Electrocardiogram (ECG) signals were acquired and the corresponding RR intervals (RRIs) were extracted. The recurrence analysis of the RRI time series suggested a more stable heart rate in the post-stimulus condition. Heart rate variability (HRV) analysis detected a dominant parasympathetic activity in the post-stimulus condition. The time-domain and the wavelet transform analyses of the ECG signals predicted an alteration in the electrical activity of the heart because of the exposure to the music stimulus. The classification of the HRV and the ECG parameters was performed using artificial neural network (ANN), which resulted in an accuracy of ≥80%.

DOI: 10.4018/978-1-5225-5149-2.ch006

INTRODUCTION

Music has been reported to arouse emotions in the human beings and can be used as a stimulus for triggering responses in the human body (Salimpoor, Benovoy, Longo, Cooperstock, & Zatorre, 2009). Music has been used in the rehabilitation, and the treatment of children and adults suffering from various diseases apart from emotional disorders (Center, Center, & Center, 2005). In recent years, the effort to analyze the effect of music on the different physiological systems of the human body like the ANS and the heart is gaining popularity (Linnemann et al., 2015; Tan, Ozdemir, Temiz, & Celik, 2015). The ANS activity can be non-invasively determined from HRV analysis of the RRIs, which are obtained by processing the ECG signals. HRV refers to the study of the variation in the time duration of the consecutive heart beats. This variation of heart rate is controlled by ANS through the sympathetic and the parasympathetic nervous systems (Nayak et al., 2016). HRV has found applications in the diagnosis of both cardiological (e.g., myocardial infarction and congestive heart failure) as well as some non-cardiological diseases (e.g., tetraplegia and diabetic neuropathy) in the last few decades. Recurrence analysis is one of the widely used non-linear signal analysis methods. Recurrence refers to the repeated occurrence of an event with time. Recurrence analysis of the RRIs has been performed in many recent studies for the diagnosis of different cardiovascular diseases. It shows the complex patterns of RRI that vary in time (Sabelli, Messer, Kovacevic, & Walthall, 2011). Analysis of the ECG signals is common for the diagnosis of the cardiovascular diseases (Wang, Chiang, Hsu, & Yang, 2013) as well as for understanding the effects of different stimuli on the cardiac electrophysiology (Nayak et al., 2016). The ECG signal analysis has been reported in the time, the frequency and the joint time-frequency domains (Chen, Ni, & Wang, 2016; Kinoshita, et al., 1995). Among the joint time-frequency domain analysis methods, wavelet transform has received special attention of the researchers. Taking a note of the above-mentioned discussion, the present work attempts to analyze the effect of an old generation music on the ANS and the heart of the Indian male volunteers.

LITERATURE REVIEW

The current section discusses some of the recent developments in the field of recurrence-based RRI time series analysis, HRV analysis, and wavelet-based joint time-frequency analysis of ECG signals. Schlenker *et al.* (2016) have proposed recurrence analysis as a tool for the diagnosis of the ANS dysfunction that is responsible for vasovagal syncope. ECG signals were recorded during orthostatic test from the patients, experiencing vasovagal syncope. Sequences of RRIs were analyzed using frequency-domain, time domain and recurrence analysis methods. Both time domain analysis and recurrence analysis showed significant changes in patients experiencing vasovagal syncope as compared to healthy patients. As the time domain HRV becomes problematic for short term ECG signal so the authors proposed that recurrence analysis can be considered as an important tool for detecting the ANS dysfunction in person having vasovagal syncope (Schlenker & Nedělka, 2013). Houshyarifar *et al.* (2017) have proposed a method to predict the sudden cardiac death, which is based on the features extracted from recurrence plot, poincarȅ plot of HRV signal. The method consisted of four stages, i.e., preprocessing, feature extraction, feature reduction and classification. Seven features were extracted from recurrence plot and poincarȅ plot. These features are then reduced to one feature by linear discrimination technique. Support vector machine (SVM) was used to classify the HRV signals. The proposed method could predict the occurrence of sudden cardiac death 5 min before the sudden cardiac death with an accuracy of 92% (Houshyarifar & Amirani, 2017).

Tarvainen *et al.* (2014) have reported that the "Kubios HRV" software can be used for easy analysis of the HRV. It employs an adaptive algorithm for the detection of the QRS complexes. The "Kubios HRV" software provides all the time-domain, the frequency-domain, and the non-linear HRV features. It supports both ECG and RRI data, provides wide variety of analysis methods and possesses a user-friendly graphical user interface (Niskanen, Tarvainen, Ranta-Aho, & Karjalainen, 2004). Thus, the authors have suggested that "Kubios HRV" software can be recommended for HRV analysis. Castaldo *et al.* (2015) have reported about the association between the intense mental stress and the HRV parameters. The frequency-domain HRV parameters suggested autonomic balance shift towards sympathetic activation during mental stress. Further, only one non-linear parameter was significant that suggested a reduced chaotic behavior during intense stress (Castaldo et al., 2015).

Yadav *et al.* (2015) have proposed a non-local wavelet transform-based denoising method for the ECG signals. ECG signals get distorted by muscle noise, baseline wander, and power-line interference. During the wireless recording of the ECG signals, the signals get corrupted by white Gaussian noise. So, in order to remove these noises, wavelet transform domain denoising method for the ECG signals was used to exploit the correlation among both non-local and local samples of the signals. The proposed method resulted in significant qualitative and quantitative performance over other ECG signal denoising methods (Yadav, Sinha, & Bora, 2015). Kumar *et al.* (2017) have proposed a mechanized method for the diagnosis of the coronary artery disease (CAD) using ECG signal analysis. ECG signals from 40 healthy persons and 7 CAD patients were segmented into beats. Flexible Analytic Wavelet Transform (FAWT) was employed to decompose these ECG beats. Cross information potential (CIP) parameter was extracted from the coefficients of decomposed signals. For

CAD patients, the mean value calculated from the CIP parameter was higher than the normal patients. Classification efficiency was calculated for each decomposition levels. Using the proposed method, the significant improvement in the classification efficiency was observed. Thus, the authors have suggested that the proposed method can be used for the diagnosis of different cardiovascular diseases (Kumar, Pachori, & Acharya, 2017).

MAIN FOCUS OF THE CHAPTER

This study was focussed on analyzing the effect of an old generation romantic music on the ANS and the heart. ECG signals were acquired from 15 Indian male volunteers in the pre- and the post-stimulus conditions. The ECG signals were processed to extract the RRIs. Recurrence and HRV analysis were performed using the RRI time series to understand the effect of the music stimulus on the ANS. The 5 sec portions of ECG signals were subjected to time-domain and wavelet transform-domain analyses to identify any alteration in the cardiac electrophysiology.

METHODOLOGY

In the present study, 15 healthy male volunteers of 18-22 years old were invited to participate in the acquisition of the ECG signals. None of the volunteers reported any symptoms of physiological or neurological disorders. They were also not involved in either smoking or any kind of physical exercises. The volunteers were made to listen to an old generation Bollywood romantic song "dooba dooba rehta hoon" (stimulus) from the Album "Boondein", which was released in 1998. The ECG signals (5 min duration) were acquired with the help of the reusable ECG clamp electrodes placed in the lead-I configuration and Vernier EKG sensor (Vernier Software & Technology, USA), before and after the stimulus. The ECG signals were saved in the laptop at the sampling rate of 1 KHz using USB 4704 DAQ (Advantech Corporation, Taiwan) and a LabVIEW (V13.0, National instruments, USA) program. The pre- and the post-stimulus ECG signals were categorized under Category WS and Category OS. The extraction of the QRS complexes (using a band-pass filter of 10-25 Hz), and the detection of R-peaks were performed using Biomedical Workbench Toolkit of LabVIEW to obtain the RRI time series.

Recurrence analysis of the RRI time series was performed using Bios Analyzer software. Bios Analyzer is a set of computer programs for time series analysis that measures the parameters of a creative phenomenon such as novelty, diversification, complexes and non-random complexity. The examples of creative processes are RRI time series, galactic distribution, meteorological time series and economic time series (Sabelli et al., 2005). Various parameters of the recurrence analysis such as isometry, consecutive isometry, radial isometry, consecutive radial isometry, and novelty were calculated, and recurrence plot was drawn to identify any variation in variation in the RRI time series due to the stimulus. The Biomedical Workbench toolkit was further used to perform HRV analysis from the RR intervals and a total of 29 HRV parameters were extracted. The HRV parameters included the time-domain, the frequency-domain and the non-linear parameters. For the HRV analysis, the 5 min ECG signals were used. The linear and non-linear statistical methods were implemented using Statistica (trial V13.2, Dell Inc., USA). These statistically important parameters were analyzed to quantify the alteration in the ANS physiology due to the music stimulus. These statistically important parameters were given as inputs to RBF and MLP ANN networks. Thereafter, the time-domain and wavelet transform analyses of the ECG signals were performed using the 5 sec recordings of the ECG signals to understand the effect of the music stimulus on the electrophysiology of the heart. In the time-domain analysis of the ECG signals, 12 statistical parameters were extracted from the ECG signals and their statistical significance was analyzed. ANN classification was performed using the statistically significant parameters as the inputs. For the wavelet analysis, the 5 sec ECG signals were subjected to wavelet decomposition up to level 8 using db06 wavelet and the signal reconstruction was performed using D7 and D8 sub-bands. The reconstructed ECG signals were analyzed similar to that of the time-domain analysis of the ECG signals.

RESULTS AND DISCUSSION

Recurrence Analysis

Cardiovascular signals have been reported to have discontinuous alterations in between deterministic trajectories and stochastic processes (Sabelli & Lawandow, 2010; Sabelli et al., 2011; Sabelli et al., 2005). Recurrence analysis is one of the important tools for analyzing non-deterministic complexity, as seen in cardiovascular signals (Sabelli et al., 2005). The non-linear, non-stationary properties of the cardiovascular system can be easily diagnosed by recurrence analysis. Recurrence analysis measures the degree of randomness, state changes as well as the degree of determinism, which characterize the signal. Recurrence-based methods demonstrate the variations in the temporal pattern by analyzing the sequences of consecutive members of the time series, and then plotting the recurrences among these vectors (Sabelli et al., 2011). However, they do not measure the amplitude of the variation.

Recurrence analysis is the central component of the bios analysis. Bios is a kind of pattern, which is found in the RRI time series (Sabelli et al., 2011). Its pattern varies continuously as the heart is subjected to the ever-changing central nervous system activity. In this study, the recurrence parameters, namely, isometry, consecutive isometry, radial isometry, consecutive radial isometry, and novelty were analyzed along with recurrence plot to find out any change in the RRI time series pattern due to the music stimulus. Isometry is defined as the recurrence of vectors having same length (Sabelli & Lawandow, 2010). This vector length is calculated from its Euclidean norm. Euclidean norm of a vector is the square root of the sum of squares of its members. Two vectors are regarded as isometric if the absolute value of the difference between their Euclidean norms is smaller than some cut-off radius. The number of time series points included in each data sequence is called embedding dimension (Sabelli & Lawandow, 2010). Embedding plots represent the variation in isometry or its derived parameters (e.g., consecutive isometry, radial isometry, consecutive radial isometry and novelty) as a function of embedding dimensions (Sabelli et al., 2005).

The embedding plot of isometry for the RRI data obtained from both Category WS and Category OS has been shown in Figure 1(a). It is clear from Figure 1(a) that isometry is more for Category WS than Category OS in lower embedding dimension (till embedding dimension 60), but was lower after that. This suggested that the amount of isometric recurrence was lower in the post-stimulus condition than the pre-stimulus condition for lower embedding dimensions. But, after a certain embedding dimension (in this study 60) the amount of isometric recurrence became higher in the post-stimulus condition than the pre-stimulus condition.

Consecutive isometry is another measure of recurrence that represents causation including periodicity. It is the number of recurrences that follow each other (Sabelli et al., 2005). In this study, the consecutive isometry was calculated for the RRI time series of both Category WS and Category OS (Figure 1(b)). However, the values of consecutive isometry did not show any specific pattern (i.e., consistent increase or decrease) in Category OS as compared to Category WS with the increase in the embedding dimension. The changes in isometry and consecutive isometry with respect to cut-off radius are regarded as radial isometry and consecutive radial isometry, respectively. The values of the radial isometry (Figure 1(c)) and the consecutive radial isometry (Figure 1(d)) did not vary significantly among Category WS and Category OS. Novelty is another important recurrence parameter, which can be defined as the property of possessing a lower isometry by a given time series data as compared to its shuffled version. It is expressed as the ratio of the isometry of the original time series to the isometry of the shuffled time series. Thus, the calculation

Figure 1. (a) Embedding plot of isometry, (b) embedding plot of consecutive isometry, (c) bar graph of radial isometry versus cut-off radius, and (d) bar graph of consecutive radial isometry versus cut-off radius

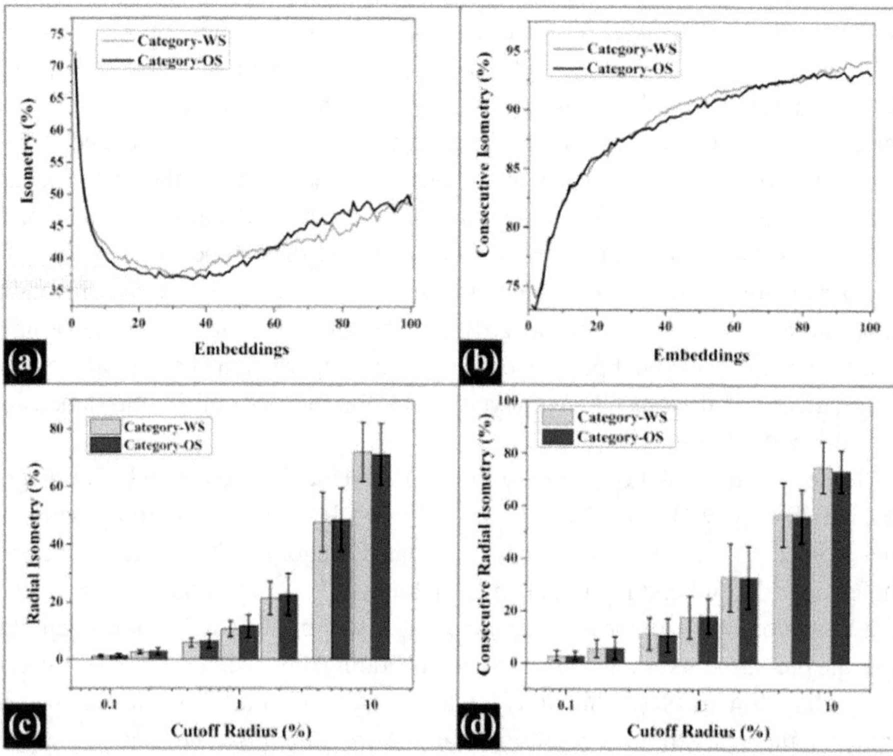

of isometry allows the computation of novelty. In this study, Category OS showed higher novelty as compared to Category WS. It was evident from the embedding plots of novelty for Category WS and Category OS (Figure 2) (Sabelli & Lawandow, 2010). Finally, the recurrence plots were drawn for both Category WS and Category OS (Figure 3). The recurrence plot portrays the variation in the patterns of RRI time series with time. In the previous studies, it has been reported that the recurrence-free regions in the recurrence plot depict acceleration or deceleration of the heart rate. On the other hand, the recurrence-rich regions in the recurrence plot depict the stable heart rate (Sabelli & Lawandow, 2010). It was evident from the recurrence plots for Category WS Category OS that more recurrence-rich regions were found in Category OS. This, in turn, suggested that the heart rate was more stable in the post-stimulus condition as compared to the pre-stimulus condition.

Figure 2. Embedding plot of novelty

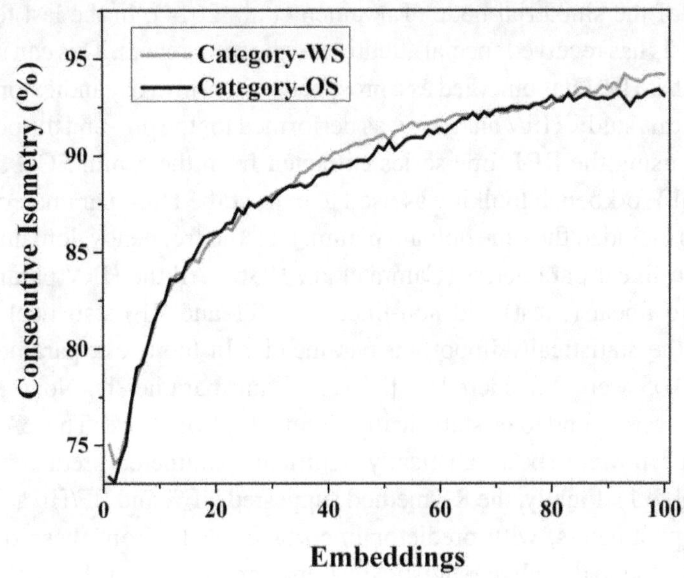

Figure 3. Recurrence Plot: (a) Category WS and (b) Category OS

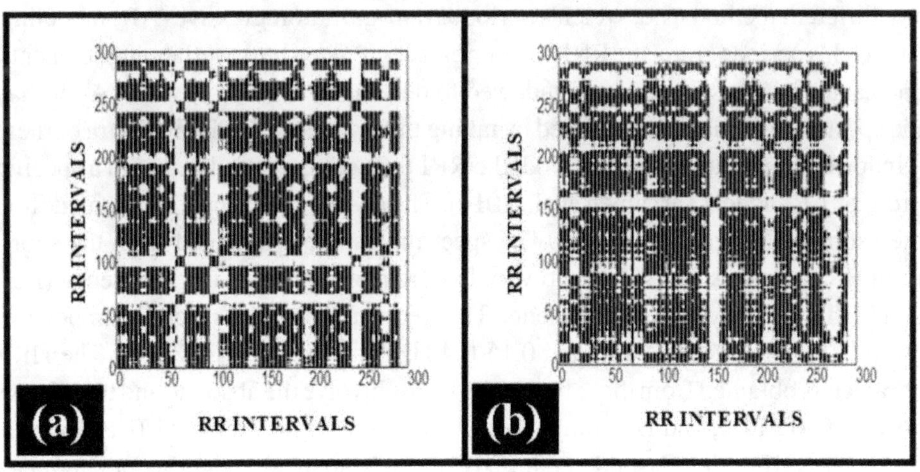

HRV Analysis

HRV is a reliable estimator of ANS functioning in different human well-being applications and cardiovascular research (Tarvainen, Niskanen, Lipponen, Ranta-Aho, & Karjalainen, 2014). HRV has been reported to be very much affected by hypertension, anxiety, stress, and any pathological state. HRV is caused by the ANS regulation of the sinoatrial node (Tarvainen et al., 2014). In the last few decades, HRV analysis has received special attention of the researchers. This can be attributed to the fact that HRV has emerged as a prospective non-invasive indicator of the ANS activity. In this study, HRV analysis was performed for the pre- and the post-stimulus conditions using the RRI time series extracted from the 5 min ECG signals. The Biomedical Workbench toolkit was used to extract the HRV parameters. The HRV parameters included the time domain parameters, the frequency domain parameters and the non-linear parameters (Camm et al., 1996). All the HRV parameters were subjected to linear (t-test) and non-linear (CART and RF) statistical methods to recognize the statistically important parameters. In the t-test, parameters having p-value ≤ 0.05 were considered as the significant parameters. None of the HRV parameters were found to be statistically significant from t-test. The CART analysis suggested LF power to be a statistically significant parameter (predictor importance ≥ 0.95) (Table 1). Finally, the RF method suggested HF% and LF/HF as statistically important parameters, with predictor importance = 1. From these decision tree methods, we found that all the statistically important parameters belong to frequency domain. These statistically important frequency-domain HRV parameters consist of the components of the power spectral density (Tarvainen et al., 2014). In the frequency domain, the power spectrum for the RRI time series can be calculated by two different methods, i.e, Welch's periodogram and autoregressive (AR) modeling. In Welch's periodogram, the RRI time series is segregated into overlapping segments, and each of these segments is windowed to decrease the leakage effect. After that, the spectrum estimate is calculated by taking the average of the FFT spectra of these windowed segments. In AR method, the RRI time series is modeled with a specific order of AR model (Tarvainen et al., 2014). The spectrum estimate is obtained from the estimated model parameters. The spectrum estimate obtained from the short-term HRV analysis is divided into very low frequency (VLF), low frequency (LF), and high frequency (HF) components. The frequency of these spectral components are 0-0.04 Hz, 0.04-0.15 Hz, and 0.15-0.4 Hz (Tarvainen et al., 2014). The HRV parameters obtained from these frequency bands involve the absolute and the relative power of VLF, LF, and HF components apart from the normalized LF, HF powers and the LF/HF ratio (Castaldo et al., 2015). The statistically significant parameter LF power was found to decrease in the post-stimulus condition as compared to the pre-stimulus condition. It has been reported that LF power is related to both sympathetic and parasympathetic activity. So, we cannot conclude any specific activity here (Guzik et al., 2007). The important predictor HF power (expressed as % of total power) exhibited an increased value in post-stimulus condition as compared to pre-stimulus condition. It has been reported by many researchers that HF power is an indicator of parasympathetic activity. Hence, HF power suggested an increase in parasympathetic activity (Kemp et al., 2014). Again, the important predictor LF/HF power was found to decrease in the post-stimulus condition. As per the reported literature, an increase in LF/HF ratio indicates sympathetic activity and the decrease in LF/HF ratio indicates parasympathetic activity (Billman, 2013). Thus, the decrease in LF/HF ratio also suggested an increase in the parasympathetic activity in the post-stimulus condition (Billman, 2013). The statistically important HRV parameters were used to classify the HRV data into Category OS and Category WS using the RBF ANN classifier. While performing the ANN classification, the RBF 3-13-2 network provided the highest classification efficiency of 86.67% with all the important parameters as categorical inputs. The details of the RBF 3-13-2 network have been given in Table 2. The ANN classification results also showed that there was alteration in the ANS activity in the post-stimulus condition as compared to the pre-stimulus condition.

Time-Domain Analysis

For the time-domain analysis, 5 sec ECG signals were extracted from the acquired 5 min ECG signals. 12 statistical parameters were computed from these ECG signals using a LabVIEW program. The parameters were kurtosis, skewness, variance, mode, arithmetic mean, median, summation, energy density (ED), Shannon entropy (SE), log energy (LE), standard deviation (SD), root mean square (RMS). Using Statistica software, several linear and non-linear tests are performed to find out the statistically important parameters as mentioned earlier. The t-test could not suggest

Table 1. Statistically significant parameters obtained from HRV analysis

Methods	Parameters	Mean ± SD		Predictor Importance
		Category-WS	Category-OS	
CART	LF POWER	22.33±2049.90	1448±797.94	1.00
RF	HF(%)	40.33±5.40	42.93±3.84	1.00
	LF/HF	0.89±0.26	0.72±0.18	1.00

Table 2. Details of RBF 3-13-2 network

Networks	Features Used	Classification Efficiency	Training Performance	Testing Performance	Algorithm	Error Function	Hidden Activation Function	Output Activation Function
RBF 3-13-2	LF POWER HF(%) LF/HF	86.67%	87.50	83.33	RBFT	SOS	Gaussian	Identity

any statistically important parameter. However, the CART and the RF analyses could find out kurtosis and mode as the statistically significant parameters, respectively (predictor importance ≥ 0.95) (Table 3). Kurtosis is a non-dimensional statistical quantity. It is used to measure the relative flatness in any random distribution. It measures the heaviness or thickness of the tail of a distribution (DeCarlo, 1997). Further kurtosis can be used for denoising of the ECG signals by ICA technique. This technique is capable to remove noise and other artifacts (Barhatte, Ghongade, & Tekale, 2016). Mode of a discrete probability distribution is defined as that value which occurs with the greatest frequency in a given data set. If the greatest frequency is 1, then there is no mode. But if the discrete quantitative variable has greatest frequency 2 or more than 2, then the value having greatest frequency is called the mode /sample mode of that variable (Parzen, 1962). The existence of the statistically significant parameters, between Category WS and Category OS, suggested the alteration in the cardiac electrophysiology due to the music stimulus. To confirm the change in the cardiac electrophysiology, ANN classification of the ECG data was performed using the statistically important parameters as the inputs. The RBF 2-10-2 network provided the highest classification efficiency of 86.67%, same as that of the HRV analysis. The details of the RBF 2-10-2 network have been given in Table 4.

Wavelet Transform Analysis

In the wavelet transform analysis, the 5 sec ECG signals were subjected to db06-based wavelet decomposition up to the level 8. The reason for selecting Daubechies wavelet as the mother wavelet was its similarity with the ECG signals (De Chazal,

Table 3. Statistically significant features obtained from time domain analysis

Methods	Parameters	Mean ± SD		Predictor Importance
		Category-WS	Category-OS	
CART	kurtosis	27.31±50.39	13.61±4.26	1.00
RF	mode	-0.00±0.03	.00±.03	1.00

Table 4. Details of the RBF 2-10-2 network

Networks	Features Used	Classification Efficiency	Training Performance	Testing Performance	Algorithm	Error Function	Hidden Activation Function	Output Activation Function
RBF 2-10-2	kurtosis, mode	86.67%	87.50	83.33	RBFT	Entropy	Gaussian	Softmax

Celler, & Reilly, 2000). This was followed by the signal reconstruction using D7 and D8 sub-bands. As a result, the R-waves of the ECG signals could be obtained as the reconstructed signals (González-Barajas, 2014). 12 statistical features were extracted from the reconstructed ECG signals, similar to that of the time domain analysis of the ECG signals and their statistical significance was analyzed using t-test, CART, and RF. No important predictors were found out from the t-test. However, the CART analysis identified RMS, SD, variance, median, and skewness as the important parameters (Table 5). ED was obtained as the statistically significant parameter from the RF method. The RMS value of a signal can be described as the square root of the mean value of the signal. Mathematically, it is given by Equation 1 (Carl Jr & De Rouffignac, 1993).

$$x_{rms} = \sqrt{\frac{1}{T}\int_{t0}^{t0+T} x^2(t)} \qquad (1)$$

where, x_{rms} is the RMS value of the signal, T is the total time period of the time slice and t_0 is the onset of the time slice.

Standard deviation is defined as the measure of the deviation of the signal from its mean value. It is expressed as the square root of the variance of the signal as given in Equation 2 (Bland & Altman, 1996).

$$\sigma^2 = \frac{1}{N-1}\sum_{i=0}^{N-1}\left(x_i - \mu\right)^2 \qquad (2)$$

where, σ is the standard deviation, μ is the average of the signal, N is the number of terms, x_i is the ith signal point.

The variance represents the power of the fluctuation of the signal from its mean value. Real world signals have noise and other short term features that prevent the existence of the signal. Taking the average of the signal will reduce the noise but it will not make any difference in the volatility of the signal (Ait-Sahalia & Yu, 2008). It can be calculated by taking the difference between the original signal and its average. The mean of the squared differences is called the signal variance. Variance of a signal is calculated by Equation 3 (Scheffe, 1999).

$$Var_s = \frac{\sum_{i=1}^{n}\left(s\left[i\right] - s_{avg}\right)^2}{\left(n-1\right)} \qquad (3)$$

where, s_i is the consequent signals, s_{avg} is the average of the signal, n is the number of terms.

The median represents the value of the middle term in any data set. The data set should be ranked in increasing order. From the definition it can be understood that it divides the data set into 2 equal halves. The median is used for skewed distribution. A median can be expressed as any real number m which satisfies the inequality represented by Equation 4 (Sheskin, 2003).

$$P\left(X \leq m\right) \geq \frac{1}{2}\ and\ P\left(X \geq m\right) \geq \frac{1}{2} \tag{4}$$

where, P(*X*) is a probability distribution function.

The skewness represents the degree of asymmetry of a distribution around its mean. Although, mean, average deviation, SD are dimensional quantities but skewness is regarded as a non-dimensional quantity (Weisstein, 2002). It is used to represent the shape of the distribution. A positive value of skewness suggests a distribution with an asymmetric tail extending more towards right, whereas a negative value suggests a distribution with an asymmetric tail extending more towards left (Weisstein, 2002). The skewness can be calculated as given in Equation 5 (Mardia, 1970).

$$Skewness = \frac{1}{N}\sum_{j=1}^{N}\left(\frac{x_j - \bar{x}}{\sigma}\right)^3 \tag{5}$$

where σ is the standard deviation of the signal, x_j is the consequent signals, $\bar{x}$ is the mean of the signal and N is the number of term.

Energy density of a one-dimensional signal may be regarded as the amount of energy contained in a signal per length. The occurrence of the statistically significant parameters suggested that there might be alterations in the R-waves of the ECG signals by exposing the volunteers to old music, which in turn, corresponding to the electrophysiological change in the heart.

By using all these significant parameters as inputs, ANN classification was done. The RBF 6-10-2 provided the highest classification efficiency 80.00%. The details of RBF 6-10-2 has been given in Table 6. In the wavelet transform analysis also, the existence of the significant parameters and the result of ANN classification showed that there might be some electrophysiological changes in heart by making the volunteers listen to old music.

Table 5. Statistically significant features obtained from wavelet transform analysis

Methods	Parameters	Mean ± SD		Predictor Importance
		Category-WS	Category-OS	
CART	RMS	0.13±0.08	0.11±.02	0.97
	SD	0.13±0.08	0.11±.02	0.97
	variance	0.02±0.04	0.01±.00	0.97
	median	0.00±0.00	0.00±.00	1.00
	skewness	0.00±1.07	0.16±.25	0.96
RF	ED	7.53E-03±1.30E-02	0.00±.00	1.00

Table 6. Details of the RBF 2-10-2 network

Networks	Features Used	Classification Efficiency	Training Performance	Testing Performance	Algorithm	Error Function	Hidden Activation Function	Output Activation Function
RBF 6-10-2	RMS,SD, variance ED, skewness	80.00%	79.17	83.33	RBFT	CE	Gaussian	Softmax

FUTURE RESEARCH DIRECTIONS

The current study used t-test and decision tree-based methods for the identification of the statistically significant parameters. ANN was implemented for the classification of the data. Future studies can be performed using other statistical methods like Chi square and Gini index for the detection of the statistically significant parameters and different classifiers like K-nearest neighbor (KNN), support vector machine (SVM) can be implemented to suggest the best classifier among them. Future studies can also be performed on investigating the effect of a music stimulus on other physiological systems of the human body.

CONCLUSION

In our present report, the effect of an old-generation romantic music (stimulus) on the cardiac electrical activity and the ANS was analyzed. The ECG signals were acquired from around 15 male volunteers in the pre- and the post-stimulus conditions, and were categorized under Category WS and Category OS. The HRV and the recurrence analyses of the RRI time series were performed to realize the effect of the music stimulus on the ANS activity. The time-domain and the wavelet transform-domain analyses of ECG signals were performed to understand the effect on electrical activity of the heart. It was observed that none of the statistically significant parameters could be detected using the linear method t-test during the HRV, the time-domain, and the wavelet transform-domain analyses. But the non-linear classifiers were able to detect some statistically significant parameters. This suggested that there might be some non-linear alteration in the ANS and the cardiac electrophysiology. The recurrence analysis suggested a more stable heart rate in the post-stimulus condition. The HRV analysis indicated towards an increase in the parasympathetic dominance due to the exposure to music stimulus. Both the time-domain and wavelet-transform domain analyses suggested an alteration the cardiac electrophysiology. The ANN classification accuracies in HRV, time-domain and wavelet transform analyses were ≥80%, acting as an evidence for the alterations proposed by HRV and ECG signal analyses (Yang & Naiman, 2014).

REFERENCES

Ait-Sahalia, Y., & Yu, J. (2008). *High frequency market microstructure noise estimates and liquidity measures*. National Bureau of Economic Research. doi:10.3386/w13825

Barhatte, A. S., Ghongade, R., & Tekale, S. V. (2016). *Noise analysis of ECG signal using fast ICA*. Paper presented at the Advances in Signal Processing (CASP), Conference on. 10.1109/CASP.2016.7746149

Billman, G. E. (2013). The LF/HF ratio does not accurately measure cardiac sympatho-vagal balance. *Frontiers in Physiology*, 4. PMID:23431279

Bland, J. M., & Altman, D. G. (1996). Statistics notes: Measurement error. *BMJ (Clinical Research Ed.)*, *313*(7059), 744. doi:10.1136/bmj.313.7059.744 PMID:8819450

Camm, A. J., Malik, M., Bigger, J., Breithardt, G., Cerutti, S., Cohen, R. J., & ... . (1996). Heart rate variability: Standards of measurement, physiological interpretation and clinical use. Task Force of the European Society of Cardiology and the North American Society of Pacing and Electrophysiology. *Circulation*, *93*(5), 1043–1065. doi:10.1161/01.CIR.93.5.1043 PMID:8598068

Carl, F. G., Jr., & De Rouffignac, E. P. (1993). *Current to power crossover heater control*. Google Patents.

Castaldo, R., Melillo, P., Bracale, U., Caserta, M., Triassi, M., & Pecchia, L. (2015). Acute mental stress assessment via short term HRV analysis in healthy adults: A systematic review with meta-analysis. *Biomedical Signal Processing and Control*, *18*, 370–377. doi:10.1016/j.bspc.2015.02.012

Center, E. I., Center, C. R., & Center, P. F. (2005). *Music therapy*. Academic Press.

Chen, K.-C. J., Ni, Y.-S., & Wang, J.-Y. (2016). *Electrocardiogram diagnosis using wavelet-based artificial neural network*. Paper presented at the Consumer Electronics, 2016 IEEE 5th Global Conference on. 10.1109/GCCE.2016.7800547

De Chazal, P., Celler, B., & Reilly, R. (2000). Using wavelet coefficients for the classification of the electrocardiogram. *Paper presented at the Engineering in Medicine and Biology Society, 2000. Proceedings of the 22nd Annual International Conference of the IEEE*. 10.1109/IEMBS.2000.900669

DeCarlo, L. T. (1997). On the meaning and use of kurtosis. *Psychological Methods*, *2*(3), 292–307. doi:10.1037/1082-989X.2.3.292

González-Barajas, J. E. (2014). Threshold calculation for R wave detection in complex cardiac. *Tecno Lógicas*, *17*(32), 47–55.

Guzik, P., Piskorski, J., Krauze, T., Schneider, R., Wesseling, K. H., Wykretowicz, A., & Wysocki, H. (2007). Correlations between the Poincare plot and conventional heart rate variability parameters assessed during paced breathing. *The Journal of Physiological Sciences; JPS*, *57*(1), 63–71. doi:10.2170/physiolsci.RP005506 PMID:17266795

Houshyarifar, V., & Amirani, M. C. (2017). Early detection of sudden cardiac death using Poincaré plots and recurrence plot-based features from HRV signals. *Turkish Journal of Electrical Engineering and Computer Sciences*, *25*(2), 1541–1553. doi:10.3906/elk-1509-149

Kemp, A. H., Brunoni, A. R., Santos, I. S., Nunes, M. A., Dantas, E. M., Carvalho de Figueiredo, R., ... Lotufo, P. A. (2014). Effects of depression, anxiety, comorbidity, and antidepressants on resting-state heart rate and its variability: An ELSA-Brasil cohort baseline study. *The American Journal of Psychiatry*, *171*(12), 1328–1334. doi:10.1176/appi.ajp.2014.13121605 PMID:25158141

Kinoshita, O., Fontaine, G., Rosas, F., Elias, J., Iwa, T., Tonet, J., ... Frank, R. (1995). Time-and frequency-domain analyses of the signal-averaged ECG in patients with arrhythmogenic right ventricular dysplasia. *Circulation*, *91*(3), 715–721. doi:10.1161/01.CIR.91.3.715 PMID:7828298

Kumar, M., Pachori, R. B., & Acharya, U. R. (2017). Characterization of coronary artery disease using flexible analytic wavelet transform applied on ECG signals. *Biomedical Signal Processing and Control*, *31*, 301–308. doi:10.1016/j.bspc.2016.08.018

Linnemann, A., Kappert, M. B., Fischer, S., Doerr, J. M., Strahler, J., & Nater, U. M. (2015). The effects of music listening on pain and stress in the daily life of patients with fibromyalgia syndrome. *Frontiers in Human Neuroscience*, 9. PMID:26283951

Mardia, K. V. (1970). Measures of multivariate skewness and kurtosis with applications. *Biometrika*, *57*(3), 519–530. doi:10.1093/biomet/57.3.519

Nayak, S. K., Shukla, R. D., Panda, I., Champaty, B., Thakur, G., Mohapatra, B., et al. (2016). Effect of Slow and Fast Music on the Autonomic Nervous System and Cardiac Health: A Preliminary Investigation. *Classification and Clustering in Biomedical Signal Processing*, 198.

Niskanen, J.-P., Tarvainen, M. P., Ranta-Aho, P. O., & Karjalainen, P. A. (2004). Software for advanced HRV analysis. *Computer Methods and Programs in Biomedicine*, *76*(1), 73–81. doi:10.1016/j.cmpb.2004.03.004 PMID:15313543

Parzen, E. (1962). On estimation of a probability density function and mode. *Annals of Mathematical Statistics*, *33*(3), 1065–1076. doi:10.1214/aoms/1177704472

Sabelli, H., & Lawandow, A. (2010). Homeobios: The pattern of heartbeats in newborns, adults, and elderly patients. *Nonlinear Dynamics Psychology and Life Sciences*, *14*(4), 381. PMID:20887687

Sabelli, H., Messer, J., Kovacevic, L., & Walthall, K. (2011). Biotic patterns of heart rate variation in depressed and psychotic subjects. *Nonlinear Dynamics Psychology and Life Sciences*, *15*(1), 11–28. PMID:21176437

Sabelli, H., Sugerman, A., Kovacevic, L., Kauffman, L., Carlson-Sabelli, L., Patel, M., & … . (2005). Bios data analyzer. *Nonlinear Dynamics Psychology and Life Sciences*, *9*(4), 505–538. PMID:16194304

Salimpoor, V. N., Benovoy, M., Longo, G., Cooperstock, J. R., & Zatorre, R. J. (2009). The rewarding aspects of music listening are related to degree of emotional arousal. *PLoS One*, *4*(10), e7487. doi:10.1371/journal.pone.0007487 PMID:19834599

Scheffe, H. (1999). *The analysis of variance* (Vol. 72). John Wiley & Sons.

Schlenker, J., & Nedělka, T. (2013). Recurrence Analysis in Patients with Vasovagal Syncopes. *Measurement*, 145–148.

Sheskin, D. J. (2003). *Handbook of parametric and nonparametric statistical procedures*. CRC Press. doi:10.1201/9781420036268

Tan, Y. Z., Ozdemir, S., Temiz, A., & Celik, F. (2015). The effect of relaxing music on heart rate and heart rate variability during ECG GATED-myocardial perfusion scintigraphy. *Complementary Therapies in Clinical Practice*, *21*(2), 137–140. doi:10.1016/j.ctcp.2014.12.003 PMID:25747187

Tarvainen, M. P., Niskanen, J.-P., Lipponen, J. A., Ranta-Aho, P. O., & Karjalainen, P. A. (2014). Kubios HRV–heart rate variability analysis software. *Computer Methods and Programs in Biomedicine*, *113*(1), 210–220. doi:10.1016/j.cmpb.2013.07.024 PMID:24054542

Wang, J.-S., Chiang, W.-C., Hsu, Y.-L., & Yang, Y.-T. C. (2013). ECG arrhythmia classification using a probabilistic neural network with a feature reduction method. *Neurocomputing*, *116*, 38–45. doi:10.1016/j.neucom.2011.10.045

Weisstein, E. W. (2002). *Skewness*. Academic Press.

Yadav, S. K., Sinha, R., & Bora, P. K. (2015). Electrocardiogram signal denoising using non-local wavelet transform domain filtering. *IET Signal Processing*, *9*(1), 88–96. doi:10.1049/iet-spr.2014.0005

Yang, S., & Naiman, D. Q. (2014). Multiclass cancer classification based on gene expression comparison. *Statistical Applications in Genetics and Molecular Biology*, *13*(4), 477–496. PMID:24918456

ADDITIONAL READING

Acharya, U. R., Fujita, H., Sudarshan, V. K., Ghista, D. N., Lim, W. J. E., & Koh, J. E. (2015). *Automated prediction of sudden cardiac death risk using Kolmogorov complexity and recurrence quantification analysis features extracted from HRV signals.* Paper presented at the Systems, Man, and Cybernetics (SMC), 2015 IEEE International Conference on. 10.1109/SMC.2015.199

Anczykowski, J., Willems, S., Hoffmann, B. A., Meinertz, T., Blankenberg, S., & Patten, M. (2016). Early Detection of Symptomatic Paroxysmal Cardiac Arrhythmias by Trans-Telephonic ECG Monitoring: Impact on Diagnosis and Treatment of Atrial Fibrillation. *Journal of Cardiovascular Electrophysiology*, *27*(9), 1032–1037. doi:10.1111/jce.13025 PMID:27257094

Chakrabarty, A., Das, N., & Das, D. (2017). *Assessment of Values of Time-Domain and Frequency-Domain Parameters for ECG Signals Through HRV Analysis Using Symlets for Arrhythmia Prediction.* Paper presented at the Advances in Computational Intelligence: Proceedings of International Conference on Computational Intelligence 2015. 10.1007/978-981-10-2525-9_41

da Silva Pinho, A. M., Pombo, N., & Garcia, N. M. (2016). *Sleep apnea detection using a feed-forward neural network on ECG signal.* Paper presented at the e-Health Networking, Applications and Services (Healthcom), 2016 IEEE 18th International Conference on. 10.1109/HealthCom.2016.7749468

Dar, M. N., Akram, M. U., Shaukat, A., & Khan, M. A. (2015). *ECG Based Biometric Identification for Population with Normal and Cardiac Anomalies Using Hybrid HRV and DWT Features.* Paper presented at the IT Convergence and Security (ICITCS), 2015 5th International Conference on. 10.1109/ICITCS.2015.7292977

Desai, U., Martis, R. J., Acharya, U. R., Nayak, C. G., Seshikala, G., & Shetty K, R. (2016). Diagnosis of multiclass tachycardia beats using recurrence quantification analysis and ensemble classifiers. *Journal of Mechanics in Medicine and Biology, 16*(01), 1640005. doi:10.1142/S0219519416400054

Falcone, C., Colonna, A., Bozzini, S., Matrone, B., Guasti, L., Paganini, E., & … . (2014). Cardiovascular risk factors and Sympatho-Vagal balance: Importance of time-domain heart rate variability. *Journal of Clinical & Experimental Cardiology, 5*(2).

Galiano, G., & Velasco, J. (2014). On a nonlocal spectrogram for denoising one-dimensional signals. *Applied Mathematics and Computation, 244*, 859–869. doi:10.1016/j.amc.2014.07.003

Gang, S., Liang, R., & Yuhan, G. (2015). *Research on the method of ECG denoising based on improved wavelet packet.* Paper presented at the Cyber Technology in Automation, Control, and Intelligent Systems (CYBER), 2015 IEEE International Conference on. 10.1109/CYBER.2015.7288152

Gang, U. J., Nalliah, C. J., Lim, T. W., Thiagalingam, A., Kovoor, P., Ross, D. L., & Thomas, S. P. (2015). Atrial ectopy predicts late recurrence of atrial fibrillation after pulmonary vein isolation. *Circulation: Arrhythmia and Electrophysiology, 8*(3), 569–574. doi:10.1161/CIRCEP.114.002052 PMID:25904494

Garg, N., & Babbar, N. (2016). Feature Extraction of Wrist Pulse Signals using Gabor Spectrogram. *Indian Journal of Science and Technology, 9*(47). doi:10.17485/ijst/2015/v8i1/101745

Hampel, K. G., Thijs, R. D., Elger, C. E., & Surges, R. (2017). Recurrence risk of ictal asystole in epilepsy. *Neurology*, *89*(8), 785–791. doi:10.1212/WNL.0000000000004266 PMID:28747444

Hassan, A. R., & Haque, M. A. (2016). Computer-aided obstructive sleep apnea identification using statistical features in the EMD domain and extreme learning machine. *Biomedical Physics & Engineering Express*, *2*(3), 035003. doi:10.1088/2057-1976/2/3/035003

Jenkal, W., Latif, R., Toumanari, A., Dliou, A., & El B'charri, O. (2015). An efficient method of ECG signals denoising based on an adaptive algorithm using mean filter and an adaptive dual threshold filter. *International Review on Computers and Software*, *10*(11), 1089–1095.

Jokanovic, B., & Amin, M. (2015). Reduced interference sparse time-frequency distributions for compressed observations. *IEEE Transactions on Signal Processing*, *63*(24), 6698–6709. doi:10.1109/TSP.2015.2477056

Joshi, S. L., Vatti, R. A., & Tornekar, R. V. (2013). *A survey on ECG signal denoising techniques.* Paper presented at the Communication Systems and Network Technologies (CSNT), 2013 International Conference on. 10.1109/CSNT.2013.22

Kanzaki, Y., Inden, Y., Ando, M., Kamikubo, Y., Ito, T., Mizutani, Y., ... Murohara, T. (2016). An ECG Index of P-Wave Force Predicts the Recurrence of Atrial Fibrillation after Pulmonary Vein Isolation. *Pacing and Clinical Electrophysiology*, *39*(11), 1191–1197. doi:10.1111/pace.12956 PMID:27723112

Lankveld, T., de Vos, C. B., Limantoro, I., Zeemering, S., Dudink, E., Crijns, H. J., & Schotten, U. (2016). Systematic analysis of ECG predictors of sinus rhythm maintenance after electrical cardioversion for persistent atrial fibrillation. *Heart Rhythm*, *13*(5), 1020–1027. doi:10.1016/j.hrthm.2016.01.004 PMID:26776554

Lee, W., Yoon, H., & Park, K. (2016). Smart ECG Monitoring Patch with Built-in R-Peak Detection for Long-Term HRV Analysis. *Annals of Biomedical Engineering*, *44*(7), 2292–2301. doi:10.100710439-015-1502-5 PMID:26558395

Li, T., Tang, H., Qiu, T., & Park, Y. (2013). Heart sound cancellation from lung sound record using cyclostationarity. *Medical Engineering & Physics*, *35*(12), 1831–1836. doi:10.1016/j.medengphy.2013.05.004 PMID:23764431

Lin, S.-L., Lin, T.-Y., Huang, C.-Y., Hsu, Y.-L., & Chang, H.-C. (2017). *The comparison study between distinct physical fitness norms and their ecg signals under graded exercise intensities and recovery.* Paper presented at the Applied System Innovation (ICASI), 2017 International Conference on. 10.1109/ICASI.2017.7988284

Lin, W.-H., Wu, D., Li, C., Zhang, H., & Zhang, Y.-T. (2014). *Comparison of heart rate variability from PPG with that from ECG.* Paper presented at the The International Conference on Health Informatics. 10.1007/978-3-319-03005-0_54

Liu, G., & Luan, Y. (2015). An adaptive integrated algorithm for noninvasive fetal ECG separation and noise reduction based on ICA-EEMD-WS. *Medical & Biological Engineering & Computing, 53*(11), 1113–1127. doi:10.100711517-015-1389-1 PMID:26429348

Lopez, A. D., & Joseph, L. A. (2013). *Classification of arrhythmias using statistical features in the wavelet transform domain.* Paper presented at the Advanced Computing and Communication Systems (ICACCS), 2013 International Conference on.

Martín-Yebra, A., Landreani, F., Casellato, C., Pavan, E., Frigo, C., Migeotte, P.-F., ... (2015). *Studying heart rate variability from ballistocardiography acquired by force platform: Comparison with conventional ECG.* Paper presented at the Computing in Cardiology Conference (CinC), 2015. 10.1109/CIC.2015.7411064

Mert, A. (2016). ECG feature extraction based on the bandwidth properties of variational mode decomposition. *Physiological Measurement, 37*(4), 530–543. doi:10.1088/0967-3334/37/4/530 PMID:26987295

Orini, M., Laguna, P., Mainardi, L. T., & Bailón, R. (2017). *Time-Frequency Analysis of Cardiovascular Signals and Their Dynamic Interactions Complexity and Nonlinearity in Cardiovascular Signals* (pp. 257–287). Springer. doi:10.1007/978-3-319-58709-7_9

Orphanidou, C., & Drobnjak, I. (2016). Quality Assessment of Ambulatory ECG Using Wavelet Entropy of the HRV signal. *IEEE Journal of Biomedical and Health Informatics.* PMID:28113529

Pathoumvanh, S., Airphaiboon, S., & Hamamoto, K. (2014). Robustness study of ECG biometric identification in heart rate variability conditions. *IEEJ Transactions on Electrical and Electronic Engineering, 9*(3), 294–301. doi:10.1002/tee.21970

Ranaware, P. N., & Deshpande, R. A. (2016). *Detection of arrhythmia based on discrete wavelet transform using artificial neural network and support vector machine.* Paper presented at the Communication and Signal Processing (ICCSP), 2016 International Conference on. 10.1109/ICCSP.2016.7754470

Sahu, N., Peng, D., & Sharif, H. (2017). *Unequal steganography with unequal error protection for wireless physiological signal transmission.* Paper presented at the Communications (ICC), 2017 IEEE International Conference on. 10.1109/ICC.2017.7996377

Sindhu, G., & Sankar, P. (2014). *Design of an ECG acquisition device for the nonlinear analysis of heart rate variability (HRV)*. Paper presented at the Information Communication and Embedded Systems (ICICES), 2014 International Conference on.

Socha, V., Schlenker, J., Hana, K., Smrcka, P., Hanakova, L., Prucha, J., ... (2016). *Prediction of atrial fibrillation and its successful termination based on recurrence quantification analysis of ECG*. Paper presented at the Telecommunications and Signal Processing (TSP), 2016 39th International Conference on. 10.1109/TSP.2016.7760898

Stanković, L., Mandić, D., Daković, M., & Brajović, M. (2017). Time-Frequency Decomposition of Multivariate Multicomponent Signals. *Signal Processing*.

Talbi, M. (2014). Electrocardiogram de-noising based on forward wavelet transform translation invariant application in bionic wavelet domain. *Sadhana*, *39*(4), 921–937. doi:10.100712046-014-0247-4

Thomas, M., Das, M. K., & Ari, S. (2015). Automatic ECG arrhythmia classification using dual tree complex wavelet based features. *AEÜ. International Journal of Electronics and Communications*, *69*(4), 715–721. doi:10.1016/j.aeue.2014.12.013

Van Leeuwen, P., Werner, L., Cysarz, D., Hatzmann, W., & Gronemeyer, D. (2014). *Evaluation of fetal heart rate variability based on automatically determined R-times in a fetal ecg monitor*. Paper presented at the Cardiovascular Oscillations (ESGCO), 2014 8th Conference of the European Study Group on. 10.1109/ESGCO.2014.6847503

Weinschenk, S. W., Beise, R. D., & Lorenz, J. (2016). Heart rate variability (HRV) in deep breathing tests and 5-min short-term recordings: Agreement of ear photoplethysmography with ECG measurements, in 343 subjects. *European Journal of Applied Physiology*, *116*(8), 1527–1535. doi:10.100700421-016-3401-3 PMID:27278521

Wu, S., Shen, Y., Zhou, Z., Lin, L., Zeng, Y., & Gao, X. (2013). Research of fetal ECG extraction using wavelet analysis and adaptive filtering. *Computers in Biology and Medicine*, *43*(10), 1622–1627. doi:10.1016/j.compbiomed.2013.07.028 PMID:24034754

Yadav, S. K., Sinha, R., & Bora, P. K. (2015). Electrocardiogram signal denoising using non-local wavelet transform domain filtering. *IET Signal Processing*, *9*(1), 88–96. doi:10.1049/iet-spr.2014.0005

KEY TERMS AND DEFINITIONS

Artificial Neural Network (ANN): An ANN is a combination of connected units known as artificial neurons that perform computation similar to the biological neurons.

Autonomic Nervous System (ANS): The ANS is a division of peripheral nervous system. The basic functions of autonomic nervous system are the control of heart rate, digestion, respiratory rate, and reflex action.

Heart Rate Variability: HRV is the study of the alteration in the time duration between successive heart beats.

Parasympathetic Nervous System: It is one of the two branches of autonomic nervous system. Its general function is to control the body's response while at rest.

Sympathetic Nervous System: It is one of the two branches of the ANS. Its general function is to mobilize the body's fight or flight response.

Chapter 7
Use of Orange Data Mining Toolbox for Data Analysis in Clinical Decision Making:
The Diagnosis of Diabetes Disease

Musa Peker
Muğla Sıtkı Koçman University, Turkey

Osman Özkaraca
Muğla Sıtkı Koçman University, Turkey

Ali Şaşar
Muğla Sıtkı Koçman University, Turkey

ABSTRACT

Diabetes is a life-long illness which occurs as a result of lack of insulin hormone or ineffectiveness of insulin hormone. Blood sugar, fructosamine, and hemoglobin A1c (HbA1c) values are widely used for diagnosis of this disease. Although the role of insulin in diagnosing diabetes is great, the HbA1c value is more accurate. This is because HbA1c value gives information about the past two or three months of blood sugar in the treatment of diabetes. This study aims to estimate the HbA1c value with high accuracy. Follow-up data of diabetic patients were used as data. The Orange data mining software is used because it is easy to use in the modeling phase and contains many methods. In this context, the chapter aims to develop an effective prediction model by using a large number of feature selection and classification methods. The results show that the proposed model successfully predicts the HbA1c parameter. In addition, determination of the parameters that are effective in the diagnosis of diabetes has been carried out with the feature selection methods.

DOI: 10.4018/978-1-5225-5149-2.ch007

INTRODUCTION

Nowadays, diabetes is becoming one of the most serious diseases. Incidence frequency of diabetes which is increasing in the world varies from one community to another based on age, gender, race, dietary habits, genetic characteristics and environmental factors. According to the data obtained from World Health Organization, 108 million diabetics are thought to be in the world in 1980, it is estimated as 422 million in 2014. The global prevalence of diabetes has almost doubled from 4.7% to 8.5% from 1980 to 2014 (World Health Organization, 2016). Unfortunately, every year, about 1.5 million people lose their lives due to diabetes. One of the most important reasons for this increase can be thought as increase in overweight or obese people resulting from malnutrition and sedentary life. According to the data obtained from the same report, 1 out of 3 adults over 18 years old are overweight and 1 out of 10 adults are obese (World Health Organization, 2016).According to the obtained data and the results obtained from the scientific studies, the risk factors of diabetes can be summarized as shown in Figure 1.

Figure 1 .Risk factors of diabetes

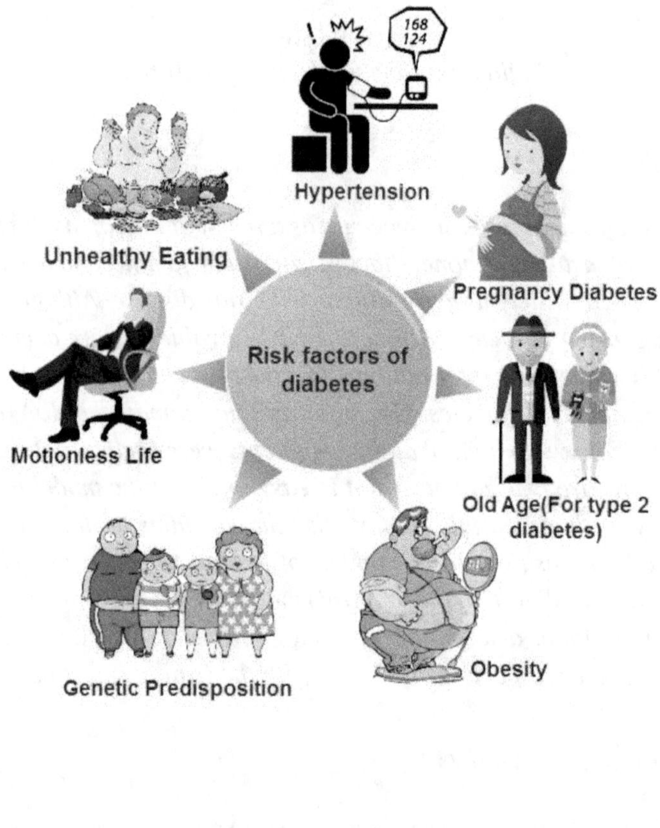

The most important reason of diabetes are the impairments occurred especially in the insulin-secreting cells of pancreas. Insulin is needed for nutrients to be transferred into the cell after the taken by a healthy person, nutrients pass into the blood from the intestines in order to be turned into glucose which is the fuel most needed by the body. If there is no insulin hormone or if the effect of insulin decreases, glucose cannot be transferred into the cell and the amount of sugar in the blood (hyperglycemia) will increase. If this high blood sugar keeps going on constantly, it causes serious damages in our organs (nerve, eye, heart, kidney etc.) over time. As can be seen from Figure 2, excessive and frequent thirst of an individual, increased fluid consumption, excessive urine production, visual impairment, unidentified weight loss, constant tiredness and exhaustion are considered as preliminary indicators of diabetes in energy metabolism (Bilous & Donnelly, 2010).

There are two types of diabetes. These are Type 1, Type 2 and Gestational diabetes. Type 1 diabetes is caused by damage to pancreatic and insulin-producing beta cells at the end of an autoimmune process, or due to unfamiliar disorders. In general, 5-10% of diabetes cases in the community constitute cases of Type 1 diabetes. Type 1 diabetes is a disease that occurs when the immune system of a healthy individual perceives pancreatic beta cells as foreign as a result of virus, vaccination, medicine, physical or psychic stress and destroy them. When this destruction reaches over 80%, disease symptoms arise. Because Patients with type 1 have insulin deficiency, they must take insulin hormone from outside for life (Durna, 2002).

Type 2 diabetes is generally associated with obesity and physical immobility. At the basis of the disease, genetically predisposed individuals have a lifestyle-related insulin resistance and decreased insulin secretion over time. More than 90% of diabetes cases diagnosed worldwide are type 2 diabetes. Type 2 diabetes is controlled using diet, antihyperglycemic drugs and insulin supplementation or combination of them in the first step treatment plan (Durna, 2002).

Gestational diabetes, the third type of diabetes, is expressed by hyperglycemia or increased blood sugar, which is normally higher during pregnancy, but below the

Figure 2. Indicators of diabetes

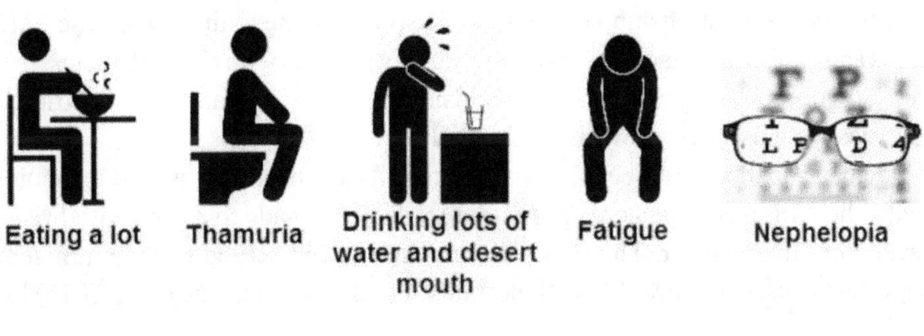
Eating a lot
Thamuria
Drinking lots of water and desert mouth
Fatigue
Nephelopia

diagnostic value of diabetes mellitus. Women with gestational diabetes are at risk of complications during pregnancy and birth. At this point, they and their children are at increased risk of type 2 diabetes in the future.

Blood sugar, fructosamine and HbA1c values are widely used for the diagnosis of diabetes. However, it is known that the HbA1c value is more accurate in the diagnosis of the disease. The reason for this is that the HbA1c value gives information about the past two or three months of blood sugar in the treatment of diabetes. Thus, this value has started to be used more in recent years. The American Diabetes Association (ADA) approved the HbA1c test in 2010 as a diabetes diagnostic test. It has been emphasized that normal range of this value is between 3% - 6% and 6.5% hasbeen chosen as the diagnostic criterion (Afarideh et al., 2016; Rau et al., 2016)

RELATED WORKS

There are many studies on diabetes in literature. Because of the quite satisfactory results obtained in recent years, technological approaches in the field of medicine are attracted by physicians. Diversification and progress of both technological and theoretical approaches in computer science have attracted attention of health professionals. In particular, technology is in serious demand for the benefits it provides in decision making of health professionals and facilitating their work.

Hypoglycaemia is very common in type 1 diabetic patients and may occur at any age. For this reason, a continuous accurate hypoglycaemia monitoring system is a very important medical device for diabetic patients. Needle measuring systems used in such patients considerably reduce patients' quality of life. Thus, Ling et al. (2016) proposed a noninvasive hypoglycaemia monitoring system using the physiological parameters of the electrocardiography (ECG) signal. In the study, an over-learning machine was used to increase the accuracy of perception in recognition of the presence of hypoglycemia.

Another study model in this area was specifically designed to explore the relationship between different parameters and disorders in diabetic patients. For example; in the study carried out by Afarideh et al. (2016), it is aimed to determine the prospective relationship between basal serum alanine aminotransferase (ALT) levels and cardiovascular diseases (CVD) among patients with type 2 diabetes. In the study, regression analysis, artificial neural network modeling, and risk classification analyzes were used to report risk ratios (HR).

Diabetes is thought to be the source of many serious problems, and technology is also helping medicine here. For example, diabetes leads to an increased risk of developing liver cancer. These two diseases are known as the most common and important causes of morbidity and mortality. For this reason, Rau et al. (2016) have developed a model to estimate the development of liver cancer 6 years after diagnosis with type II diabetes using data mining techniques. The data obtained from Taiwan National Health Insurance Research Database (NHIRD) have been divided into two groups: patients diagnosed with cancer after diabetes (case group) and patients with diabetes but no liver cancer (control group). Risk factors have been determined from the literature review and from the physician's recommendation. A chi square test has been used for each independent variable (or potential risk factor) to compare non-significant findings with patients with liver cancer. Artificial neural network (ANN) and logistic regression (LR) methods have been used in the classification phase.

When we look at the studies carried out in the literature in the past, it is seen that the existing expert-based identification algorithms are no longer preferred because of the low recall rate and the loss of a large number of valuable data under strict filtering standards. For this reason, the recent studied on machine learning, which is becoming increasingly important, has begun to draw attention. Zheng et al. (2017) have attempted to reveal several genotypic phenotype associations related to Type 2 Diabetes Mellitus (T2DM) through genome-wide association studies (GWAS) and phenomenon-wide association studies (PheWAS). In their study, they used patients with or without Type 2 diabetes from their Electronic Health Records. In their study, they have evaluated and compared the performance of commonly used machine learning models including the nearest neighbors algorithm, Naive Bayes, Decision Tree, Random Forest, Support Vector Machine and Logistic Regression. In the study, from the data obtained from the electronic registration system, it is emphasized that machine learning is effective in separating subjects with and without Type 2 diabetes.

The analysis of data on the symptoms of a person with many diseases at the same time and taking into account all the factors is not possible by a person (doctor). In such cases, an intelligent system can take into account various factors, and the determination of a suitable model among different parameters can provide tremendous convenience. Heydari et al. (2016) have applied a variety of data mining methods and algorithms to screening data for type 2 diabetes. Performance of methods such as support vector machine, artificial neural networks, decision tree, nearest neighbors and Bayesian networks have been compared to find the best algorithm in diagnosing of this disease. In the study, artificial neural networks have the best performance with an accuracy rate of 97.44% on the selected dataset. The accuracy rates for support vector machine, decision tree, k-nearest neighbors and Bayesian methods are 81.19%, 95.03%, 90.85% and 91.60%, respectively.

The estimation of the results is significant in the clinical decision-making process. ANNs have been used to forecast the risk of post-operative events including survival, and are increasingly being used in complex medical decision making. In a study conducted by Lopez-de-Andres et al. (2016), they have designed an observational study using ANN analysis to calculate prognostic factors of in-hospital mortality in patients with type 2 diabetes (T2DM) after major lower extremity amputation (LEA).

Soltani and Jafarian (2016) have emphasized the necessity of using methods with a minimum error rate in order to better diagnose a dangerous disease such as diabetes. They have used the probabilistic artificial neural network approach to diagnose type II diabetes. As a result, training accuracy and test accuracy have been found as 89.56% and 81.49%, respectively.

Amato et al. (2013) examined the abilities and limitations of artificial neural networks by applying a medical diagnosis on cancer and diabetes data. As a result, they have mentioned that artificial neural networks are a powerful aid for diagnosis, and they have also mentioned the advantages of artificial neural networks such as ability for processing large data and rapid diagnosis. However, it has been emphasized that the decision of expert physicians is important in establishing a definite diagnosis.

In another study conducted by Leema et al. (2016)., they have developed a computer-assisted diagnostic system. In this system, artificial neural networks, particle swarm optimization and gradient descent based backpropagation algorithms are proposed for classification of clinical data sets. The study used Pima Indian Diabetes, Wisconsin Breast Cancer and Cleveland Heart Disease datasets obtained from the California Irvine (UCI) machine learning repository. As a method, a backpropagation based differential variation algorithm based on universal knowledge has been chosen. The results show that the proposed method achieves an accuracy of 85.71% for diabetes, 98.52% for breast cancer and 86.66% for heart disease.

Choubey and Paul (2016) have compared various techniques used to classify the diagnosis of medical diabetes on various data sets. These techniques have been analyzed and compared based on advantages, problems and performance of success.

Wang et al. (2013) have used artificial neural networks to classify type 2 diabetes. The verification ability of the different models has been compared using the ROC curve. In diagnosis of diabetes, it has been seen that classification success of artificial neural networks is high and it has been accepted as an effective classification method.

In their study, Rajesh and Sangeetha (2012), have stated that the data mining has been applied to find useful patterns in determining medical diagnosis and treatment. In the study, several classification algorithms have been applied to classify the diabetes data set and performance analyzes of these algorithms have been carried out. With the C4.5 decision tree algorithm, 91% classification success has achieved in the diagnosis of diabetes mellitus.

In this study, it is explained that follow-up data of diabetes obtained from the hospitals in Turkey/Muğla region is processed by ORANGE program which is anew data visualization, machine learning and data mining software with open source code (Demšar et al., 2013). This study differs from the other studies in terms of originality especially in terms of the data used and the usage of ORANGE software in the field of data mining applications. Using this software, data from different hospitals are combined. After that, a method for diagnosis of diabetes is proposed with the possibilities offered by this software. The proposed method involves data mining processes.

MATERIALS AND METHODS

Dataset

The data used in the study are diabetes follow-up data obtained from Köyceğiz and Dalaman State Hospitals of Mugla province in Turkey. Table 1 includes 27 features that constitute our data set and their explanations. There are 2252 records of patients (963 male and 1289 female) in the data set. Their age range is between 6 and 89.

Table 1. Short explanations of attributes

LN	Attribute	Values
1	SEX	Male:963, Female:1289
2	AGE	Min Value: 6, Max Value: 89
3	BODY MASS INDEX	Min Value: 15, Max Value: 57
4	WAIST CIRCUMFERENCE	Min Value: 50, Max Value:160
5	EXERCISE 1	(1) Easy, (2) Medium, (3) Hard, (4) Three times a week or more, at least 20 minutes, (5) Five times a week or more, at least 30 minutes, (6) More than the first two options.
6	MEDICAL NUTRITION	(1) Not Conform, (2) Conform, (3) Change List, (4) Carbohydrate Count
7	SISTOLIC BLOOD PRESSURE	Min Value: 60, Max Value:180
8	DIASTOLIC BLOOD PRESSURE	Min Value: 60, Max Value:130
9	THYROID INSPECTION	(1)Troid diffuse is feeled by hand, (2) Troid is not feeled by hand,(3) Troid nodular is feeled by hand.
10	DIAGNOSIS	(1) Type 1, (2) Type 2, (3) Other
11	MEDICAL NUTRITION TREATMENT	(1) The patient obey the medical nutrition, (2) The patient sometimes obey the medical nutrition, (3) The patient doesn't obey the medical nutrition, (4) Medical nutrition recommended but we don't know to the patient obey the medical nutrition or not, (5) Medical nutrition is not recommended, (6) Nothing is know about the patient.

continued on following page

Table 1. Continued

LN	Attribute	Values
12	EXERCISE 2	(1) Exercise is recommended, patient conforms, (2) Exercise is recommended, patient sometimes conforms, (3) Exercise recommended, patient doesn't conform, (4) Not a suitable patient for exercise, (5) Exercise is recommended but we don't know to the patient obey the exercise or not. (6) Exercise isn't recommended, (7) Nothing is know about the patient.
13	REASON OF APPLICATION 1	(1) General control, (2) Routine examination, (3) Acute metabolic complication related to the disease, (4) Acute chronic complication related to the disease
14	CORONARY HEART DISEASE	(0) Yes, (1) No
15	CEREBROVASCULER	(0) Yes, (1) No
16	DIABETES EDUCATION	(1) Yes, (2) No
17	GLUKOMETER	(0) Yes, (1) No
18	FASTİNG BLOOD GLUCOSE	Min Value: 38, Max Value:673
19	POSTPRANDIAL BLOOD GLUCOSE	Min Value: 83, Max Value:688
20	TRIGLISERIT: The Main Component of Vegetable and Animal Oils	Min Value: 25, Max Value:885
21	HDL: High Density Lipoprotein	Min Value: 14, Max Value:109
22	LDL: Lov Density Lipoprotein	Min Value: 12, Max Value:467
23	ALT: An alanine aminotransferase	Min Value: 1, Max Value:116
24	HIP ENVIRONMENT	Min Value: 60, Max Value:200
25	REASON OF APPLICATION 2	(1) Asymptomatic, (2) Other, (3) Diabetic ketoacidos, (4) Kadiabetic ketosis, (5) Hyperglycemia, (6) Hypoglycemia coma
26	EXERCISE_PROPOSITION	(1) Not recommended, (2) Contraindicated, (3) Recommended
27	HBA1C: Hemoglobin A_{1C} Value	(0) HBA1C value less than 6.5, (1) HBA1C value more than 6.5

Orange Data Mining Software

ORANGE data mining software was originally developed by scientists at the University of Ljubljana in 1997 using the Python, Cython, C++ and C programming languages. The software's graphical environment and interfaces have been developed using the Python and Qt3 libraries (Demšar et al., 2013). This software, with the latest version presented on March 6, 2017 with ORANGE 3.4.0 has a simple interface on which users create a data analysis workflow by placing graphical components (widgets).

The graphical components (Widget) of this software which is user friendly provide basic functions to the user such as data reading, displaying the data tables, selecting the features, learning estimators, comparison of learning algorithms and visualization of data items. User can explore the visualizations interactively. User can also observe the results visually. The comparison of different algorithms with different criteria in the performance evaluation phase is one of the important advantages of this program. The user interface of the Orange program is shown in Figure 3.

Orange is designed to work with a .tab extensioned dataset. But it can also open commonly used dataset extensions such as txt, basket, .csv, .arff. In this study, short but effective examples related to the ORANGE program are given.

Feature Selection Methods

Features extracted from the data set are usually used as input to the classification method that will be used in data mining applications. In some applications, the number of features is limited to a few, while some of them may have too much. The extracted features for each data item are stored in a feature matrix. Hence, both the dataset size and the number of features will affect the size of the matrix, i.e. the duration of the process. It is important how well the extracted features represent the dataset and the classes corresponding to the dataset. Features that can better distinguish between classes are called high-level features and are more important in

Figure 3.Orange Canvas 2.7

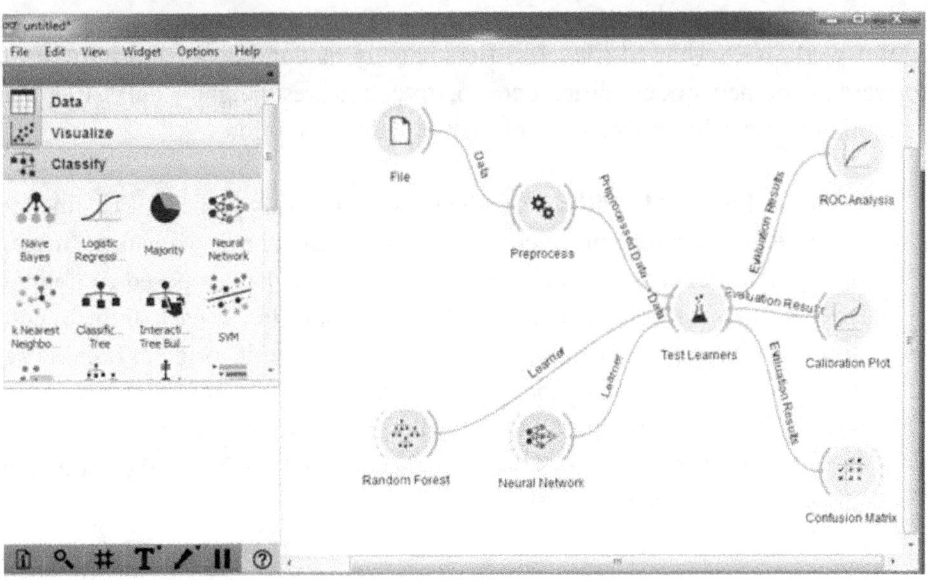

terms of classifier performance. Rather than using all features, only the use of some high-level features can reduce the number of operations performed. In addition, performance increases can be provided by cleaning up noisy features.

In this study, experiments have been performed using 4 different feature selection algorithms. These algorithms are ReliefF, Information Gain, Chi-Square and Gain Ratio. ReliefF is an improved version of the Relief statistical model (Kononenko, 1994). The ReliefF method handles an example from the dataset. And, it performs the feature selection by creating a model based on this example's proximity to other samples in its class and its distance from the different classes. Compared to Relief, ReliefF is a more robust algorithm. It processes missing and noisy data better, can be applicable in all situations, less biased, allow interaction between features, and can catch local dependencies missed by other methods. Information Gain: This method is commonly used in feature selection operations. The main purpose of this method is to find the feature set with the most knowledge of classes. It is an entropy-based feature selection algorithm and the information gain coefficient is calculated for each attribute, and the feature sets with the highest coefficient are selected. The chi-square method is statistics based and it is commonly used in feature selection. This method calculates the chi-square of all attributes and evaluates them one by one according to the class of attributes. Gain Ratio is a different version of Information Gain. Information gain favors features that have a large number of values. But, the Gain Ratio method is to maximize the feature information gain while minimizing the number of its values.

Classification Methods

In this work, we have used five classifiers namely random forest algorithm, Feed forward neural network classifier, decision tree, k-nearest neighbors classifier and support vector machines which are briefly explained as follows.

- **Random Forest Algorithm:** During the classification process, it is aimed to increase the classification value by using more than one decision tree. Instead of producing a single decision tree, Breiman (2001) has proposed combining the decisions of a large number of multivariate trees, each trained with different training sets. Training sets are created from the original training set with random feature selection and bootstrap. First, each decision tree gives its own decision, and the class with the maximum number of votes in the decision forest is regarded as the final decision and the incoming test data is included in that class.

- **Feed-Forward Artificial Neural Networks:** This algorithm is a mathematical system consisting of several processing units linked together in a weighted fashion. This processing unit receives signals from other neurons; combines them, transforms them, and generates a numerical result. In general, the processing units correspond roughly to real neurons and are interconnected within a network; this structure constitutes neural networks. In this study, feed-forward neural network is used among neural network models. There are basically three different layers in feed-forward artificial neural networks. These layers are respectively; an input layer that holds input data to the artificial neural network, a hidden layer or layers on which operations are performed and trains itself according to the desired result, and finally an output layer that shows output values.
- **K-Nearest Neighbors Classifier (KNN):** This is a supervised learning method where a new coming sample is classified based on the closest training samples present in feature field. When the test data is given, it is mapped to the class that is most common among the k neighbors (Acharya et al., 2012).
- **Support Vector Machines (SVM):** This is a supervised classification algorithm which constructs a separating hyperplane in high dimensional space that can be used for classification. A good separation is obtained by the hyperplane that has largest distance to the nearest training data point of any class (Acharya et al., 2012).
- **Decision Tree (DT):** In this algorithm, the input features are used to construct a tree. A set of rules representing the different classes is then derived from the tree. These rules are used to forecast the class of a new instance with an unknown class (Acharya et al., 2012).

Performance Evaluation Criteria

In this study, five different performance evaluation criteria have been used during the performance evaluation phase. These are; accuracy, sensitivity, specificity, AUC and ROC curves, respectively.

$$Accuracy = \frac{TP + TN}{TP + FP + FN + TN} x100\% \tag{1}$$

$$Sensitivity = \frac{TP}{TP + FN} x100\% \tag{2}$$

$$Specificity = \frac{TN}{FP + TN} x100\% \tag{3}$$

$$Area\,under\,curve\left(AUC\right) = \frac{1}{2}\left(\frac{TP}{TP + FN} + \frac{TN}{FP + TN}\right) \tag{4}$$

True Positive (TP) refers to the number of correct classification of diseased data, false negative (FN) refers to the number of incorrect classification of healthy data. True Negative (TN) indicates the correct classification number of healthy data, while False Positive (FP) indicates the number of incorrect classification of diseased data.

The ROC curve is often used to allow the diagnostic test to define its own correctness and to make a reliable comparison between the tests. The area under the ROC for a diagnostic test can range from 0.50 to 1.00 depending on the activity level. The larger this area, the more distinction ability the diagnostic test will have.

EXPERIMENTAL RESULTS AND DISCUSSION

Case Study 1: Comparison of Classification Algorithms in the Estimation of Three-Level HbA1c Value

In this application, an estimation of the level of HbA1c which is an important parameter for the diagnosis of diabetes is aimed. In this context, a 3-level estimation system has been realized. The level classification has been carried out as follows: If HbA1c <6.5, "normal (Level 0)", if 6.5≤HbA1c <9, "high (Level 1)" and if HbA1c≥9, "very high (Level 2)".

The block diagram of the proposed system is presented in Figure 4. In the first step, in order to make the classification process more efficient, normalization process is applied to the data between 0-1. The Min-Max method given in Equation 5 is used as the normalization method.

$$x' = \frac{x_i - x_{min}}{x_{max} - x_{min}} \tag{5}$$

In this equation, x' denotes the normalized data; x_i denotes the input value; x_{min} denotes smallest number in the input set; x_{max} denotes the largest number in the input set. After the normalization phase, values are assigned to the missing data using the "Change with Random Values" method in the missing data analysis module of the Orange program.

After the data selection and pre-processing stages, the Training-Test data distribution phase has been carried out. In this phase, 10 layered cross validation method is used. Classification operations have been performed at the next stage. In this stage, experiments were carried out with 5 different classification algorithms to evaluate the performance of the feed-forward neural networks. These algorithms include; Artificial neural networks, Random Forest, k-nearest-neighbors, support vector machines and decision tree learning. The number of trees in the Random Forest algorithm has been determined as 10. In the neural network algorithm, the hidden layer neuron number is 20, the hidden layer activation function is sigmoid, the number of iterations is 1000 and the learning rate is determined as 0.5. In the SVM algorithm, the RBF function is used as the kernel function. In the kNN algorithm, the k-value is determined as 6.

The generated classification model has been created in Orange program. The model developed in the Orange program is shown in Figure 5.

Figure 4. Graph of the methodology followed in this study

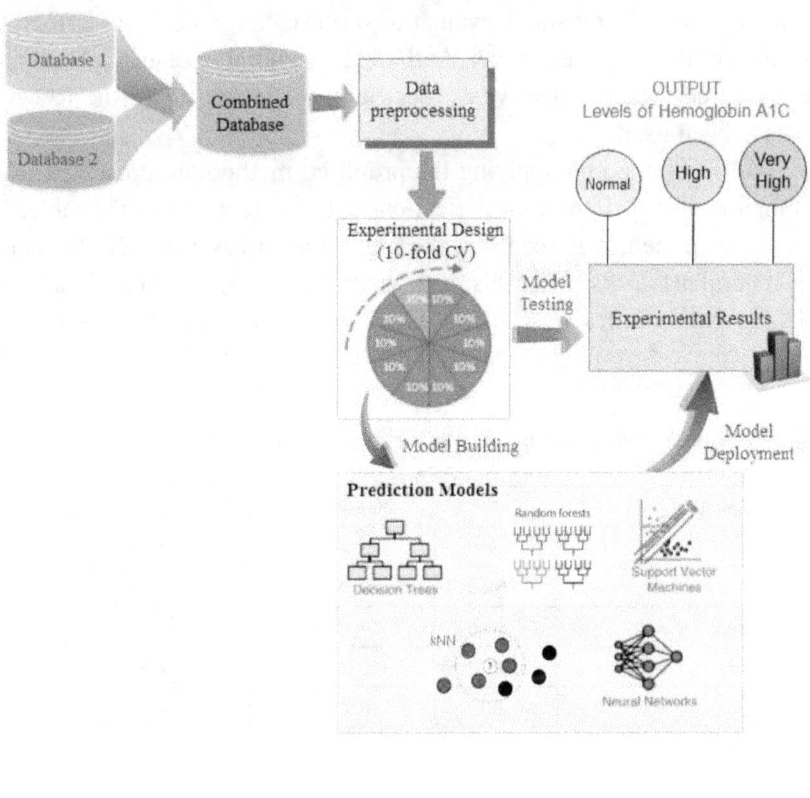

Figure 5. Orange application of 5 classification methods

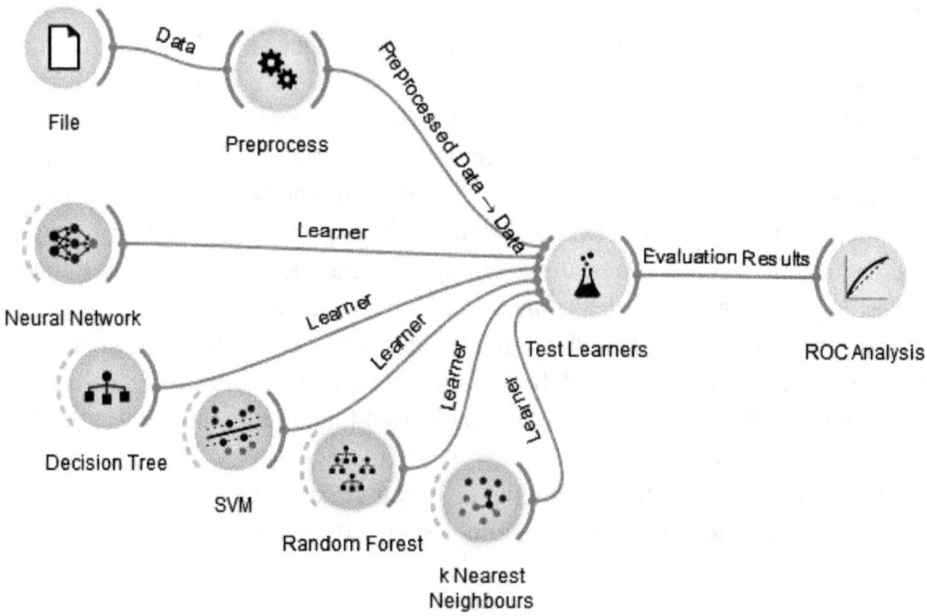

At the last stage, statistical evaluation criteria have been used to test the effectiveness of the proposed model. At this stage, a number of evaluation methods such as Accuracy Rate, Sensitivity, Specificity and Area under the ROC curve (AUC) have been used.

The results obtained by applying the proposed method are presented in Table 2. A comparison of different classification methods is given in the table. When the table is examined, it is seen that the highest accuracy value is obtained with artificial neural networks. After this method, the highest success rate is obtained by the kNN algorithm. The lowest success is achieved by the support vector machines

Table 2. The results obtained in the Phase of application 1

Algorithm	CA	Sensitivity	Specificity	AUC
kNN	0.8939	0.9284	0.9690	0.9406
SVM	0.6466	0.7881	0.9254	0.8542
Random Forest	0.8686	0.9194	0.9709	0.9767
Neural Network	0.9027	0.9269	0.9760	0.9599
DecisionTree	0.8912	0.9254	0.9747	0.9495

algorithm. It is also seen that artificial neural networks generally give better results in other statistical parameters besides the accuracy rate. It is seen that the Random Forest algorithm gives better results only in AUC values.

The success of the proposed method has also been assessed with different evaluation criteria. At this stage, ROC curves have been utilized. The ROC curves obtained are presented in Figure 6. When the figure is examined, it is seen that the area value under ROC is the largest with Random Forest (AUC: 0.9767) and artificial neural networks (AUC: 0.9599) for 3 different classes. The worst result has been obtained with SVM method (AUC: 0.8542).

Figure 6.ROC curves

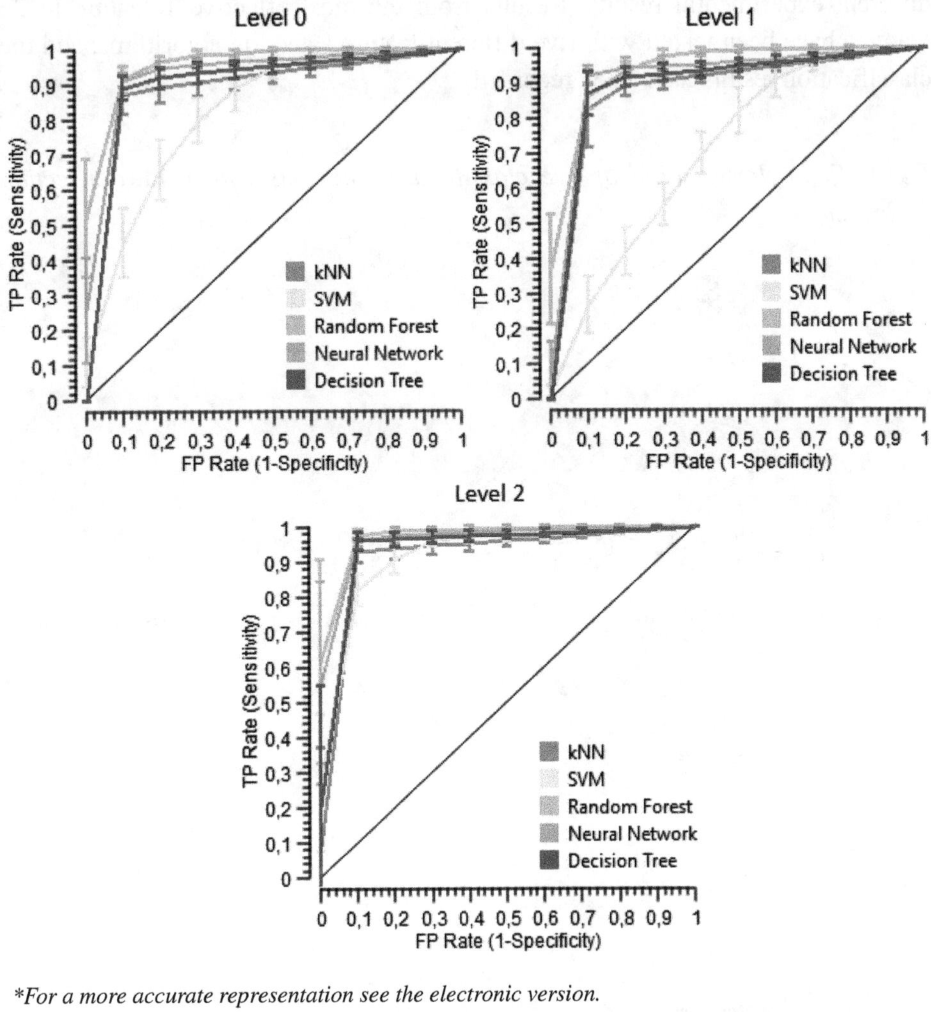

**For a more accurate representation see the electronic version.*

Case Study 2: The Use of Feature Selection Methods in Estimating the Two-Level HbA1c Value

In this application, a 2-level prediction of HbA1c is aimed. Level classification is performed as follows: If HbA1c is <6.5 then "normal" and if HbA1c≥6.5, "high". In this application, classification algorithms are compared by applying feature selection algorithms to the cleansed and filtered data. The model established in the Orange program is presented in Figure 7. In addition, the workflow carried out in this application is given in Figure 8. In the model, 4 feature selection algorithms are applied to 5 classification algorithms. The feature selection algorithms used in the study are ReliefF, information gain, gain ratio and chi-square.

By applying the model, the most effective feature sets have been obtained in different experimental results. Results from the most effective 1 feature to 26 features have been tested with five different feature selection algorithms, and the classification results have been recorded.

Figure 7. Implementation of five classification methods with feature selection algorithms

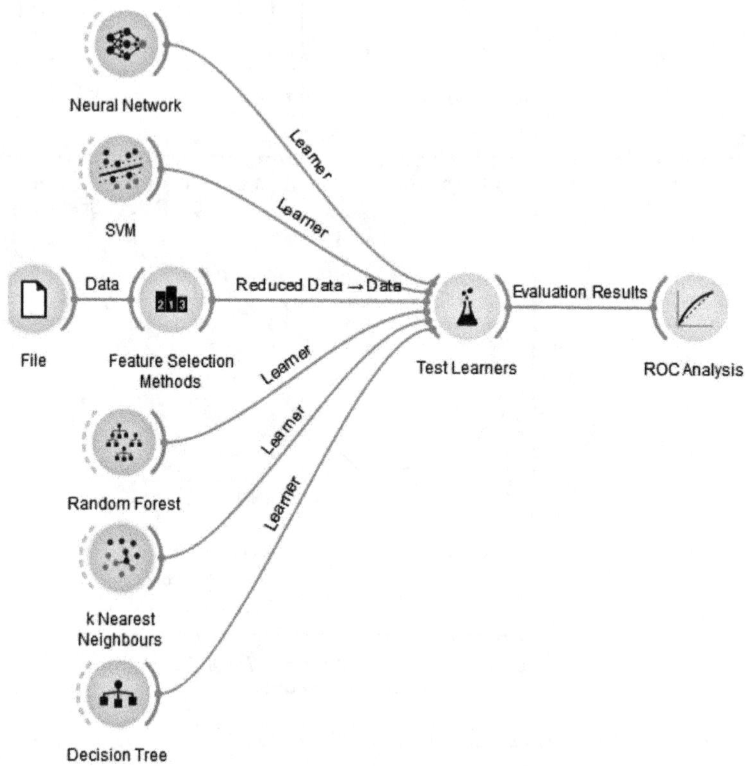

Figure 8. The proposed method for Case Study 2

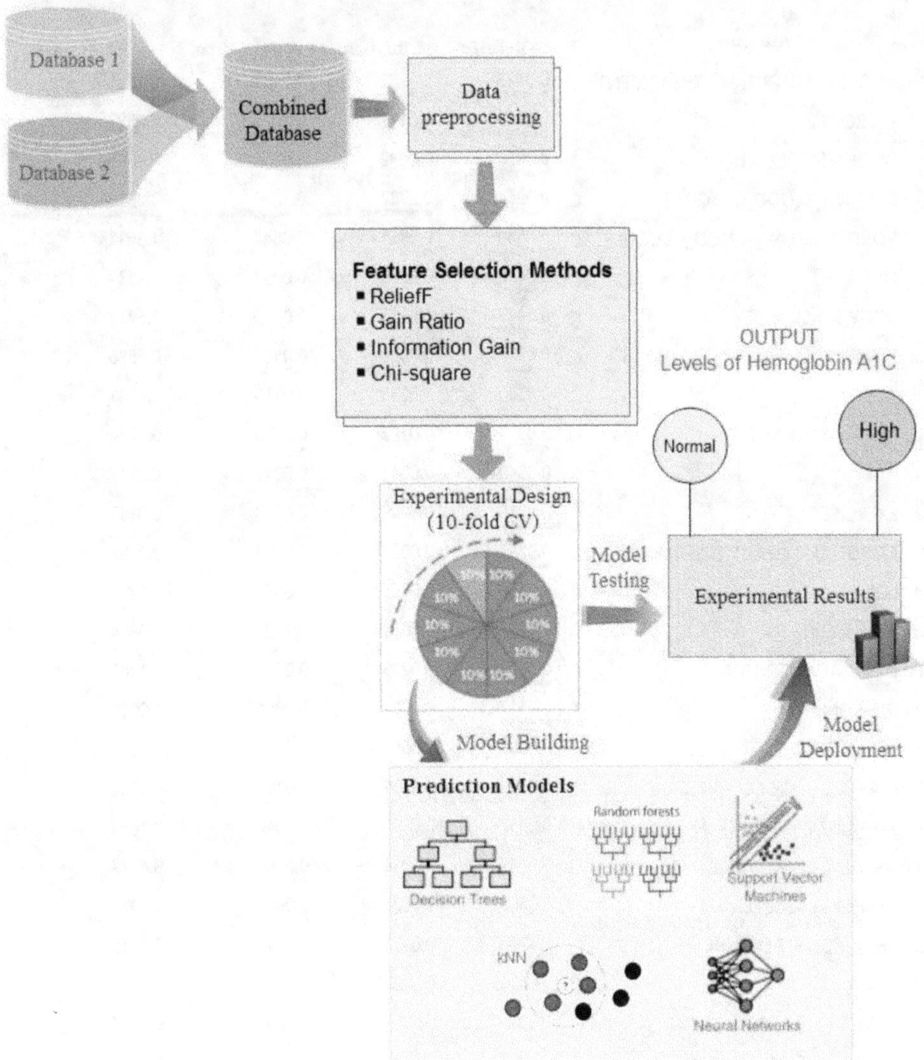

The order of the effective features obtained by different feature selection methods is given in Figure 9. In this figure, the features are scored for each algorithm. For example, according to ReliefF algorithm, the most effective feature is MEDICAL_NUTRITION_TREATMENT. The least effective feature according to ReliefF algorithm is the REASON_OF_APPLICATION_1. The most effective feature according to information gain algorithm is FASTING_BLOOD_GLUCOSE, and the least effective feature according to same algorithm is GLUKOMETER. The most effective feature according to Gain Ratio algorithm is FASTING_BLOOD_

Figure 9. Effective feature orders obtained according to different feature selection algorithms

	Attribute	#	ReliefF	Inf. Gain	Gain Ratio	Chi-Square
1	MEDICAL_NUTRITION_TREATMENT	C	0.0925	0.0282	0.0140	0.1265
2	EXERCISE 2	C	0.0882	0.0152	0.0071	0.0527
3	DIABETES_EDUCATION	2	0.0866	0.0032	0.0155	0.0085
4	FASTING_BLOOD_GLUCOSE	C	0.0844	0.2787	0.1200	38.3182
5	POSTPRANDIAL_BLOOD_GLUCOSE	C	0.0548	0.0861	0.0647	4.8611
6	HDL	C	0.0470	0.0074	0.0032	0.3537
7	BODY_MASS_INDEX	C	0.0447	0.0115	0.0050	1.5712
8	DIAGNOSIS	C	0.0396	0.0088	0.0583	0.6586
9	ALT	C	0.0380	0.0255	0.0116	0.0841
10	HIP_ENVIRONMENT	C	0.0353	0.0122	0.0053	0.2734
11	AGE	C	0.0349	0.0041	0.0018	0.0117
12	EXERCISE 1	C	0.0310	0.0009	0.0027	0.0107
13	CORONARY_HEART_DISEASE	2	0.0233	0.0021	0.0137	0.0303
14	LDL	C	0.0182	0.0067	0.0029	0.0339
15	TRIGLISERIT	C	0.0133	0.0059	0.0026	0.0854
16	MEDICAL NUTRITION	C	0.0119	0.0223	0.0193	0.1308
17	GLUKOMETER	2	0.0117	0.0001	0.0001	0.0016
18	WAIST_CIRCUMFERENCE	C	0.0086	0.0069	0.0030	0.3915
19	DIASTOLIC_BLOOD_PRESSURE	C	0.0059	0.0251	0.0161	0.0007
20	EXERCISE_PROPOSITION	C	0.0052	0.0260	0.0340	0.1854
21	SISTOLIC_BLOOD_PRESSURE	C	0.0047	0.0336	0.0167	0.4277
22	CEREBROVASCULER	2	0.0000	0.0002	0.0031	0.0071
23	THYROID_INSPECTION	C	-0.0000	0.0023	0.0024	0.0016
24	SEX	2	-0.0045	0.0002	0.0002	0.0003
25	REASON_OF_APPLICATION_2	C	-0.0069	0.0067	0.0063	0.0000
26	REASON_OF_APPLICATION_1	C	-0.0094	0.0047	0.0037	0.0105

GLUCOSE and the least effective one is GLUKOMETER. Finally, the most effective feature according to Chi-Square algorithm is FASTING_BLOOD_GLUCOSE and the least effective one is REASON_OF_APPLICATION_2.

Once effective feature sequences have been identified, these features are classified by different classification algorithms. In the first step, the ReliefF algorithm is applied to the feature. Figure 10 displays the classification accuracy rates of the feature clusters identified by the ReliefF algorithm. As can be seen, the highest

Figure 10. Classification results of ReliefF feature selection algorithm

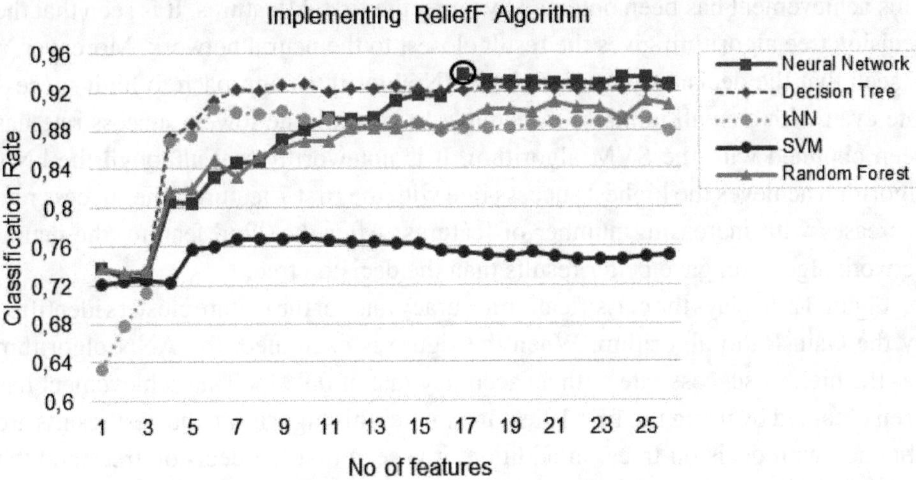

success rate was obtained with the ANN algorithm with an accuracy of 0.9385. This achievement has been obtained by using the first 17 features. The closest result to neural networks is given by the Decision trees algorithm. Moreover, it seems that the decision trees and the CNN algorithm are approaching a higher success rate with fewer features. In general, the lowest success rate has been obtained with the SVM algorithm.

Figure 11 displays the classification accuracy of the feature clusters identified by the information Gain algorithm. As can be seen from the figure, the highest

Figure 11. Classification results of information gain feature selection algorithm

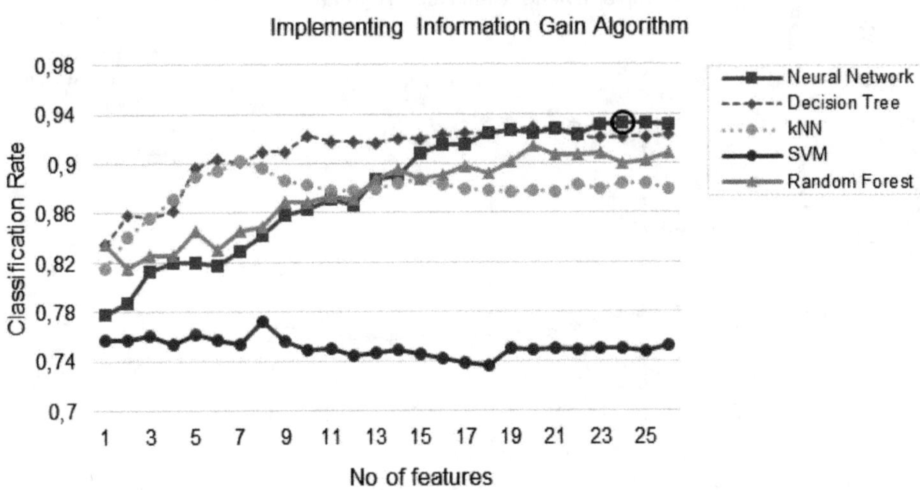

success rate has been obtained with the ANN algorithm with an accuracy of 0.9325. This achievement has been obtained by using the first 24features. It is seen that the decision tree algorithm gives the result closest to the neural network. Moreover, it is seen that the decision trees and the KNN algorithms approach to high success rate even with a small number of features. In general, the lowest success rate has been obtained with the SVM algorithm. It is noteworthy that although the kNN algorithm achieves the highest success rate with the first 7 features, the success rate decreases with increasing number of features. After the 22nd feature, the neural network algorithm gave better results than the decision tree.

Figure 12 displays the classification accuracy rates of the feature clusters identified by the Gain Ratio algorithm. When the figure is examined, the ANN algorithm has the highest success rate with an accuracy rate of 0.9345. This achievement has been obtained by using the first 19features. After this algorithm, the best results are obtained with decision trees. In addition, it is seen that the decision trees and the KNN algorithms approach to high success rate even with a small number of features. In general, the lowest success rate has been obtained with the SVM algorithm.

Figure 13 shows the results obtained using the chi-square algorithm. When the figure is examined, the ANN algorithm has the highest success rate of 0.9316. This achievement has been obtained by using the first 17features. The closest competitive algorithm is the decision tree with 16 features and a success rate of 0.9303. Moreover, it is seen that the decision tree algorithm approaches to a higher success rate with less features up to 17. In general, the lowest success rate has been obtained with the SVM algorithm.

Figure 12. Classification results of the gain ratio feature selection algorithm

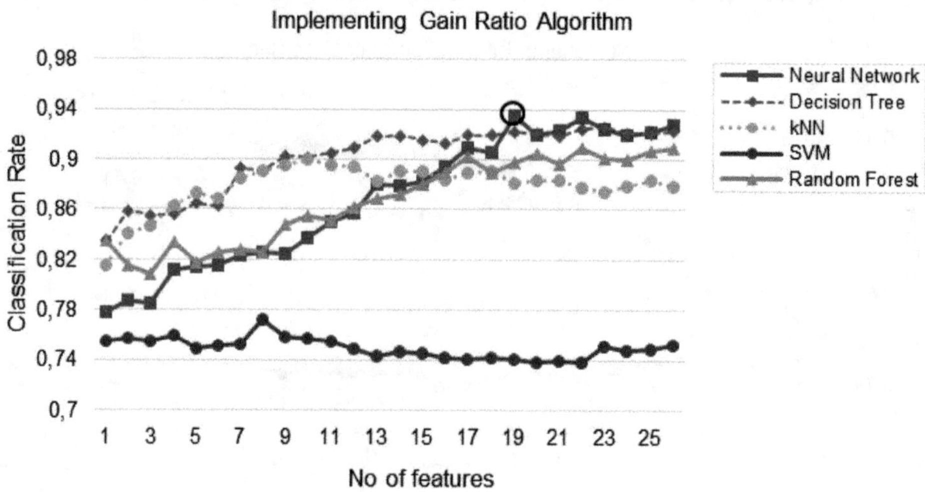

Figure 13. Classification results of the chi-square feature selection algorithm

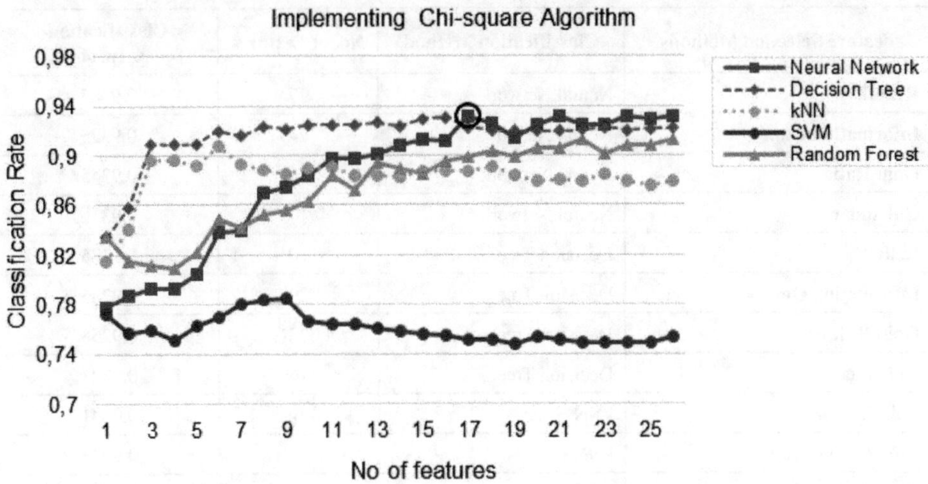

Best results obtained by applying all the classification algorithms and all feature selection algorithms are given in Table 3. When the table is examined, the highest accuracy is obtained by the first 17 features obtained by the ReliefF algorithm and the classification of these attributes by the ANN algorithm.

CONCLUSION

The study carried out is generally a clinical decision support system. In this study, predictions have been made for diagnosis and treatment, and tried to help decision-makers with recommendations by using clinical data stack and patient-specific data of diabetes patients especially created by internal medicine specialists.

In the study, a comparison has been made between different algorithms that could be used for the component of inference mechanism which is the brain of the clinical decision support systems.

From the results obtained, it is seen that artificial neural networks generally generate the best result among these classification algorithms. The performance impact of the selected features with the feature selection algorithms is more positive and more favorable than the use of all the features. When studies on the diagnosis of diabetes are examined in the literature, it is seen that many features are used. But, it is seen as an important problem that which features are effective. The study has also a great importance in this respect. It will be an important guide for researchers working on this subject.

Table 3. The number of features and success rates for the best results obtained

Feature Selection Methods	Classification Method	No. of Features	Classification Accuracy
ReliefF	Neural Network	17	0,9385
Information Gain	Neural Network	24	0.9325
Gain Ratio	Neural Network	19	0,9345
Chi-square	Neural Network	17	0,9316
ReliefF	Decision Tree	10	0,9285
Information Gain	Decision Tree	20	0,9285
Gain Ratio	Decision Tree	23	0.9258
Chi-square	Decision Tree	16	0,9303
ReliefF	kNN	6	0.9041
Information Gain	kNN	7	0.9023
Gain Ratio	kNN	10	0.9006
Chi-square	kNN	6	0.9085
ReliefF	SVM	10	0,7691
Information Gain	SVM	8	0.7727
Gain Ratio	SVM	8	0.7727
Chi-square	SVM	9	0.7851
ReliefF	Random Forest	25	0.9103
Information Gain	Random Forest	20	0.9134
Gain Ratio	Random Forest	22	0.9090
Chi-square	Random Forest	22	0.9130

Orange data mining software has been introduced in the scope of the study and an application in the field of medicine has been presented.

The developed system can help to the experts in the cases in which it is difficult for physicians to make decisions due to the increased amount of medical data and the number of patients or where multi-directional thinking is necessary. In addition, this system can be very helpful especially for diabetes patients in the early diagnosis warnings, drug recommendations or prevention of mistakes due to negligence.

ACKNOWLEDGMENT

The authors are grateful to Muğla Sıtkı Koçman University Research Projects Coordination Office (BAP- 17/202) for the financial support.

REFERENCES

Acharya, U. R., Molinari, F., Sree, S. V., Chattopadhyay, S., Ng, K. H., & Suri, J. S. (2012). Automated diagnosis of epileptic EEG using entropies. *Biomedical Signal Processing and Control, 7*(4), 401–408. doi:10.1016/j.bspc.2011.07.007

Afarideh, M., Aryan, Z., Ghajar, A., Noshad, S., Nakhjavani, M., Baber, U., ... Esteghamati, A. (2016). Complex association of serum alanine aminotransferase with the risk of future cardiovascular disease in type 2 diabetes. *Atherosclerosis, 254*, 42–51. doi:10.1016/j.atherosclerosis.2016.09.009 PMID:27684605

Amato, F., López, A., Peña-Méndez, E. M., Vaňhara, P., Hampl, A., & Havel, J. (2013). *Artificial neural networks in medical diagnosis*. Academic Press.

Bilous, R., & Donnelly, R. (2010). *Handbook of diabetes*. John Wiley & Sons. doi:10.1002/9781444391374

Breiman, L. (2001). Random forests. *Machine Learning, 45*(1), 5–32. doi:10.1023/A:1010933404324

Choubey, D. K., & Paul, S. (2016). Classification techniques for diagnosis of diabetes: A review. *International Journal of Biomedical Engineering and Technology, 21*(1), 15–39. doi:10.1504/IJBET.2016.076730

Demšar, J., Curk, T., Erjavec, A., Gorup, Č., Hočevar, T., Milutinovič, M., ... Štajdohar, M. (2013). Orange: Data mining toolbox in Python. *Journal of Machine Learning Research, 14*(1), 2349–2353.

Durna, Z. (2002). DiyabetinSınıflandırılmasıveTanıKriteleri.İçinde: Edit. Erdoğan S. DiyabetHemşireliğiTemelBilgiler. YüceYayım, İstanbul, 11-21.

Heydari, M., Teimouri, M., Heshmati, Z., & Alavinia, S. M. (2016). Comparison of various classification algorithms in the diagnosis of type 2 diabetes in Iran. *International Journal of Diabetes in Developing Countries, 36*(2), 167–173. doi:10.100713410-015-0374-4

Kononenko, I. (1994). Estimating attributes: analysis and extensions of RELIEF. In *European conference on machine learning* (pp. 171-182). Springer. 10.1007/3-540-57868-4_57

Leema, N., Nehemiah, H. K., & Kannan, A. (2016). Neural network classifier optimization using differential evolution with global information and back propagation algorithm for clinical datasets. *Applied Soft Computing, 49*, 834–844. doi:10.1016/j.asoc.2016.08.001

Ling, S. H., San, P. P., & Nguyen, H. T. (2016). Non-invasive hypoglycemia monitoring system using extreme learning machine for Type 1 diabetes. *ISA Transactions*, *64*, 440–446. doi:10.1016/j.isatra.2016.05.008 PMID:27311357

Lopez-de-Andres, A., Hernandez-Barrera, V., Lopez, R., Martin-Junco, P., Jimenez-Trujillo, I., Alvaro-Meca, A., ... Jimenez-Garcia, R. (2016). Predictors of in-hospital mortality following major lower extremity amputations in type 2 diabetic patients using artificial neural networks. *BMC Medical Research Methodology*, *16*(1), 160. doi:10.118612874-016-0265-5 PMID:27876006

Rajesh, K., & Sangeetha, V. (2012). Application of data mining methods and techniques for diabetes diagnosis. *International Journal of Engineering and Innovative Technology*, *2*(3).

Rau, H. H., Hsu, C. Y., Lin, Y. A., Atique, S., Fuad, A., Wei, L. M., & Hsu, M. H. (2016). Development of a web-based liver cancer prediction model for type II diabetes patients by using an artificial neural network. *Computer Methods and Programs in Biomedicine*, *125*, 58–65. doi:10.1016/j.cmpb.2015.11.009 PMID:26701199

Soltani, Z., & Jafarian, A. (2016). A New Artificial Neural Networks Approach for Diagnosing Diabetes Disease Type II. *International Journal of Advanced Computer Science and Applications*, *7*(6), 89–94. doi:10.14569/IJACSA.2016.070611

Wang, C., Li, L., Wang, L., Ping, Z., Flory, M. T., Wang, G., ... Li, W. (2013). Evaluating the risk of type 2 diabetes mellitus using artificial neural network: An effective classification approach. *Diabetes Research and Clinical Practice*, *100*(1), 111–118. doi:10.1016/j.diabres.2013.01.023 PMID:23453177

World Health Organization. (2016). *Global report on diabetes*. World Health Organization.

Zheng, T., Xie, W., Xu, L., He, X., Zhang, Y., You, M., ... Chen, Y. (2017). A machine learning-based framework to identify type 2 diabetes through electronic health records. *International Journal of Medical Informatics*, *97*, 120–127. doi:10.1016/j.ijmedinf.2016.09.014 PMID:27919371

KEY TERMS AND DEFINITIONS

Classification: It is a kind of supervised machine learning in which an algorithm "learns" to classify novel observations from samples of labeled data.

Diabetes: This is a life-long illness which occurs as a result of lack of insulin hormone or ineffectiveness of insulin hormone.

Feature Selection: This is the process of reducing the inputs for processing and analysis, or of finding the most meaningful inputs.

Hemoglobin A1c: This is a protein on the surface of red blood cells that sugar molecules stick to, usually for the life of the red blood cell (about three months).

Medical Diagnosis: It is a classification operation including the decision-making process based on available medical data.

Orange Data Mining Toolbox: This is an open source data mining toolbox developed for novice and expert.

ROC Curve: It is a graphical method that assesses the success of a binary classifier system.

Chapter 8
Wavelet Packet Analysis of ECG signals to Understand the Effect of a Motivating Song on Heart of Indian Male Volunteers

Gitika Yadu
National Institute of Technology Rourkela, India

Debasisha Panigrahi
National Institute of Technology Rourkela, India

Suraj Kumar Nayak
National Institute of Technology Rourkela, India

Anilesh Dey
Kaziranga University, India

Kunal Pal
National Institute of Technology Rourkela, India

ABSTRACT

This chapter investigates the effect of a motivational song (acting as a stimulus) on the electrical activity of the heart using wavelet packet analysis of electrocardiogram (ECG) signals. ECG signals were acquired from 18 healthy male volunteers during the pre- and the post-stimulus conditions. Wavelet packet decomposition of the ECG signals was performed up to level 3 using db04 wavelet, which resulted in the formation of 8 wavelet packet coefficients. Linear (t-test) and nonlinear (classification and regression tree [CART], boosted tree [BT], and random forest [RF]) methods were used to identify the statistically significant parameters. The statistically significant parameters were used as categorical inputs for multilayer perceptron (MLP)-based artificial neural network (ANN) classification of the ECG signals. A classification efficiency of ≥ 80% was obtained, suggesting an alteration in the cardiac electrophysiology of the volunteers caused by the music stimulus.

DOI: 10.4018/978-1-5225-5149-2.ch008

INTRODUCTION

Music has been reported to have an advantageous impression on the human health (MacDonald, Kreutz, & Mitchell, 2013). It has been reported to arouse the emotions (Juslin & Sloboda, 2001) and can be used as a stimulus for triggering the emotional responses for the person. Recent studies have suggested that listening to the music is also associated with a change in the physical states (e.g., promotes sleep, reduces anxiety, increases positive attitude towards exercise, and increases brain activities) of the person (Lai, 2001) . Therefore, it can be told that a temporary change occurs in both the physiological and the psychological states of the person while listening to the music (Levenson, 2014; Yen et al., 2010). Apart from exploring the above-mentioned physiological effects of the music, research is going on to establish the effect of music on the heart. The electrical activity of the heart can be analyzed non-invasively using electrocardiogram (ECG) signals, obtained from electrocardiography test. Electrocardiography is a painless and uncomplicated test (Clark, 2015; De Mello, 2013). It records the electrical activity of the heart as a function of time through the placement of the electrodes on the skin. As the ECG signal is acquired in a non-invasive condition, its classification has been extensively studied by the researchers for the diagnosis of the cardiac diseases as well as for identifying any alteration in the cardiac electrophysiology due to a stimulus (Yaman et al., 2013). The classification of the ECG signals usually comprises of four stages, i.e., preprocessing, segmentation, feature extraction, and classification. The pre-processing level typically performs artefact removal, signal enhancement and normalization. Then, segmentation fragments the signal into smaller segments that indicate the electrical activity of the heart in a better way (Da S Luz, Nunes, De Albuquerque, Papa, & Menotti, 2013). From these two stages, good results can be obtained using some prevalent features (Li & Zhou, 2016; Da S Luz, Merschmann, Menotti, & Moreira, 2017). Feature extraction is essential for the ECG signal classification and can be performed using the raw or segmented ECG signals. Various types of methods have been proposed for the extraction of the ECG signal features, such as, the extraction of the sample points at some frequency from the ECG signal, statistical and/or morphological methods, and transformed domain methods. Amongst the transformed domain methods, wavelet-based methods such as discrete wavelet transform (DWT) and its extension to wavelet packet decomposition (WPD) have gained significance because of their ability to capture the centralized spatial-frequency information of the ECG signals (Li & Zhou, 2016). However, WPD has been reported to provide better results than DWT. This may be because of the fact that it decomposes both the approximation and the detail coefficients of the ECG signals. Over the years, classification of the ECG signals has been attempted by numerous methods such as support vector machine (SVM), K-nearest neighbour (KNN) and ANN in different studies. Amongst the supervised learning-based classification methods, ANN has received special attention of the researchers because of the multi-parametric nature of its architecture (Alexakis et al., 2003). Taking the motivation from the above-mentioned discussion, the current study proposes the use of WPD analysis and ANN classification of ECG signals to understand the effect of a motivational song on the cardiac electrophysiology.

BACKGROUND

An important step for the classification of any signal is the extraction of suitable features from it that contains all the relevant information about the signal. The features are used as input to any classification algorithm instead of the original signal (Li & Zhou, 2016). Among the different feature extraction methods, wavelet transform-based methods such as continuous wavelet transform (CWT) and DWT have received wide-spread applications (Addison, 2017; Aguiar-Conraria & Soares, 2014). The wavelet transform-based methods have been regarded as some of the most appropriate tools for the analysis of the signals by many researchers (Alfaouri & Daqrouq, 2008). Wavelet transform-based methods decompose a signal in such a way that the location of the features and the frequency characteristics in the temporal series can be highlighted at the same time (Addison et al., 2000). For the implementation of the DWT, Mallat (1989) proposed an efficient algorithm for the computation of DWT, which decomposes the signal using the decomposition filters (Mallat, 1989). The algorithm has received wide-spread acceptance in the scientific community. The DWT method decomposes the signal at each level using a set of filters, having the properties of high pass and low pass filters, peculiar for each mother wavelet (Van Fleet, 2011). The outputs of these filters are an approximation coefficient and a detail coefficient. In the next level, the approximation coefficient further split into approximation and detail coefficients. Hence, successive detail coefficients are not analyzed further. This results in the loss of high-frequency information. However, with the introduction of wavelet packet decomposition (WPD), all the sub-bands of frequency can be analyzed (Hu, Li, & Chen, 2011). WPD is a special kind of DWT. In WPD, each detail coefficient is also decomposed in the same manner as the decomposition of the approximation coefficients (Antoniadis & Oppenheim, 2012). Figure 1 and Figure 2 show the 3-layer binary trees for DWT and WPD, respectively. In these figures, S represents the signal, "L" represents the low-pass filter and "H" represents the high-pass filter. A and D represents the approximation coefficient and the detail coefficient, respectively.

Figure 1. 3-level decomposition tree for DWT

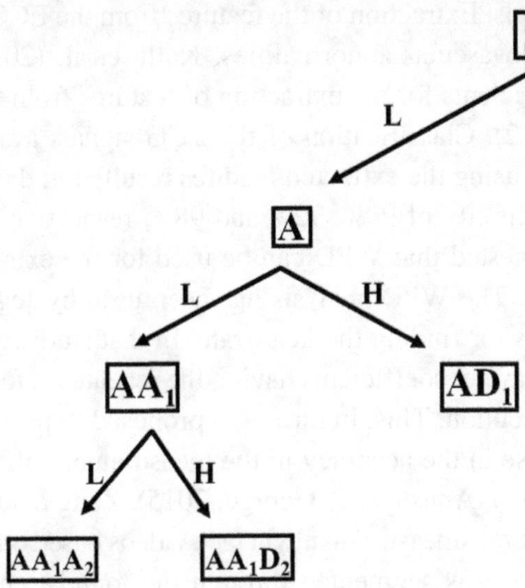

Figure 2. 3-level decomposition tree for WPT

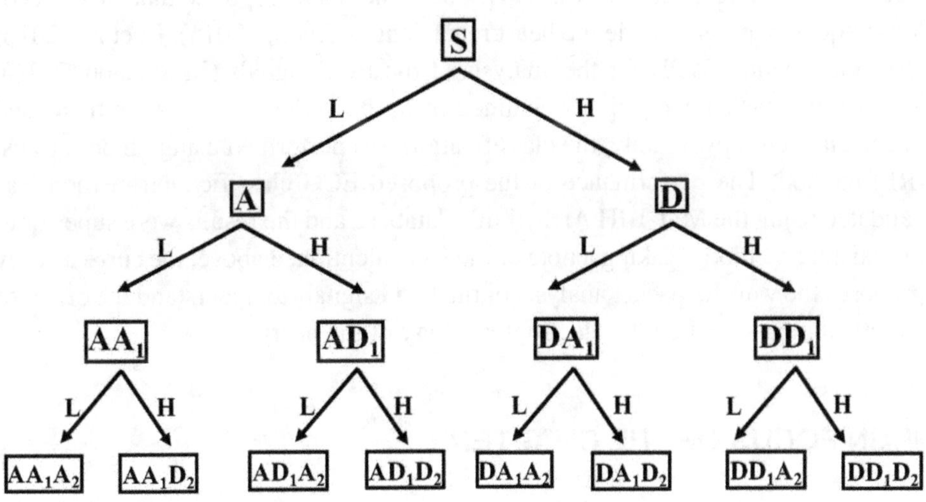

In the last few decades, researchers have proposed the applications of WPD in various fields of research like hydrolic systems (Liu, Su, Qin, & Li, 2016), wind speed forecasting (Meng, Ge, Yin, & Chen, 2016), river stage prediction (Seo, Kim, Kisi, Singh, & Parasuraman, 2016), and biomedical signal processing (Fujita et al., 2017). In recent years, WPD has been used in the analysis of the biosignals, e.g., electromyogram (EMG) (Abdullah, Subasi, & Qaisar, 2017), electroencephalogram

(EEG) (Puri, Ingle, Kachare, Patil, & Awale, 2017), respiratory signals (lung sound) (He et al., 2016) and ECG signals. Extraction of the features from the ECG signals is requisite for detecting cardiovascular abnormalities. Kutlu et al. (2012) have reported the use of WPD coefficients for the extraction of features from the ECG signals (Kutlu & Kuntalp, 2012). Classification of the ECG signals available in MIT-BIH arrhythmia database using the extracted features resulted in the average sensitivity, selectivity and specificity of 90%, 92% and 98%, respectively. Based on the results, the authors suggested that WPD can be used for the extraction of features from the ECG signals. The WPD analysis has been used by Jegan et al. (2015) to detect the ECG peaks for finding the heart rate. In that study, the WPD tree was used for eliminating wavelet coefficients having the repeated information, thus optimizing the time of execution. This, in turn, was proposed to provide high temporal resolution and increase in the accuracy in the measurement of the heart rate from the ECG signals (Jegan, Anusuya, & George, 2015). Zeng et al. (2015) presented a method for the heart rate measurement via face videos based on wavelet packet decomposition. The face was segmented through the foundation of skin model in each frame, segregated into 3 RGB channels and then was averaged over all pixels to obtain 3 signals. Then the independent signals were chosen, and the frequency parts were acquired by WPD. The authors have reported that the peaks of low-frequency parts provide the heart rate (Zeng & Zhong, 2015). Li et al. (2016) also implemented WPD for the analysis of the ECG signals (Li & Zhou, 2016). The wavelet packet coefficients obtained from the WPD analysis were then used to calculate entropy. Finally, the classification was performed using random forest (RF) method. The performance of the proposed ECG classification method was validated using the MIT-BIH Arrhythmia database and the results were superior to the existing methods. Taking a note of the facts mentioned above, the current study proposes the wavelet packet analysis of the ECG signals to understand the effect of a motivational signal on the electrophysiology of the heart.

MAIN FOCUS OF THE CHAPTER

The current study used a motivational song as the stimulus and aimed to understand its effect on the electrical activity of the heart. ECG signals were acquired from 19 healthy male volunteers and subjected to WPD. Statistical features were extracted from the wavelet packet coefficients. Statistically significant features were identified using linear and non-linear methods, and finally, ANN based classification was implemented.

METHODOLOGY

In this study, 19 healthy male volunteers in the age group of 21 to 23 years, with no medical complications, were invited to participate. Also, the selected volunteers were nonsmokers. These shortlisted volunteers were asked to report at the ECG recording station. They were advised not to take food within 1 hour before the recording of the ECG signals. The ECG signals were recorded in the lead-1 configuration for 5 min with a sampling frequency of 1000 Hz, which were considered as the pre-stimulus ECG signals. The volunteers were then advised to relax for 30 min. After the resting stage, the volunteers were allowed to listen to the motivational song (stimulus). Then the ECG signals were again recorded for 5 min, considered as the post-stimulus ECG signals. The 5 sec ECG signals were extracted from 5 min of the recorded ECG data by using a program developed in LabVIEW (Version 13.0 National Instruments, USA). The 5 sec ECG data were then band-limited using a low-pass filter (LPF) of cut-off frequency 50 Hz. The band-limited ECG signals were resampled at 360 Hz using another program developed in LabVIEW (Li & Zhou, 2016). We know that by Nyquist sampling theory (Gang, Jiapin, HongHui, & Lu, 2004):where, the maximum frequency of the signal is denoted by f_m and f_s is the sampling frequency.

This 5 sec of ECG signals were subjected to WPD. The decomposition of the pre-stimulus and the post-stimulus ECG signals was done up to the level 3 using Daubechies 04 wavelet (db04). The wavelets from the Daubechies family are considered to be the best ones for the analysis of the ECG signals because of their good correlation with the ECG signals (De Chazal, Celler, & Reilly, 2000). The WPD of each of the ECG signals resulted in the formation of 8 wavelet packet coefficients.

12 statistical parameters were then extracted for each wavelet packet coefficients using a program developed in LabVIEW. These extracted features were arithmetic mean (AM), root mean square (RMS), standard deviation (SD), variance (VAR), kurtosis (KUR), median (MED), mode (MOD), skewness (SKW), summation (SUM), energy density (ED), Shannon entropy (SE), and log energy (LE). This resulted in the extraction of 96 statistical parameters from each ECG signal, which were tabulated in the excel spreadsheet. This excel spreadsheet was imported as a Statistica (trial version 13.0, Dell Inc., USA) spreadsheet. Statistica is an analytics software that was used for statistical analysis. Linear and non-linear methods were used to identify the statistically significant parameters of the ECG signals. The only linear method we performed was t-test and the non-linear methods were Classification and Regression Tree (CART), Boosted Tree (BT) and Random Forest (RF). These statistical parameters were used as the categorical inputs for ANN based classification.

ANN is inspired by biological neural networks (Jain, Mao, & Mohiuddin, 1996). For the analysis of the ECG signals, we have used MLP neural networks. The flow chart of the proposed method is provided in Figure 3.

RESULTS AND DISCUSSION

ECG signal is used to record the electrical activities of the heart. The analysis of the ECG signal has been widely explored to detect the changes in the heart physiology. In this study, 5 sec portions of the acquired ECG signals were used for investigating the effect of the music stimulus on the heart. The preprocessing of the pre- and the post-stimulus ECG signals was done, and the resulting ECG signals were subjected to WPD before feature extraction. As mentioned earlier, WPD is an extension of

Figure 3. Flow chart of proposed framework

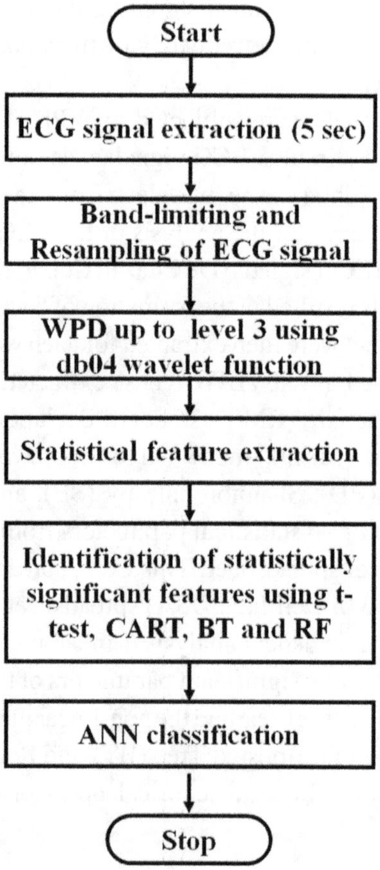

the DWT that decomposes both the approximation and the detail coefficients of a given signal. This is in contrary to the decomposition of the approximate coefficients in case of DWT. This property makes the WPD not to lose any information (from the original ECG signal) during the feature extraction process of the signal, which may occur in case of DWT as the detail coefficients are not decomposed (Li & Zhou, 2016). Mathematically, WPD of a signal $s(t)$ can be defined as in Equation 1 (Li & Zhou, 2016).

$$\begin{aligned} c_{0,0}(t) &= s(t) \\ c_{i,2j-1}(t) &= \sqrt{2}\sum_k h(k)\,c_{i-1,j}(2t-k) \\ c_{i,2j}(t) &= \sqrt{2}\sum_k l(k)\,c_{i-1,j}(2t-k) \end{aligned} \tag{1}$$

where, $h(k)$ is high pass filter, $l(k)$ is low pass filter, $c_{i,j}$ is the coefficient (reconstructed signal) of WPD, i represents the level index, and j represents the node index.

There are various types of wavelets and the selection of a particular wavelet depends on the type of the application (Mahmoodabadi, Ahmadian, & Abolhasani, 2005). In the current study, db04 mother wavelet was used for the decomposition of the ECG signals. Many researchers have reported that although the Daubechies family of wavelets is more complex it shows good correlation with the ECG signals (Raeiatibanadkooki, Quchani, KhalilZade, & Bahaadinbeigy, 2016). It has a shape similar to that of the QRS complex and the energy spectrum is concentrated around the low-frequency regions (Mahmoodabadi et al., 2005).

Figure 4 represents the level 3 WPD of a 5 sec ECG signal. In the 1st level of decomposition, the signal was split into A (left) and D (right), which corresponded to the approximation and detail coefficients, respectively.

The approximation coefficient of 1st level (A) was further split into the approximation coefficient (AA_1) and the detail coefficient (AD_1) in the 2nd level of decomposition. Similarly, the detail coefficient (D) of 1st level was split into approximation coefficient (DA_1) and detail coefficient (DD_1) in the 2nd level of decomposition. In the third level decomposition, the approximate coefficient AA_1 was split into approximation coefficient AA_1A_2 and detail coefficient AA_1D_2. Similarly, all the other coefficients of the 2nd level of decomposition were decomposed into approximation and detail coefficients in the third level decomposition. All these wavelet coefficients were named as "P/ (X-Y) Hz" in Figure 4, where P indicated whether the coefficient was an approximation or detail coefficient, and (X-Y) Hz indicated the range of the coefficient frequency in Hertz. After the 3 levels of

Figure 4. Wavelet packet decomposition tree for a normal heartbeat

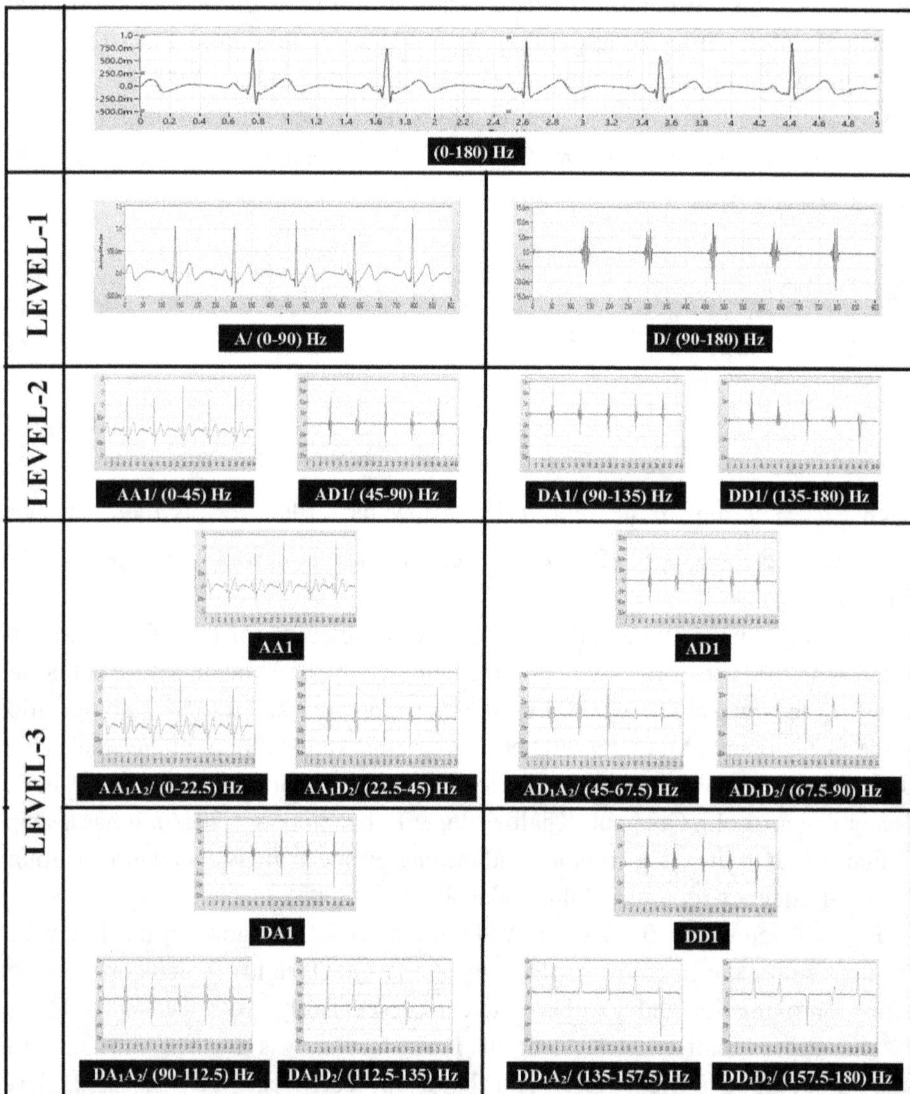

decomposition, a combined total of 8 approximation and detail coefficients were obtained, which were given binary nomenclature, i.e., 000, 001, 010, 011, 100, 101, 110, 111.

The statistical features of ECG signal usually change over time. The major concern for the ECG signals is to extract important features from it and its proper detection. So WPD method provides a good range of possibilities for the analysis of the ECG signals (Haque, Ali, Kiber, & Hasan, 2009).

For detecting the variations in the ECG signals, acquired during the pre- and the post-stimulus conditions, 12 statistical features of their corresponding wavelet packet coefficients were extracted. The features were arithmetic mean (AM), root mean square (RMS), variance (VAR), standard deviation (SD), kurtosis (KUR), median (MED), mode (MOD), skewness (SKW), summation (SUM), energy density (ED), Shannon entropy (SE) and log energy (LE). Thus, for 8 wavelet packet coefficients, 96 statistical parameters were obtained. These features were labeled as "P-Q", where P denotes the name of the statistical parameter and Q denotes the binary name of the wavelet packet coefficient.

Arithmetic mean (AM) is the statistical parameter that represents the average elevation of a given signal from its baseline (Equation 2).

$$S_m = E\{X\} = \mu \tag{2}$$

where, S_m denotes the mean of the signal and E{X} is the expectation of the signal. AM is also indicated by μ.

Kurtosis provides the idea about the distribution of the signal values relative to the normal distribution (Aubert et al., 1999). Mode provides the information regarding the signal value that occurs most often in a particular set of values of the signal. Mode of a continuous signal is calculated from the grouped distribution of frequency. It has been reported that the value of mode of a signal is considerably lesser than the other statistical parameters of the signal (Lane).

Skewness is the parameter that represents the extent of asymmetry of the distribution of the signal values. If a signal has a symmetric probability density function, then skewness will be zero. If the skewness value is high, then the signal has a sharp transition either from high to low or low to high. In other words, it detects the edges of signal (Ghaffari, Homaeinezhad, Khazraee, & Daevaeiha, 2010). When the skewness is positive, the AM is greater than the median of the signal (Lane).

$$S_{skw} = \frac{\sigma_1^{\ 3}}{\sigma_2^{\ 3/2}} \frac{E\{(X-\mu)^3\}}{\sqrt{(E\{(X-\mu)^2\})^3}} \tag{3}$$

Shannon entropy is the average information content in the signal. It is a measure of uncertainty in information contained by the signal due to the random variables. It helps in the characterization of the chaotic signals (Aydın, Saraoğlu, & Kara, 2009). Suppose x is the random variable with a finite range $x_1, x_2, \ldots, x_n$. Let p_k be the probability of the information s, therefore, the Shannon entropy (SE) (Hammer, Romashchenko, Shen, & Vereshchagin, 2000) of s can be defined as

$$SE(s) = -\sum_k p_k \log_2 p_k \tag{3}$$

Log energy is a parameter (a measure of entropy) used to describe the information contained in a signal. It is used for attaining higher classification accuracy. Log energy is sensitive to the degree of complexity of the signals (Li & Zhou, 2016).

$$LE(s) = \sum_k \log(p_k^2) \tag{4}$$

Entropy provides the knowledge about the information contained by the signal (Aydın et al., 2009). Summation is the statistical parameter used to measure the sum of all the values of the signal (Meharrar, Tioursi, Hatti, & Stambouli, 2011).

The statistical methods used for identifying the statistically significant parameters included t-test, CART, BT and RF. The t-test analysis resulted that the parameters AM110 and SUM110 were statistically important (p-value ≤ 0.05) (Hare, Schultz, Camerer, O'Doherty, & Rangel, 2011). AM110 had a negative mean value for the post-stimulus signal, whereas, it had a positive value for the pre-stimulus signal (Table 1). Similarly, SUM110 was also negative valued for the post-stimulus signals and positive valued for the pre-stimulus signals (Table 1). This was suggestive of the fact that the music stimulus might have an effect on the heart activity. CART is a primitive decision tree-based non-linear method useful for the analysis of the complex data (Friedl & Brodley, 1997). It provides an informative way to represent the results in the form of decision trees (Speybroeck, 2012). It is competent in handling the missed values in response as well as explanatory parameters (Speybroeck, 2012). Missing data are treated as a special category (Speybroeck, 2012). CART determines the best possible parameter for splitting a node of the decision tree into two sub-nodes (Speybroeck et al., 2004). In this study, MED101 was found to be a statistically significant parameter with a predictor importance of 1 (≥ 0.95) from the CART analysis. Similar to that of AM110 and SUM110, MED101 is a negative-valued for pre-stimulus and positive-valued for post-stimulus (Table 1). Therefore, there was a marked decrement in the value during the post-stimulus.

Boosted tree is another widely used decision tree-based method. Training in boosted tree automatically detects feature interactions. In this study, the statistically significant parameters obtained from boosted tree analysis were AM000, SUM000, MOD011, and KUR101 with a predictor importance of 1. In this study, kurtosis for the post-stimulus signal was very high, which suggested that the deviation of the signal values from the mean value was large (Table 1). In 2001, Leo Breiman developed random forest (RF) and it has been reported to provide excellent performance among the non-linear decision tree (Chen, Wang, Cao, Chen, & Gu, 2014). Randomness is

Table 1. Statistically significant features

Methods	Parameters	Mean ± SD		Predictor Importance	p-value
		Category-N	Category-H		
t-test	AM110	3.29E-05 ± 0.000076	-3.04972E-05 ± 7.59422E-05		0.02
	SUM110	0.008 ± 0.017	-0.007 ± 0.018		0.02
CART	MED101	9.03E-06 ± 2.83E-05	-8.44E-06 ± 6.24506E-05	1.00	
BT	AM000	0.004 ± 0.019	0.005 ± 0.026	1.00	
	SUM000	0.89 ± 4.47	127.42 ± 535.54	1.00	
	MOD011	-0.0007 ± 0.0012	-0.0002 ± 0.0018	0.98	
	KUR101	22.00 ± 4.60	7633.17 ± 31505.31	0.99	
RF	VAR000	0.34 ± 0.31	0.38 ± 0.40	1.00	

injected by growing each tree on different random subsamples and determining splitter partly at random (Chen et al., 2014). For RF, there is a combination of decision trees. In the combination of tree predictors, each tree depends on random vectors, which are sampled independently with the same distribution for all trees in the forest. RF has its application in many fields like microarray data, remote sensing (Pal, 2005), Alzheimer's disease detection (Gray et al., 2013) etc. In this study, VAR000 was the only important parameter found from the RF method.

The statistically important parameters obtained using the above methods suggested an alteration in the cardiac electrophysiology due to the motivation song. These statistically important parameters were applied as input to the MLP-based ANN classifier. ANN is the computational model that imitates the functioning of the human brain (Graupe, 2013). It comprises of highly interconnected computing devices, which mimic the biological neurons. Its capability is obtained from the training phase and the performance is obtained from the testing phase (Vargas, Lettnin, de Castro, & Macarthy, 2002). ANN can solve nonlinear and complicated problems in various fields (Pandya & Macy, 1995; Vargas et al., 2002). The MLP network, used in this study, was a feed-forward neural network, employing a back-propagation learning method for the training purpose. It had 4 neurons in the input layer and 2 neurons in the output layer. The number of input neurons was nothing but the number of the self-organizing networks (Engin, 2004). The MLP algorithm was named as 8-N-2 network, where N was the number of hidden layer neurons that were optimized for better classification efficiency (Li & Zhou, 2016). For classification of the ECG signals, MLP (8-13-2) network provided the highest classification efficiency of 80.55%. The confusion matrix of the MLP (8-13-2) network has been shown in

Table 2. The training algorithm for the MLP 8-13-2 network was Broyden–Fletcher–Goldfarb–Shanno 17 (BFGS 17), and the error function was Entropy (Table 3). The hidden activation function and the output activation function were Exponential and Softmax, respectively. For the classification of ECG signals, an accuracy of ≥80% is regarded as significant (Yang & Naiman, 2014). Therefore, the ANN classification result indicated towards a change in the cardiac electrophysiology of the volunteers in the post-stimulus condition as compared to the pre-stimulus condition.

CONCLUSION

This study was aimed at understanding the effect of a motivational song on the cardiac electrophysiology. The ECG signals were acquired from 18 male volunteers in the pre-stimulus and the post-stimulus conditions. The pre- and the post-stimulus ECG signals were preprocessed and subjected to WPD up to level 3 using db04 wavelet so as to obtain 8 wavelet packet coefficients. Then, the statistical feature extraction of both the pre- and the post-stimulus ECG signals were performed, which resulted in 96 features for each ECG signal. The extracted features were exposed

Table 2. Classification summary of MLP 8-13-2 network

	CATEGORY-N	CATEGORY-H	OVERALL
Total	18.00	18.00	36.00
Correct	14.00	15.00	29.00
Incorrect	4.00	3.00	7.00
Correct (%)	77.78	83.33	80.55
Incorrect (%)	22.22	16.67	19.45

Table 3. Details of MLP 8-13-2 network

Networks	Parameters	Classification Efficiency	Algorithm	Error Function	Hidden Activation Function	Output Activation Function
MLP 8-13-2	AM000 SUM000 MOD011 KUR101 AM110 SUM110 MED101 VAR000	80.55%	BFGS 17	Entropy	Exponential	Softmax

to t-test, CART, BT and RF to get the statistically important features. 8 features were found to be statistically significant, suggesting the alteration in the cardiac electrophysiology due to the music stimulus. The statistically important features were used to classify the pre- and the post-stimulus ECG signals by the implementation of ANN. The results of the MLP 8-13-2 network further confirmed that there was a marked alteration in the cardiac electrophysiology.

FUTURE RESEARCH DIRECTIONS

The current study implemented WPD-based feature extraction and ANN-based classification of ECG signals. Future studies may be performed using other feature extraction and classification techniques to improve the classification accuracy. Studies can also be performed using different types of music signals as the stimuli to analyze their effects on heart and other physiological systems.

REFERENCES

Abdullah, A. A., Subasi, A., & Qaisar, S. M. (2017). Surface EMG Signal Classification by Using WPD and Ensemble Tree Classifiers. In CMBEBIH 2017 (pp. 475-481). Springer. doi:10.1007/978-981-10-4166-2_73

Addison, P. S. (2017). *The illustrated wavelet transform handbook: introductory theory and applications in science, engineering, medicine and finance*. CRC Press.

Addison, P. S., Watson, J. N., Clegg, G. R., Holzer, M., Sterz, F., & Robertson, C. E. (2000). Evaluating arrhythmias in ECG signals using wavelet transforms. *IEEE Engineering in Medicine and Biology Magazine*, *19*(5), 104–109. doi:10.1109/51.870237 PMID:11016036

Aguiar-Conraria, L., & Soares, M. J. (2014). The continuous wavelet transform: Moving beyond uni-and bivariate analysis. *Journal of Economic Surveys*, *28*(2), 344–375. doi:10.1111/joes.12012

Alexakis, C., Nyongesa, H., Saatchi, R., Harris, N., Davies, C., & Emery, C. (2003). *Feature extraction and classification of electrocardiogram (ECG) signals related to hypoglycaemia.* Paper presented at the Computers in Cardiology.

Alfaouri, M., & Daqrouq, K. (2008). ECG signal denoising by wavelet transform thresholding. *American Journal of Applied Sciences*, *5*(3), 276–281. doi:10.3844/ajassp.2008.276.281

Antoniadis, A., & Oppenheim, G. (2012). *Wavelets and statistics* (Vol. 103). Springer Science & Business Media.

Aubert, A. E., Ramaekers, D., Beckers, F., Breem, R., Denef, C., Van de Werf, F., & Ector, H. (1999). The analysis of heart rate variability in unrestrained rats. Validation of method and results. *Computer Methods and Programs in Biomedicine*, *60*(3), 197–213. doi:10.1016/S0169-2607(99)00017-6 PMID:10579513

Aydın, S., Saraoğlu, H. M., & Kara, S. (2009). Log energy entropy-based EEG classification with multilayer neural networks in seizure. *Annals of Biomedical Engineering*, *37*(12), 2626–2630. doi:10.100710439-009-9795-x PMID:19757057

Chen, W., Wang, Y., Cao, G., Chen, G., & Gu, Q. (2014). A random forest model based classification scheme for neonatal amplitude-integrated EEG. *Biomedical Engineering Online*, *13*(2Suppl 2), S4. doi:10.1186/1475-925X-13-S2-S4 PMID:25560269

Clark, A. J. (2015). *Comparative physiology of the heart*. Cambridge University Press.

De Chazal, P., Celler, B., & Reilly, R. (2000). Using wavelet coefficients for the classification of the electrocardiogram. *Paper presented at the Engineering in Medicine and Biology Society, 2000. Proceedings of the 22nd Annual International Conference of the IEEE*. 10.1109/IEMBS.2000.900669

De Mello, W. C. (2013). *Electrical phenomena in the heart*. Academic Press.

Engin, M. (2004). ECG beat classification using neuro-fuzzy network. *Pattern Recognition Letters*, *25*(15), 1715–1722. doi:10.1016/j.patrec.2004.06.014

Friedl, M. A., & Brodley, C. E. (1997). Decision tree classification of land cover from remotely sensed data. *Remote Sensing of Environment*, *61*(3), 399–409. doi:10.1016/S0034-4257(97)00049-7

Fujita, H., Sudarshan, V. K., Adam, M., Oh, S. L., Tan, J. H., & Hagiwara, Y. (2017). *Characterization of Cardiovascular Diseases Using Wavelet Packet Decomposition and Nonlinear Measures of Electrocardiogram Signal*. Paper presented at the International Conference on Industrial, Engineering and Other Applications of Applied Intelligent Systems. 10.1007/978-3-319-60042-0_30

Gang, R., Jiapin, X., HongHui, W., & Lu, J. (2004). *A new quadrature sampling and reconstruction technique and computer simulation of its performances*. Paper presented at the Communications, Circuits and Systems, 2004. ICCCAS 2004. 2004 International Conference on.

Ghaffari, A., Homaeinezhad, M., Khazraee, M., & Daevaeiha, M. (2010). Segmentation of holter ECG waves via analysis of a discrete wavelet-derived multiple skewness–kurtosis based metric. *Annals of Biomedical Engineering*, *38*(4), 1497–1510. doi:10.100710439-010-9919-3 PMID:20087769

Graupe, D. (2013). *Principles of artificial neural networks* (Vol. 7). World Scientific. doi:10.1142/8868

Gray, K. R., Aljabar, P., Heckemann, R. A., Hammers, A., & Rueckert, D. (2013). Random forest-based similarity measures for multi-modal classification of Alzheimer's disease. *NeuroImage*, *65*, 167–175. doi:10.1016/j.neuroimage.2012.09.065 PMID:23041336

Hammer, D., Romashchenko, A., Shen, A., & Vereshchagin, N. (2000). Inequalities for Shannon entropy and Kolmogorov complexity. *Journal of Computer and System Sciences*, *60*(2), 442–464. doi:10.1006/jcss.1999.1677

Haque, A., Ali, M. H., Kiber, M. A., & Hasan, M. T. (2009). Detection of small variations of ECG features using wavelet. *Journal of Engineering and Applied Sciences (Asian Research Publishing Network)*, *4*(6), 27–30.

Hare, T. A., Schultz, W., Camerer, C. F., O'Doherty, J. P., & Rangel, A. (2011). Transformation of stimulus value signals into motor commands during simple choice. *Proceedings of the National Academy of Sciences of the United States of America*, *108*(44), 18120–18125. doi:10.1073/pnas.1109322108 PMID:22006321

He, Q.-H., Yu, B., Hong, X., Lv, B., Liu, T., & Ran, J. (2016). An Improved Lung Sound De-noising Method by Wavelet Packet Transform with Pso-Based Threshold Selection. *Intelligent Automation & Soft Computing*, 1-7.

Hu, D., Li, W., & Chen, X. (2011). *Feature extraction of motor imagery EEG signals based on wavelet packet decomposition.* Paper presented at the Complex Medical Engineering (CME), 2011 IEEE/ICME International Conference on. 10.1109/ICCME.2011.5876829

Jain, A. K., Mao, J., & Mohiuddin, K. M. (1996). Artificial neural networks: A tutorial. *Computer*, *29*(3), 31–44. doi:10.1109/2.485891

Jegan, R., Anusuya, K., & George, E. M. (2015). Real-time ECG peak detection for heart rate measurement using wavelet packet transform. *International Journal of Biomedical Engineering and Technology*, *19*(3), 244–254. doi:10.1504/IJBET.2015.072994

Juslin, P. N., & Sloboda, J. A. (2001). *Music and emotion: Theory and research.* Oxford University Press.

Kutlu, Y., & Kuntalp, D. (2012). Feature extraction for ECG heartbeats using higher order statistics of WPD coefficients. *Computer Methods and Programs in Biomedicine*, *105*(3), 257–267. doi:10.1016/j.cmpb.2011.10.002 PMID:22055998

Lai, H.-L. (2001). *The Effects of Music Therapy on Sleep Quality in Elderly Peopl.* Case Western Reserve University. Retrieved from http://onlinestatbook.com/Online_Statistics_Education.pdf

Levenson, R. W. (2014). The autonomic nervous system and emotion. *Emotion Review*, *6*(2), 100–112. doi:10.1177/1754073913512003

Li, T., & Zhou, M. (2016). ECG classification using wavelet packet entropy and random forests. *Entropy (Basel, Switzerland)*, *18*(8), 285. doi:10.3390/e18080285

Liu, Z., Su, J., Qin, C., & Li, Z. (2016). *Wavelet packet decomposition and grey relational analysis application in fault diagnosis of aero hydraulic pump.* Paper presented at the Aircraft Utility Systems (AUS), IEEE International Conference on. 10.1109/AUS.2016.7748150

Luz, E. J. D. S., Merschmann, L. H., Menotti, D., & Moreira, G. J. (2017). Evaluating a hierarchical approach for heartbeat classification from ECG. *International Journal of Bioinformatics Research and Applications*, *13*(2), 146–160. doi:10.1504/IJBRA.2017.083148

Luz, E. J. D. S., Nunes, T. M., De Albuquerque, V. H. C., Papa, J. P., & Menotti, D. (2013). ECG arrhythmia classification based on optimum-path forest. *Expert Systems with Applications*, *40*(9), 3561–3573. doi:10.1016/j.eswa.2012.12.063

MacDonald, R., Kreutz, G., & Mitchell, L. (2013). *Music, health, and wellbeing.* Oxford University Press.

Mahmoodabadi, S., Ahmadian, A., & Abolhasani, M. (2005). ECG feature extraction using Daubechies wavelets. *Proceedings of the fifth IASTED International conference on Visualization, Imaging and Image Processing.*

Mallat, S. G. (1989). A theory for multiresolution signal decomposition: The wavelet representation. *IEEE Transactions on Pattern Analysis and Machine Intelligence*, *11*(7), 674–693. doi:10.1109/34.192463

Meharrar, A., Tioursi, M., Hatti, M., & Stambouli, A. B. (2011). A variable speed wind generator maximum power tracking based on adaptative neuro-fuzzy inference system. *Expert Systems with Applications*, *38*(6), 7659–7664. doi:10.1016/j.eswa.2010.12.163

Meng, A., Ge, J., Yin, H., & Chen, S. (2016). Wind speed forecasting based on wavelet packet decomposition and artificial neural networks trained by crisscross optimization algorithm. *Energy Conversion and Management*, *114*, 75–88. doi:10.1016/j.enconman.2016.02.013

Pal, M. (2005). Random forest classifier for remote sensing classification. *International Journal of Remote Sensing*, *26*(1), 217–222. doi:10.1080/01431160412331269698

Pandya, A. S., & Macy, R. B. (1995). *Pattern recognition with neural networks in C*. CRC press.

Puri, D., Ingle, R., Kachare, P., Patil, M., & Awale, R. (2017). *Wavelet Packet Sub-band Based Classification of Alcoholic and Controlled State EEG Signals*. Academic Press.

Raeiatibanadkooki, M., Quchani, S. R., KhalilZade, M. M., & Bahaadinbeigy, K. (2016). Compression and encryption of ECG signal using wavelet and chaotically Huffman code in telemedicine application. *Journal of Medical Systems*, *40*(3), 73. doi:10.100710916-016-0433-5 PMID:26779641

Seo, Y., Kim, S., Kisi, O., Singh, V. P., & Parasuraman, K. (2016). River stage forecasting using wavelet packet decomposition and machine learning models. *Water Resources Management*, *30*(11), 4011–4035. doi:10.100711269-016-1409-4

Speybroeck, N. (2012). Classification and regression trees. *International Journal of Public Health*, *57*(1), 243–246. doi:10.100700038-011-0315-z PMID:22015650

Speybroeck, N., Berkvens, D., Mfoukou-Ntsakala, A., Aerts, M., Hens, N., Van Huylenbroeck, G., & Thys, E. (2004). Classification trees versus multinomial models in the analysis of urban farming systems in Central Africa. *Agricultural Systems*, *80*(2), 133–149. doi:10.1016/j.agsy.2003.06.006

Van Fleet, P. J. (2011). *Discrete wavelet transformations: An elementary approach with applications*. John Wiley & Sons.

Vargas, F., Lettnin, D., de Castro, M. C. F., & Macarthy, M. (2002). Electrocardiogram pattern recognition by means of MLP network and PCA: A case study on equal amount of input signal types. *Paper presented at the Neural Networks, 2002. SBRN 2002. Proceedings. VII Brazilian Symposium on.* 10.1109/SBRN.2002.1181474

Yaman, A., Pamir, I., Yarali, N., Karademir, S., Cetinkaya, S., & Ali, B. (2013). Common complications in beta-thalassemia patients. *International Journal of Hematologic Oncology*, *27*(1), 193–199. doi:10.4999/uhod.12005

Yang, S., & Naiman, D. Q. (2014). Multiclass cancer classification based on gene expression comparison. *Statistical Applications in Genetics and Molecular Biology*, *13*(4), 477–496. PMID:24918456

Yen, B. S., Wang, H.-M., Hou, M. C., Tcm, D., Huang, S.-C., & Chou, L.-C. (2010). The relationship between music processing and electrocardiogram (ECG) in vegetative state (VS). *Circuits and Systems (ISCAS), Proceedings of 2010 IEEE International Symposium on*. 10.1109/ISCAS.2010.5537211

Zeng, S.-d., & Zhong, Q.-h. (2015). Heart-rate Measurement via Face-video Base on FastICA and Wavelet Packet Decomposition. *Laser Journal, 11*, 13.

ADDITIONAL READING

Addison, P. S. (2005). Wavelet transforms and the ECG: A review. *Physiological Measurement*, *26*(5), R155–R199. doi:10.1088/0967-3334/26/5/R01 PMID:16088052

Alexakis, C., Nyongesa, H., Saatchi, R., Harris, N., Davies, C., & Emery, C. (2003). *Feature extraction and classification of electrocardiogram (ECG) signals related to hypoglycaemia.* Paper presented at the Computers in Cardiology, 2003.

Alfaouri, M., & Daqrouq, K. (2008). ECG signal denoising by wavelet transform thresholding. *American Journal of Applied Sciences*, *5*(3), 276–281. doi:10.3844/ajassp.2008.276.281

Avci, E., Turkoglu, I., & Poyraz, M. (2005). Intelligent target recognition based on wavelet packet neural network. *Expert Systems with Applications*, *29*(1), 175–182. doi:10.1016/j.eswa.2005.01.016

Bahoura, M., Hassani, M., & Hubin, M. (1997). DSP implementation of wavelet transform for real time ECG wave forms detection and heart rate analysis. *Computer Methods and Programs in Biomedicine*, *52*(1), 35–44. doi:10.1016/S0169-2607(97)01780-X PMID:9034668

Banerjee, S., & Mitra, M. (2014). Application of cross wavelet transform for ECG pattern analysis and classification. *IEEE Transactions on Instrumentation and Measurement*, *63*(2), 326–333. doi:10.1109/TIM.2013.2279001

Chen, W., Wang, Y., Cao, G., Chen, G., & Gu, Q. (2014). A random forest model based classification scheme for neonatal amplitude-integrated EEG. *Biomedical Engineering Online, 13*(2Suppl 2), S4. doi:10.1186/1475-925X-13-S2-S4 PMID:25560269

Colombet, I., Ruelland, A., Chatellier, G., Gueyffier, F., Degoulet, P., & Jaulent, M.-C. (2000). *Models to predict cardiovascular risk: comparison of CART, multilayer perceptron and logistic regression.* Paper presented at the Proceedings of the AMIA Symposium.

Cvetkovic, D., Übeyli, E. D., & Cosic, I. (2008). Wavelet transform feature extraction from human PPG, ECG, and EEG signal responses to ELF PEMF exposures: A pilot study. *Digital Signal Processing, 18*(5), 861–874. doi:10.1016/j.dsp.2007.05.009

Di Virgilio, V., Francaiancia, C., Lino, S., & Cerutti, S. (1995). *ECG fiducial points detection through wavelet transform.* Paper presented at the Engineering in Medicine and Biology Society, 1995., IEEE 17th Annual Conference. 10.1109/IEMBS.1995.579466

Djohan, A., Nguyen, T. Q., & Tompkins, W. J. (1995). *ECG compression using discrete symmetric wavelet transform.* Paper presented at the Engineering in Medicine and Biology Society, 1995., IEEE 17th Annual Conference. 10.1109/IEMBS.1995.575053

Emanet, N. (2009). *ECG beat classification by using discrete wavelet transform and Random Forest algorithm.* Paper presented at the Soft Computing, Computing with Words and Perceptions in System Analysis, Decision and Control, 2009. ICSCCW 2009. Fifth International Conference on. 10.1109/ICSCCW.2009.5379457

Fucai, Z., Yihua, H., & Shiqi, H. (2008). Classification using wavelet packet decomposition and support vector machine for digital modulations. *Journal of Systems Engineering and Electronics, 19*(5), 914–918. doi:10.1016/S1004-4132(08)60174-7

Ghaffari, A., Homaeinezhad, M., Khazraee, M., & Daevaeiha, M. (2010). Segmentation of holter ECG waves via analysis of a discrete wavelet-derived multiple skewness–kurtosis based metric. *Annals of Biomedical Engineering, 38*(4), 1497–1510. doi:10.100710439-010-9919-3 PMID:20087769

Gokgoz, E., & Subasi, A. (2015). Comparison of decision tree algorithms for EMG signal classification using DWT. *Biomedical Signal Processing and Control, 18*, 138–144. doi:10.1016/j.bspc.2014.12.005

Haque, A., Ali, M. H., Kiber, M. A., & Hasan, M. T. (2009). Detection of small variations of ECG features using wavelet. *Journal of Engineering and Applied Sciences (Asian Research Publishing Network), 4*(6), 27–30.

He, Q.-H., Yu, B., Hong, X., Lv, B., Liu, T., Ran, J. (2016). An Improved Lung Sound De-noising Method by Wavelet Packet Transform with Pso-Based Threshold Selection. *Intelligent Automation & Soft Computing*, 1-7.

Hosseini, H. G., Reynolds, K., & Powers, D. (2001). *A multi-stage neural network classifier for ECG events.* Paper presented at the Engineering in Medicine and Biology Society, 2001. Proceedings of the 23rd Annual International Conference of the IEEE.

Ingale, V., & Nalbalwar, S. (2016). ECG Classification using Dynamic High Pass Filtering and Statistical Framework (HRV). *Signal Processing: An International Journal, 10*(2), 12.

Jegan, R., Anusuya, K., & George, E. M. (2015). Real-time ECG peak detection for heart rate measurement using wavelet packet transform. *International Journal of Biomedical Engineering and Technology, 19*(3), 244–254. doi:10.1504/IJBET.2015.072994

Karvounis, E., Papaloukas, C., Fotiadis, D., & Michalis, L. (2004). *Fetal heart rate extraction from composite maternal ECG using complex continuous wavelet transform.* Paper presented at the Computers in Cardiology, 2004. 10.1109/CIC.2004.1443044

Kottaimalai, R., Rajasekaran, M. P., Selvam, V., & Kannapiran, B. (2013). *EEG signal classification using principal component analysis with neural network in brain computer interface applications.* Paper presented at the Emerging Trends in Computing, Communication and Nanotechnology (ICE-CCN), 2013 International Conference on. 10.1109/ICE-CCN.2013.6528498

Krishnamurthy, N., Kresch, E., Rao, S., & Kresh, Y. (1995). *Adaptive wavelet packet decomposition for ECG data compression.* Paper presented at the Engineering in Medicine and Biology Society, 1995., IEEE 17th Annual Conference. 10.1109/IEMBS.1995.575071

Kumari, P., & Vaish, A. (2014). *Brainwave's energy feature extraction using wavelet transform.* Paper presented at the Electrical, Electronics and Computer Science (SCEECS), 2014 IEEE Students' Conference on. 10.1109/SCEECS.2014.6804433

Kutlu, Y., & Kuntalp, D. (2012). Feature extraction for ECG heartbeats using higher order statistics of WPD coefficients. *Computer Methods and Programs in Biomedicine, 105*(3), 257–267. doi:10.1016/j.cmpb.2011.10.002 PMID:22055998

Labate, D., La Foresta, F., Occhiuto, G., Morabito, F. C., Lay-Ekuakille, A., & Vergallo, P. (2013). Empirical mode decomposition vs. wavelet decomposition for the extraction of respiratory signal from single-channel ECG: A comparison. *IEEE Sensors Journal*, *13*(7), 2666–2674. doi:10.1109/JSEN.2013.2257742

Levenson, R. W. (2014). The autonomic nervous system and emotion. *Emotion Review*, *6*(2), 100–112. doi:10.1177/1754073913512003

Li, T., & Zhou, M. (2016). ECG Classification Using Wavelet Packet Entropy and Random Forests. *Entropy (Basel, Switzerland)*, *18*(8), 285. doi:10.3390/e18080285

Liang, H., & Nartimo, I. (1998). *A feature extraction algorithm based on wavelet packet decomposition for heart sound signals.* Paper presented at the Time-Frequency and Time-Scale Analysis, 1998. Proceedings of the IEEE-SP International Symposium on. 10.1109/TFSA.1998.721369

Lu, Z., Kim, D. Y., & Pearlman, W. A. (2000). Wavelet compression of ECG signals by the set partitioning in hierarchical trees algorithm. *IEEE Transactions on Biomedical Engineering*, *47*(7), 849–856. doi:10.1109/10.846678 PMID:10916255

Luz, E. J. D. S., Nunes, T. M., De Albuquerque, V. H. C., Papa, J. P., & Menotti, D. (2013). ECG arrhythmia classification based on optimum-path forest. *Expert Systems with Applications*, *40*(9), 3561–3573. doi:10.1016/j.eswa.2012.12.063

Luz, E. J. S., Schwartz, W. R., Cámara-Chávez, G., & Menotti, D. (2016). ECG-based heartbeat classification for arrhythmia detection: A survey. *Computer Methods and Programs in Biomedicine*, *127*, 144–164. doi:10.1016/j.cmpb.2015.12.008 PMID:26775139

Mahmoodabadi, S., Ahmadian, A., Abolhasani, M., Eslami, M., & Bidgoli, J. (2006). *ECG feature extraction based on multiresolution wavelet transform.* Paper presented at the Engineering in Medicine and Biology Society, 2005. IEEE-EMBS 2005. 27th Annual International Conference of the.

Mallat, S. G. (1989). A theory for multiresolution signal decomposition: The wavelet representation. *IEEE Transactions on Pattern Analysis and Machine Intelligence*, *11*(7), 674–693. doi:10.1109/34.192463

Martis, R. J., Acharya, U. R., & Min, L. C. (2013). ECG beat classification using PCA, LDA, ICA and discrete wavelet transform. *Biomedical Signal Processing and Control*, *8*(5), 437–448. doi:10.1016/j.bspc.2013.01.005

Melillo, P., De Luca, N., Bracale, M., & Pecchia, L. (2013). Classification tree for risk assessment in patients suffering from congestive heart failure via long-term heart rate variability. *IEEE Journal of Biomedical and Health Informatics*, *17*(3), 727–733. doi:10.1109/JBHI.2013.2244902 PMID:24592473

Meng, A., Ge, J., Yin, H., & Chen, S. (2016). Wind speed forecasting based on wavelet packet decomposition and artificial neural networks trained by crisscross optimization algorithm. *Energy Conversion and Management*, *114*, 75–88. doi:10.1016/j.enconman.2016.02.013

Nagendra, H., Mukherjee, S., & Kumar, V. (2011). Application of wavelet techniques in ECG signal processing: An overview. *International Journal of Engineering Science and Technology*, *3*(10), 7432–7443.

Nayak, S. K., Shukla, R. D., Panda, I., Champaty, B., Thakur, G., & Mohapatra, B. (2016). Effect of Slow and Fast Music on the Autonomic Nervous System and Cardiac Health: A Preliminary Investigation. In *Classification and Clustering in Biomedical Signal Processing* (pp. 198–218). IGI Global. doi:10.4018/978-1-5225-0140-4.ch009

Noorollahi, Y., Jokar, M. A., & Kalhor, A. (2016). Using artificial neural networks for temporal and spatial wind speed forecasting in Iran. *Energy Conversion and Management*, *115*, 17–25. doi:10.1016/j.enconman.2016.02.041

Ozbay, Y., & Karlik, B. (2001). *A recognition of ECG arrhytihemias using artificial neural networks.* Paper presented at the Engineering in Medicine and Biology Society, 2001. Proceedings of the 23rd Annual International Conference of the IEEE. 10.1109/IEMBS.2001.1020538

Puri, D., Ingle, R., Kachare, P., Patil, M., & Awale, R. (2017). Wavelet Packet Sub-band Based Classification of Alcoholic and Controlled State EEG Signals.

Rajoub, B. A. (2002). An efficient coding algorithm for the compression of ECG signals using the wavelet transform. *IEEE Transactions on Biomedical Engineering*, *49*(4), 355–362. doi:10.1109/10.991163 PMID:11942727

Ranjith, P., Baby, P., & Joseph, P. (2003). ECG analysis using wavelet transform: Application to myocardial ischemia detection. *ITBM-RBM*, *24*(1), 44–47. doi:10.1016/S1297-9562(03)00003-2

Safara, F., Doraisamy, S., Azman, A., Jantan, A., & Ramaiah, A. R. A. (2013). Multi-level basis selection of wavelet packet decomposition tree for heart sound classification. *Computers in Biology and Medicine*, *43*(10), 1407–1414. doi:10.1016/j.compbiomed.2013.06.016 PMID:24034732

Sayadi, O., & Shamsollahi, M. B. (2007). Multiadaptive bionic wavelet transform: Application to ECG denoising and baseline wandering reduction. *EURASIP Journal on Advances in Signal Processing*, *2007*(1), 041274. doi:10.1155/2007/41274

Shyu, L.-Y., Wu, Y.-H., & Hu, W. (2004). Using wavelet transform and fuzzy neural network for VPC detection from the Holter ECG. *IEEE Transactions on Biomedical Engineering*, *51*(7), 1269–1273. doi:10.1109/TBME.2004.824131 PMID:15248543

Silipo, R., & Marchesi, C. (1998). Artificial neural networks for automatic ECG analysis. *IEEE Transactions on Signal Processing*, *46*(5), 1417–1425. doi:10.1109/78.668803

Speybroeck, N. (2012). Classification and regression trees. *International Journal of Public Health*, *57*(1), 243–246. doi:10.100700038-011-0315-z PMID:22015650

Speybroeck, N., Berkvens, D., Mfoukou-Ntsakala, A., Aerts, M., Hens, N., Van Huylenbroeck, G., & Thys, E. (2004). Classification trees versus multinomial models in the analysis of urban farming systems in Central Africa. *Agricultural Systems*, *80*(2), 133–149. doi:10.1016/j.agsy.2003.06.006

Tetschke, F., Schneider, U., Schleussner, E., Witte, O. W., & Hoyer, D. (2016). Assessment of fetal maturation age by heart rate variability measures using random forest methodology. *Computers in Biology and Medicine*, *70*, 157–162. doi:10.1016/j.compbiomed.2016.01.020 PMID:26848727

Ting, W., Guozheng, Y., & Banghua, Y. (2007). EEG feature extraction in brain computer interface based on wavelet packet decomposition. *Yiqi Yibiao Xuebao*, *28*(12), 2230.

Vijaya, G., Kumar, V., & Verma, H. (1998). ANN-based QRS-complex analysis of ECG. *Journal of Medical Engineering & Technology*, *22*(4), 160–167. doi:10.3109/03091909809032534 PMID:9680599

Yang, S., & Naiman, D. Q. (2014). Multiclass cancer classification based on gene expression comparison. *Statistical Applications in Genetics and Molecular Biology*, *13*(4), 477–496. PMID:24918456

Yen, B. S., Wang, H.-M., Hou, M. C., Tcm, D., Huang, S.-C., & Chou, L.-C. (2010). *The relationship between music processing and electrocardiogram (ECG) in vegetative state (VS)*. Paper presented at the Circuits and Systems (ISCAS), Proceedings of 2010 IEEE International Symposium on. 10.1109/ISCAS.2010.5537211

ZENG, S.-d., & ZHONG, Q.-h. (2015). Heart-rate Measurement via Face-video Base on FastICA and Wavelet Packet Decomposition. *Laser Journal, 11*, 013.

Zhang, Y., Liu, B., Ji, X., & Huang, D. (2017). Classification of EEG signals based on autoregressive model and wavelet packet decomposition. *Neural Processing Letters*, *45*(2), 365–378. doi:10.100711063-016-9530-1

Zhao, Q., & Zhang, L. (2005). *ECG feature extraction and classification using wavelet transform and support vector machines.* Paper presented at the Neural Networks and Brain, 2005. ICNN&B'05. International Conference on.

KEY TERMS AND DEFINITIONS

Artificial Neural Network (ANN): ANN is a nonlinear computational model that tries to mimic the functionalities of the biological neural networks. It consists of a layer of input neurons, one or more layers of hidden neurons, and one layer of output neurons. Back-propagation is the most commonly used training algorithm in many ANN networks.

Classification and Regression Tree (CART): CART is a widely used primitive decision-tree algorithm.

Electrocardiogram (ECG): ECG is the transthoracic interpretation of the electrical activity of the heart over time, captured and externally recorded by skin electrodes.

Multilayer Perceptron (MLP): MLP is a type of feed-forward ANN, consisting of three or more layers of neurons.

Wavelet Packet Decomposition (WPD): WPD is a joint time-frequency analysis method derived from discrete wavelet transform that divides the frequency space into various parts and allows better frequency localization of signals.

Conclusion

In this book, techniques related to biomedical science, expert system and application of expert system in biomedical science have been described. The necessities of expert system in biomedical science have been also described. Some of the applications of the expert system in different problems of biomedical science have been discussed in various chapters. In the Introduction, the importance of biomedical science and usefulness of expert system in biomedical science has been discussed. In Chapter 1 the dual aspects of spiritual intelligence as self-knowledge and then theology correlated with commitment organization is discussed. Also, the main hypothesis of this study is to examine the relationship between organizational commitment and spiritual intelligence is concerned, remains the highest correlation with intellectual intelligence and emotional commitment.

In Chapter 2 aimed to improve the performance of classification in computer-aided medical diagnosis. First, all features obtained from these datasets were converted into complex-valued number format using phase encoding method. After complex-valued feature set was obtained, these features were then classified by an ensemble of complex-valued radial basis function method. In order to test the performance and the effectiveness of the medical diagnostic system; ROC analysis, classification accuracy, specificity, sensitivity, kappa statistic value and f-measure were used. In Chapter 3 a novel kernel based fuzzy clustering approach to enhance the contrast of masses has been discussed. Local entropy and intensity mean of each kernel position play the key role to enhance masses. A kernel is moved across the mammograms to collect all possible values of those features and hence they are exploited as the input data of fuzzy clustering technique. Moreover, unwanted enhancement of obscured tissues is also suppressed in this approach.

In Chapter 4 design of a capacitance sensor array for analyzing and imaging the non-homogeneity in biological materials has been discussed. Further, tissue mimicking phantoms are developed using Agar-Agar and Polyacrylamide gels for testing the developed sensor. Also, the sensor employs an unsupervised learning algorithm for automated analysis of non-homogeneity. The reconstructed capacitance image can also be sensitive to topographical and morphological variations in the sample. In Chapter 5 system for measuring EGG signals along with the decision support system developed for automated classification of digestive disorders has been proposed. The normal and abnormal EGG signals were acquired at Balaji Medical Hospital, Chennai. Further, the features were extracted using descriptive statistics and Empirical Mode Decomposition algorithm. Finally, an automated classification system was developed using k-means algorithm. This chapter explains the recording of electrogastrograms and a method for classification of normal and abnormal EGG signals.

In Chapter 6 effect of an old generation romantic music on the autonomic nervous system activity and the cardiac electrophysiology of Indian male volunteers were investigated. Electrocardiogram signals were acquired and the corresponding RR intervals were extracted. The recurrence analysis of the RRI time series suggested a more stable heart rate in the post-stimulus condition. The time- domain and the wavelet transform analyses of the ECG signals predicted an alteration in the electrical activity of the heart because of the exposure to the music stimulus. In Chapter 7 the HbA1c value is estimated with high accuracy. The Orange data mining software is used because it is easy to use in the modelling phase and contains many methods. In this context, it is aimed to develop an effective prediction model by using a large number of feature selection and classification methods. The results show that the proposed model successfully predicts the HbA1c parameter. In Chapter 8 effect of a motivational song on the electrical activity of the heart using wavelet packet analysis of electrocardiogram signals has been discussed. ECG signals were acquired from 18 healthy male volunteers during the pre- and the post-stimulus conditions. Wavelet packet decomposition of the ECG signals was performed up to level 3 using db04 wavelet, which resulted in the formation of 8 wavelet packet coefficients. Linear (t-test) and nonlinear (classification and regression tree, boosted tree and random forest) methods were used to identify the statistically significant parameters.

Expert systems are today, widely increasing the acceptance among the industries for commercialization of health care and non-clinical applications. Our goal in this edited book was to make available a comprehensible, responsive outline to expert system application to biomedical science. However, this book intended to share many aspects of biomedical research work. We wish the chapters, and this book, express not only some significant information about biomedical research but also the keenness that authors share about promising and expeditious research field.

Glossary

Adaptive Neighborhood Contrast Enhancement (ANCE): ANCE is another conventional image enhancement method to improve the medical image quality. This is an automatic method, which starts its operation with each image pixel to be processed, considering as a seed.

Agar-Agar: A substance obtained from polysaccharide agarose. Agar is a polysaccharide complex which has the capacity to hold water within its structure due to the presence of hydrophilic groups. Agar is mostly used in microbiology and plant biology. Agar is a promising material for preparing tissue phantoms since it doesn't require refrigeration. It resists melting and spoilage and can be reused. Agar models provide images similar to real tissue and they are one of the commonly used models.

APS: Ammonium Per-Sulphate.

Artificial Neural Network (ANN): ANN is a nonlinear computational model that tries to mimic the functionalities of the biological neural networks. It consists of a layer of input neurons, one or more layers of hidden neurons and one layer of output neurons. Back-propagation is the most commonly used training algorithm in many ANN networks.

Average Signal to Noise Ratio (ASNR): ASNR is an important quantitative measuring parameter for evaluation of image enhancement performance. This ASNR can be defined as the ratio of difference of mean gray level value of foreground portion and background portion of the image to the standard deviation of the background portion of image.

BIRADS (Breast Imaging-Reporting and Data System): BIRADS is a quality assurance tool mainly designed for study, research and use with Mammography. The system is a collaborative effort of many health groups but this is published and trademarked only by the American College of Radiology (ACR). The system is mainly used by medical professionals to communicate a patient's risk for developing Breast Cancer.

CAD (Computer-Aided Diagnosis): CAD framework is used to improve subsequent image segmentation and feature extraction processes or for manual reading.

Capacitive Sensors: Capacitive sensors are constructed from many different media, such as copper, Indium tin oxide (ITO) and printed ink. Copper capacitive sensors can be implemented on standard PCBs too. Size and spacing of the capacitive sensor are very important to the sensor's performance.

Classification: It is a kind of supervised machine learning in which an algorithm "learns" to classify novel observations from samples of labeled data.

Classification and Regression Tree (CART): CART is a widely used primitive decision-tree algorithm.

Complex-Valued Neural Network: It is a variety of neural network and its parameters such as input, output, weight and bias values consist of complex numbers.

Complex-Valued Radial Basis Function Networks (CVRBF): CVRBF was first proposed by Chen et al. (1994). Initially, it was applied to a non-linear signal processing, which includes complex signals.

DAQ: Data acquisition (DAQ) is the process of measuring an electrical phenomenon with computer system.

Decision Support System: It is a computer-based information system that supports organizational or business decision-making activities.

Descriptive Statistics: Descriptive Statistics are the basic features of a given data set, which can be either a representation of the entire population or a sample of it.

Diabetes: This is a life-long illness which occurs as a result of lack of insulin hormone or ineffectiveness of insulin hormone.

Digestive Diseases: Digestive diseases are disorders of the digestive tract.

EGG: Electrogastrography (EGG) is an efficient and noninvasive technique for diagnosis of digestive disorders.

Electrocardiogram (ECG): ECG is the transthoracic interpretation of the electrical activity of the heart over time, captured and externally recorded by skin electrodes.

EMD: Empirical mode decomposition (EMD) is a technique to decompose a given signal into a set of elemental signals called intrinsic mode functions.

Emotional Commitment: Refers to identification, participation, and affective attachment to an organization, meaning that staff that have strong Emotional commitment remain because they want to keep their jobs.

Ensemble Methods: It is a set of classifiers whose individual decisions are integrated in some way to classify novel examples.

Ensemble of CVRBF: When ensemble learning methods are used, a single decision is made for the ensemble by gathering the results revealed by multiple classifiers. These methods put the class estimations made by the many different classifiers through voting. As a result of this voting, the best rated class is then presented as class estimation of the ensemble.

Feature Selection: This is the process of reducing the inputs for processing and analysis, or of finding the most meaningful inputs.

Feature Selection Methods: Features extracted from the data set are usually used as input to the classification method that will be used in data mining applications.

Fiber Optic Sensor: A sensor that uses optical fiber either as the sensing element or as a means of relaying signals from a remote sensor to the electronics.

Fuzzy C-Means (FCM) Clustering Algorithm: It is one type of fuzzy clustering method which is based on the minimization of a quadratic criterion.

Hemoglobin A1c: This is a protein on the surface of red blood cells that sugar molecules stick to, usually for the life of the red blood cell (about three months).

Image Defuzzification: It is decoding of resulting enhanced image after image fuzzification, to obtain the output image for clear human perception.

ITO: Indium tin oxide.

Jaccard Similarity Coefficient: A statistic used for comparing the similarity and diversity of different sample sets.

K-Means: K-means is an unsupervised learning algorithm used to solve the well-known clustering problem based on vector quantization.

LABVIEW: Laboratory Virtual Instrumentation Engineering Workbench (LABVIEW) is a platform and development environment for a visual programming language from National Instruments.

Machine Learning: It is the notion that a computer program can learn and adapt to novel data without human interference.

Mammographic Image Analysis Society (MIAS): MIAS is an organization of UK research groups interested only in the understanding of mammograms and it has produced a large database of digital mammograms.

Mammography: Mammography is considered to be one of the best radiological screening methods for early detection of breast cancer.

Medical Diagnosis: It is a classification operation including the decision-making process based on available medical data.

Morphology: Form, shape, or structure of a material.

Multilayer Perceptron (MLP): MLP is a type of feed-forward ANN, consisting of three or more layers of neurons.

Normative Commitment: is based on sense of commitment to the organization. Employees with strong normative commitment who remain in the organization feel obligated to stay. Those with a stronger affective commitment accept changes in instances where these changes would not alter the organization's goals, but rather benefit the organization.

Orange Data Mining Toolbox: This is an open source data mining toolbox developed for novice and expert.

PAUS Imaging: Photoacoustic and ultrasonic imaging.

PCB: Printed circuit board.

Peak Signal to Noise Ratio (PSNR): PSNR is another important quantitative measuring parameter for evaluation of image enhancement performance. PSNR is defined as the ratio of difference of maximum gray-level value of foreground portion and mean gray-level value of background portion of the image to the standard deviation of the background portion of image.

Polyacrylamide: A polymer formed from acrylamide subunits.

Rational Commitment: Refers to a commitment based on the staffs' awareness of the loss that they incur if they leave. Therefore, the staff remains in the company with a strong commitment either by force or due to personal sacrifices related to leaving the organization.

ROC Curve: It is a graphical method which assess the success of a binary classifier system.

Spiritual Intelligence (SI): There is so many description of spiritual intelligence but all these flexibility of these against changes and learning form faults, meaning and targets in work, self-awareness, creation, and developing organization.

Target to Background Contrast Enhancement Based on Standard Deviation (TBC_s): TBC_s is such type of measuring parameter which can measure this improvement of enhancement technique with the help of the ratio of standard deviation of the target region before and after the enhancement respectively.

Tissue Mimicking Phantoms: Artificial materials that reproduces the properties of the natural biological tissues.

Topography: The distribution of parts or features on the surface of a material.

Wavelet Packet Decomposition (WPD): WPD is a joint time-frequency analysis method derived from discrete wavelet transform that divides the frequency space into various parts and allows better frequency localization of signals.

Related References

To continue our tradition of advancing information science and technology research, we have compiled a list of recommended IGI Global readings. These references will provide additional information and guidance to further enrich your knowledge and assist you with your own research and future publications.

Aas, I. H. (2013). Improving patient safety with telemedicine: Exploring organizational factors. In A. Moumtzoglou & A. Kastania (Eds.), *E-health technologies and improving patient safety: Exploring organizational factors* (pp. 56–70). Hershey, PA: IGI Global. doi:10.4018/978-1-4666-2657-7.ch004

Aboelfotoh, M. H., Martin, P., & Hassanein, H. (2013). Ubiquitous multimedia data access in electronic health care systems. In D. Tjondronegoro (Ed.), *Tools for mobile multimedia programming and development* (pp. 191–227). Hershey, PA: IGI Global. doi:10.4018/978-1-4666-4054-2.ch011

Abreu, J. F., Almeida, P., & Silva, T. (2013). iNeighbour TV: A social TV application to promote wellness of senior citizens. In R. Martinho, R. Rijo, M. Cruz-Cunha, & J. Varajão (Eds.), Information systems and technologies for enhancing health and social care (pp. 1-19). Hershey, PA: IGI Global. doi:10.4018/978-1-4666-3667-5.ch001

Aceti, V., & Luppicini, R. (2013). Exploring the effect of mhealth technologies on communication and information sharing in a pediatric critical care unit: A case study. In J. Tan (Ed.), *Healthcare information technology innovation and sustainability: Frontiers and adoption* (pp. 88–108). Hershey, PA: IGI Global. doi:10.4018/978-1-4666-2797-0.ch006

Adami, I., Antona, M., & Stephanidis, C. (2014). Ambient assisted living for people with motor impairments. In G. Kouroupetroglou (Ed.), *Disability informatics and web accessibility for motor limitations* (pp. 76–104). Hershey, PA: IGI Global. doi:10.4018/978-1-4666-4442-7.ch003

Adeyemo, O. (2013). The nationwide health information network: A biometric approach to prevent medical identity theft. In I. Management Association (Ed.), User-driven healthcare: Concepts, methodologies, tools, and applications (pp. 1636-1649). Hershey, PA: IGI Global. doi:10.4018/978-1-4666-2770-3.ch081

Åkerberg, A., Lindén, M., & Folke, M. (2013). Pedometer cell phone applications and future trends in measuring physical activity. In R. Martinho, R. Rijo, M. Cruz-Cunha, & J. Varajão (Eds.), *Information systems and technologies for enhancing health and social care* (pp. 324–339). Hershey, PA: IGI Global. doi:10.4018/978-1-4666-3667-5.ch021

Al Hamouche, V. (2014). Making quality control decisions in radiology department: A decision support system for radiographers' performance appraisal using PACS. In C. El Morr (Ed.), *Research perspectives on the role of informatics in health policy and management* (pp. 48–61). Hershey, PA: IGI Global. doi:10.4018/978-1-4666-4321-5.ch004

Al-Khudairy, S. (2014). Caring for our aging population: Using CPOE and telehomecare systems as a response to health policy concerns. In C. El Morr (Ed.), *Research perspectives on the role of informatics in health policy and management* (pp. 153–166). Hershey, PA: IGI Global. doi:10.4018/978-1-4666-4321-5.ch010

Albuquerque, C. (2013). The study of social needs as a strategic tool for the innovation of the social care sector: The contribution of new technologies. In M. Cruz-Cunha, I. Miranda, & P. Gonçalves (Eds.), *Handbook of research on ICTs for human-centered healthcare and social care services* (pp. 347–365). Hershey, PA: IGI Global. doi:10.4018/978-1-4666-3986-7.ch018

Alexandrou, D. A., & Pardalis, K. V. (2013). SEMantic PATHways: Modeling, executing, and monitoring intra-organizational healthcare business processes towards personalized treatment. In A. Moumtzoglou & A. Kastania (Eds.), *E-health technologies and improving patient safety: Exploring organizational factors* (pp. 98–123). Hershey, PA: IGI Global. doi:10.4018/978-1-4666-2657-7.ch007

Algarín, A. D., Demurjian, S. A., Ziminski, T. B., Sánchez, Y. K., & Kuykendall, R. (2014). Securing XML with role-based access control: Case study in health care. In A. Ruiz-Martinez, R. Marin-Lopez, & F. Pereniguez-Garcia (Eds.), *Architectures and protocols for secure information technology infrastructures* (pp. 334–365). Hershey, PA: IGI Global. doi:10.4018/978-1-4666-4514-1.ch013

Alhaqbani, B., & Fidge, C. (2013). A medical data trustworthiness assessment model. In I. Management Association (Ed.), User-driven healthcare: Concepts, methodologies, tools, and applications (pp. 1425-1445). Hershey, PA: IGI Global. doi:10.4018/978-1-4666-2770-3.ch071

Almeida, L., Menezes, P., & Dias, J. (2013). Augmented reality framework for the socialization between elderly people. In M. Cruz-Cunha, I. Miranda, & P. Gonçalves (Eds.), *Handbook of research on ICTs for human-centered healthcare and social care services* (pp. 430–448). Hershey, PA: IGI Global. doi:10.4018/978-1-4666-3986-7.ch023

Amer, M. B., Amawi, M., & El-Khatib, H. (2013). A novel neural fuzzy approach for diagnosis of potassium disturbances. In J. Tan (Ed.), *Healthcare information technology innovation and sustainability: Frontiers and adoption* (pp. 208–218). Hershey, PA: IGI Global. doi:10.4018/978-1-4666-2797-0.ch013

Andersen, S. T., & Jansen, A. (2013). Innovation in ICT-based health care provision. In J. Tan (Ed.), *Healthcare information technology innovation and sustainability: Frontiers and adoption* (pp. 58–72). Hershey, PA: IGI Global. doi:10.4018/978-1-4666-2797-0.ch004

Angjellari-Dajci, F., Lawless, W. F., Stachura, M. E., Wood, E. A., & DiBattisto, C. (2013). Economic evaluations for service delivery in autism spectrum disorders: benefit-cost analysis for emerging telehealth systems. In M. Cruz-Cunha, I. Miranda, & P. Gonçalves (Eds.), *Handbook of research on ICTs and management systems for improving efficiency in healthcare and social care* (pp. 16–42). Hershey, PA: IGI Global. doi:10.4018/978-1-4666-3990-4.ch002

Archibald, D., MacDonald, C. J., Hogue, R., & Mercer, J. (2013). Accessing knowledge from the bedside: Introducing the tablet computer to clinical teaching. In C. Rückemann (Ed.), *Integrated information and computing systems for natural, spatial, and social sciences* (pp. 96–109). Hershey, PA: IGI Global. doi:10.4018/978-1-4666-2190-9.ch005

Archondakis, S. (2013). Static telecytological applications for proficiency testing. In V. Gulla, A. Mori, F. Gabbrielli, & P. Lanzafame (Eds.), *Telehealth networks for hospital services: New methodologies* (pp. 228–239). Hershey, PA: IGI Global. doi:10.4018/978-1-4666-2979-0.ch015

Arling, P. A., Doebbeling, B. N., & Fox, R. L. (2013). Improving the implementation of evidence-based practice and information systems in healthcare: A social network approach. In J. Tan (Ed.), *Healthcare information technology innovation and sustainability: Frontiers and adoption* (pp. 247–270). Hershey, PA: IGI Global. doi:10.4018/978-1-4666-2797-0.ch016

Arriaga, P., Esteves, F., & Fernandes, S. (2013). Playing for better or for worse?: Health and social outcomes with electronic gaming. In M. Cruz-Cunha, I. Miranda, & P. Gonçalves (Eds.), *Handbook of research on ICTs for human-centered healthcare and social care services* (pp. 48–69). Hershey, PA: IGI Global. doi:10.4018/978-1-4666-3986-7.ch003

Arslan, P. (2014). Collaborative participation in personalized health through mobile diaries. In K. Rızvanoğlu & G. Çetin (Eds.), *Research and design innovations for mobile user experience* (pp. 150–181). Hershey, PA: IGI Global. doi:10.4018/978-1-4666-4446-5.ch009

Assis-Hassid, S., Reychav, I., Pliskin, J. S., & Heart, T. H. (2013). The effects of electronic medical record (EMR) use in primary care on the physician-patient relationship. In M. Cruz-Cunha, I. Miranda, & P. Gonçalves (Eds.), *Handbook of research on ICTs for human-centered healthcare and social care services* (pp. 130–150). Hershey, PA: IGI Global. doi:10.4018/978-1-4666-3986-7.ch007

Azar, A. T. (2013). Overview of biomedical engineering. In I. Management Association (Ed.), Bioinformatics: Concepts, methodologies, tools, and applications (pp. 1-28). Hershey, PA: IGI Global. doi:10.4018/978-1-4666-3604-0.ch001

Azar, A. T., & Eljamel, M. S. (2014). Medical robotics. In I. Management Association (Ed.), Robotics: Concepts, methodologies, tools, and applications (pp. 1116-1147). Hershey, PA: IGI Global. doi:10.4018/978-1-4666-4607-0.ch054

Baladrón, C., Aguiar, J. M., Calavia, L., Carro, B., & Sánchez-Esguevillas, A. (2014). Learning on the move in the web 2.0: New initiatives in m-learning. In *K-12 education: Concepts, methodologies, tools, and applications* (pp. 1693–1714). Hershey, PA: IGI Global. doi:10.4018/978-1-4666-4502-8.ch097

Bauer, K. A. (2013). Caught in the web: The internet and the demise of medical privacy. In I. Management Association (Ed.), User-driven healthcare: Concepts, methodologies, tools, and applications (pp. 1252-1272). Hershey, PA: IGI Global. doi:10.4018/978-1-4666-2770-3.ch063

Belsis, P., Skourlas, C., & Gritzalis, S. (2013). Secure electronic healthcare records management in wireless environments. In M. Khosrow-Pour (Ed.), *Interdisciplinary advances in information technology research* (pp. 202–219). Hershey, PA: IGI Global. doi:10.4018/978-1-4666-3625-5.ch015

Benito, R. V., Vega-Colado, C., Coco, M. B., Cuadrado, R., Torres-Zafra, J. C., Sánchez-Pena, J. M., ... López-Miguel, A. (2013). New electro-optic and display technology for visually disabled people. In M. Cruz-Cunha, I. Miranda, & P. Gonçalves (Eds.), *Handbook of research on ICTs for human-centered healthcare and social care services* (pp. 687–718). Hershey, PA: IGI Global. doi:10.4018/978-1-4666-3986-7.ch036

Bergenti, F., Poggi, A., & Tomaiuolo, M. (2013). Using multi-agent systems to support e-health services. In M. Cruz-Cunha, I. Miranda, & P. Gonçalves (Eds.), *Handbook of research on ICTs for human-centered healthcare and social care services* (pp. 549–567). Hershey, PA: IGI Global. doi:10.4018/978-1-4666-3986-7.ch029

Berler, A., & Apostolakis, I. (2014). Normalizing cross-border healthcare in Europe via new e-prescription paradigms. In C. El Morr (Ed.), *Research perspectives on the role of informatics in health policy and management* (pp. 168–208). Hershey, PA: IGI Global. doi:10.4018/978-1-4666-4321-5.ch011

Bernardi, R. (2013). Information technology and resistance to public sector reforms: A case study in Kenya. In I. Management Association (Ed.), User-driven healthcare: Concepts, methodologies, tools, and applications (pp. 14-33). Hershey, PA: IGI Global. doi:10.4018/978-1-4666-2770-3.ch002

Bernhard, S., Al Zoukra, K., & Schtte, C. (2013). From non-invasive hemodynamic measurements towards patient-specific cardiovascular diagnosis. In *Data mining: Concepts, methodologies, tools, and applications* (pp. 2069–2093). Hershey, PA: IGI Global. doi:10.4018/978-1-4666-2455-9.ch106

Best, C., O'Neill, B., & Gillespie, A. (2013). Assistive technology for cognition: Enabling activities of daily living. In M. Cruz-Cunha, I. Miranda, & P. Gonçalves (Eds.), *Handbook of research on ICTs for human-centered healthcare and social care services* (pp. 112–129). Hershey, PA: IGI Global. doi:10.4018/978-1-4666-3986-7.ch006

Bhattacharya, P., Asanga, A. P., & Biswas, R. (2013). Stomodeum to proctodeum: Email narratives on clinical problem solving in gastroenterology. In I. Management Association (Ed.), User-driven healthcare: Concepts, methodologies, tools, and applications (pp. 1073-1091). Hershey, PA: IGI Global. doi:10.4018/978-1-4666-2770-3.ch054

Boboc, C., & Ţiţan, E. (2014). Migration of medical doctors, health, medical education, and employment in eastern and central Europe. In A. Driouchi (Ed.), *Labor and health economics in the Mediterranean region: Migration and mobility of medical doctors* (pp. 158–191). Hershey, PA: IGI Global. doi:10.4018/978-1-4666-4723-7.ch007

Botella, C., Baños, R. M., Etchemendy, E., Castilla, D., García-Palacios, A., & Alcañiz, M. (2013). An e-health system for promoting wellbeing in the elderly: The butler system. In I. Management Association (Ed.), User-driven healthcare: Concepts, methodologies, tools, and applications (pp. 838-852). Hershey, PA: IGI Global. doi:10.4018/978-1-4666-2770-3.ch042

Bradai, N., Chaari, L., & Kamoun, L. (2013). A comprehensive overview of wireless body area networks (WBAN). In J. Rodrigues (Ed.), *Digital advances in medicine, e-health, and communication technologies* (pp. 1–32). Hershey, PA: IGI Global. doi:10.4018/978-1-4666-2794-9.ch001

Brown, K. E., Bayley, J., & Newby, K. (2013). Serious game for relationships and sex education: Application of an intervention mapping approach to development. In S. Arnab, I. Dunwell, & K. Debattista (Eds.), *Serious games for healthcare: Applications and implications* (pp. 135–166). Hershey, PA: IGI Global. doi:10.4018/978-1-4666-1903-6.ch007

Brown, M. (2013). Will comparative effectiveness research lead to healthcare rationing? In I. Management Association (Ed.), User-driven healthcare: Concepts, methodologies, tools, and applications (pp. 1487-1507). Hershey, PA: IGI Global. doi:10.4018/978-1-4666-2770-3.ch074

Burlamaqui, A. M., Azevedo, S. O., Silva, I. R., Silva, S. R., Souto da Silva, G. H., & Benjamim, X. C. … Felix de Castro, A. (2013). Low cost t-health and t-social with ginga: Experience with mime TV, ImFine, and iFunnyCube interactive TV programs. In M. Cruz-Cunha, I. Miranda, & P. Gonçalves (Eds.), Handbook of research on ICTs for human-centered healthcare and social care services (pp. 303-318). Hershey, PA: IGI Global. doi:10.4018/978-1-4666-3986-7.ch015

Burns, J., Blanchard, M., & Metcalf, A. (2013). Bridging the digital divide in Australia: The potential implications for the mental health of young people experiencing marginalisation. In *Digital literacy: Concepts, methodologies, tools, and applications* (pp. 772–793). Hershey, PA: IGI Global. doi:10.4018/978-1-4666-1852-7.ch040

Buyurgan, N., Rardin, R. L., Jayaraman, R., Varghese, V. M., & Burbano, A. (2013). A novel GS1 data standard adoption roadmap for healthcare providers. In J. Tan (Ed.), *Healthcare information technology innovation and sustainability: Frontiers and adoption* (pp. 41–57). Hershey, PA: IGI Global. doi:10.4018/978-1-4666-2797-0.ch003

Cabrita, M. D., & Cabrita, M. (2014). Applying social marketing to healthcare: Challenges and opportunities. In A. Kapoor & C. Kulshrestha (Eds.), *Dynamics of competitive advantage and consumer perception in social marketing* (pp. 78–97). Hershey, PA: IGI Global. doi:10.4018/978-1-4666-4430-4.ch004

Carroll, J. M., & Rosson, M. B. (2013). Community networks: Infrastructure and models for therapeutic support. In M. Cruz-Cunha, I. Miranda, & P. Gonçalves (Eds.), *Handbook of research on ICTs for human-centered healthcare and social care services* (pp. 187–207). Hershey, PA: IGI Global. doi:10.4018/978-1-4666-3986-7.ch010

Castiglioni, I., Gilardi, M. C., & Gallivanone, F. (2013). E-health decision support systems for the diagnosis of dementia diseases. In A. Moumtzoglou & A. Kastania (Eds.), *E-health technologies and improving patient safety: Exploring organizational factors* (pp. 84–97). Hershey, PA: IGI Global. doi:10.4018/978-1-4666-2657-7.ch006

Catley, C., Smith, K., McGregor, C., James, A., & Eklund, J. M. (2013). A framework for multidimensional real-time data analysis: A case study for the detection of apnoea of prematurity. In A. Gangopadhyay (Ed.), *Methods, models, and computation for medical informatics* (pp. 16–35). Hershey, PA: IGI Global. doi:10.4018/978-1-4666-2653-9.ch002

Chaari, L., & Kamoun, L. (2013). QoS concepts and architecture over wireless body area networks for healthcare applications. In J. Rodrigues (Ed.), *Digital advances in medicine, e-health, and communication technologies* (pp. 114–130). Hershey, PA: IGI Global. doi:10.4018/978-1-4666-2794-9.ch007

Chamberlin, B., Maloney, A., Gallagher, R. R., & Garza, M. L. (2013). Active video games: Potential for increased activity, suggestions for use, and guidelines for implementation. In S. Arnab, I. Dunwell, & K. Debattista (Eds.), *Serious games for healthcare: Applications and implications* (pp. 191–212). Hershey, PA: IGI Global. doi:10.4018/978-1-4666-1903-6.ch009

Charisi, A., Korvesis, P., & Megalooikonomou, V. (2013). Similarity searching of medical image data in distributed systems: Facilitating telemedicine applications. In A. Gangopadhyay (Ed.), *Methods, models, and computation for medical informatics* (pp. 58–77). Hershey, PA: IGI Global. doi:10.4018/978-1-4666-2653-9.ch004

Chattopadhyay, A., Malhotra, K., & Chatterjee, S. (2013). Ethical guidelines for the quality assessment of healthcare. In I. Management Association (Ed.), User-driven healthcare: Concepts, methodologies, tools, and applications (pp. 1332-1347). Hershey, PA: IGI Global. doi:10.4018/978-1-4666-2770-3.ch066

Chen, J. Y., Xu, H., Shi, P., Culbertson, A., & Meslin, E. M. (2013). Ethics and privacy considerations for systems biology applications in predictive and personalized medicine. In I. Management Association (Ed.), Bioinformatics: Concepts, methodologies, tools, and applications (pp. 1378-1404). Hershey, PA: IGI Global. doi:10.4018/978-1-4666-3604-0.ch071

Chen, Y. (2013). Construction of digital statistical atlases of the liver and their applications to computer-aided diagnosis. In J. Wu (Ed.), *Technological advancements in biomedicine for healthcare applications* (pp. 68–79). Hershey, PA: IGI Global. doi:10.4018/978-1-4666-2196-1.ch008

Cheng, B., Stanley, R. J., De, S., Antani, S., & Thoma, G. R. (2013). Automatic detection of arrow annotation overlays in biomedical images. In J. Tan (Ed.), *Healthcare information technology innovation and sustainability: Frontiers and adoption* (pp. 219–236). Hershey, PA: IGI Global. doi:10.4018/978-1-4666-2797-0.ch014

Cherian, E. J., & Ryan, T. W. (2014). Incongruent needs: Why differences in the iron-triangle of priorities make health information technology adoption and use difficult. In C. El Morr (Ed.), *Research perspectives on the role of informatics in health policy and management* (pp. 209–221). Hershey, PA: IGI Global. doi:10.4018/978-1-4666-4321-5.ch012

Chowdhry, N., Ashraf, A., Chowdhry, B., Baloch, A., Ansari, A., & De Meer, H. (2013). Grid for post operative care through wireless sensor networks. In I. Management Association (Ed.), User-driven healthcare: Concepts, methodologies, tools, and applications (pp. 514-531). Hershey, PA: IGI Global. doi:10.4018/978-1-4666-2770-3.ch026

Chun, S. A., Kwon, J. H., & Lee, H. (2013). Social credential-based role recommendation and patient privacy control in medical emergency. In A. Gangopadhyay (Ed.), *Methods, models, and computation for medical informatics* (pp. 215–237). Hershey, PA: IGI Global. doi:10.4018/978-1-4666-2653-9.ch013

Cohen, J. F., Bancilhon, J., & Sergay, S. (2013). An empirical study of patient willingness to use self-service technologies in the healthcare context. In M. Cruz-Cunha, I. Miranda, & P. Gonçalves (Eds.), *Handbook of research on ICTs and management systems for improving efficiency in healthcare and social care* (pp. 378–395). Hershey, PA: IGI Global. doi:10.4018/978-1-4666-3990-4.ch019

Constantinides, P. (2013). The development of the English national health information infrastructure. In I. Management Association (Ed.), User-driven healthcare: Concepts, methodologies, tools, and applications (pp. 968-991). Hershey, PA: IGI Global. doi:10.4018/978-1-4666-2770-3.ch049

Constantinides, P. (2013). The development of a regional health information infrastructure in Greece. In I. Management Association (Ed.), User-driven healthcare: Concepts, methodologies, tools, and applications (pp. 992-1017). Hershey, PA: IGI Global. doi:10.4018/978-1-4666-2770-3.ch050

Corrigan, D., Hederman, L., Khan, H., Taweel, A., Kostopoulou, O., & Delaney, B. (2013). An ontology-driven approach to clinical evidence modelling implementing clinical prediction rules. In A. Moumtzoglou & A. Kastania (Eds.), *E-health technologies and improving patient safety: Exploring organizational factors* (pp. 257–284). Hershey, PA: IGI Global. doi:10.4018/978-1-4666-2657-7.ch016

Corritore, C. L., Kracher, B., Wiedenbeck, S., & Marble, R. (2013). Foundations of trust for e-health. In I. Management Association (Ed.), User-driven healthcare: Concepts, methodologies, tools, and applications (pp. 1167-1193). Hershey, PA: IGI Global. doi:10.4018/978-1-4666-2770-3.ch059

Costa, Â., Andrade, F., & Novais, P. (2013). Privacy and data protection towards elderly healthcare. In M. Cruz-Cunha, I. Miranda, & P. Gonçalves (Eds.), *Handbook of research on ICTs for human-centered healthcare and social care services* (pp. 330–346). Hershey, PA: IGI Global. doi:10.4018/978-1-4666-3986-7.ch017

Coughlan, J., & Brinkman, W. (2013). Design considerations for delivering e-learning to surgical trainees. In J. Rodrigues (Ed.), *Digital advances in medicine, e-health, and communication technologies* (pp. 341–350). Hershey, PA: IGI Global. doi:10.4018/978-1-4666-2794-9.ch020

D'Abundo, M. L. (2013). Electronic health record implementation in the United States healthcare industry: Making the process of change manageable. In V. Wang (Ed.), *Handbook of research on technologies for improving the 21st century workforce: Tools for lifelong learning* (pp. 272–286). Hershey, PA: IGI Global. doi:10.4018/978-1-4666-2181-7.ch018

D'Abundo, M. L. (2013). Electronic health record implementation in the United States healthcare industry: Making the process of change manageable. In I. Management Association (Ed.), User-driven healthcare: Concepts, methodologies, tools, and applications (pp. 382-395). Hershey, PA: IGI Global. doi:10.4018/978-1-4666-2770-3.ch019

D'Andrea, A., Ferri, F., & Grifoni, P. (2013). RFID technologies in the health sector. In A. Moumtzoglou & A. Kastania (Eds.), *E-health technologies and improving patient safety: Exploring organizational factors* (pp. 140–147). Hershey, PA: IGI Global. doi:10.4018/978-1-4666-2657-7.ch009

D'Astolfo, C. (2014). Investing in a "rehabilitation model" to improve the decision-making process in long-term care. In C. El Morr (Ed.), *Research perspectives on the role of informatics in health policy and management* (pp. 37–47). Hershey, PA: IGI Global. doi:10.4018/978-1-4666-4321-5.ch003

Daniel, V. M. (2013). Genomics and genetic engineering: Playing God? In I. Management Association (Ed.), Bioinformatics: Concepts, methodologies, tools, and applications (pp. 249-267). Hershey, PA: IGI Global. doi:10.4018/978-1-4666-3604-0.ch013

Dasgupta, S. S. (2013). Cyber capability framework: A tool to evaluate ICT for development projects. In M. Cruz-Cunha, I. Miranda, & P. Gonçalves (Eds.), *Handbook of research on ICTs for human-centered healthcare and social care services* (pp. 399–406). Hershey, PA: IGI Global. doi:10.4018/978-1-4666-3986-7.ch021

Davis, S. A. (2013). Global telemedicine and ehealth: Advances for future healthcare – Using a systems approach to integrate healthcare functions. In V. Gulla, A. Mori, F. Gabbrielli, & P. Lanzafame (Eds.), *Telehealth networks for hospital services: New methodologies* (pp. 15–32). Hershey, PA: IGI Global. doi:10.4018/978-1-4666-2979-0.ch002

Deng, M., Petkovic, M., Nalin, M., & Baroni, I. (2013). Home healthcare in cloud computing. In M. Cruz-Cunha, I. Miranda, & P. Gonçalves (Eds.), *Handbook of research on ICTs and management systems for improving efficiency in healthcare and social care* (pp. 614–634). Hershey, PA: IGI Global. doi:10.4018/978-1-4666-3990-4.ch032

DeVany, M., Knobloch-Ludwig, K., Penticoff, M., Assimacopoulos, A., & Speedie, S. (2013). Telehealth implementation: The voice of experience. In S. Sarnikar, D. Bennett, & M. Gaynor (Eds.), *Cases on healthcare information technology for patient care management* (pp. 126–139). Hershey, PA: IGI Global. doi:10.4018/978-1-4666-2671-3.ch008

Ding, W., Qiu, P., Liu, Y., & Feng, W. (2013). Current omics technologies in biomarker discovery. In I. Management Association (Ed.), Bioinformatics: Concepts, methodologies, tools, and applications (pp. 465-497). Hershey, PA: IGI Global. doi:10.4018/978-1-4666-3604-0.ch027

Dingli, A., Abela, C., & D'Ambrogio, I. (2013). PINATA: Taking e-health a step forward. In A. Moumtzoglou & A. Kastania (Eds.), *E-health technologies and improving patient safety: Exploring organizational factors* (pp. 173–195). Hershey, PA: IGI Global. doi:10.4018/978-1-4666-2657-7.ch012

Dogra, D. P., Nandam, K., Majumdar, A. K., Sural, S., Mukhopadhyay, J., Majumdar, B., ... Mukherjee, S. (2013). A tool for automatic hammersmith infant neurological examination. In J. Rodrigues (Ed.), *Digital advances in medicine, e-health, and communication technologies* (pp. 301–311). Hershey, PA: IGI Global. doi:10.4018/978-1-4666-2794-9.ch017

Doyle, J., Bertolotto, M., & Wilson, D. (2013). Towards multimodal mobile GIS for the elderly. In *Digital literacy: Concepts, methodologies, tools, and applications* (pp. 590–609). Hershey, PA: IGI Global. doi:10.4018/978-1-4666-1852-7.ch031

Dragoni, A. F. (2013). Health services through digital terrestrial television. In V. Gulla, A. Mori, F. Gabbrielli, & P. Lanzafame (Eds.), *Telehealth networks for hospital services: New methodologies* (pp. 207–227). Hershey, PA: IGI Global. doi:10.4018/978-1-4666-2979-0.ch014

Dragoni, A. F. (2013). Virtual carer: A first prototype. In V. Gulla, A. Mori, F. Gabbrielli, & P. Lanzafame (Eds.), *Telehealth networks for hospital services: New methodologies* (pp. 290–299). Hershey, PA: IGI Global. doi:10.4018/978-1-4666-2979-0.ch019

Driouchi, A. (2014). Introduction to labor and health economics: Mobility of medical doctors in the Mediterranean region. In A. Driouchi (Ed.), *Labor and health economics in the Mediterranean region: Migration and mobility of medical doctors* (pp. 1–22). Hershey, PA: IGI Global. doi:10.4018/978-1-4666-4723-7.ch001

Driouchi, A. (2014). Medical knowledge, north-south cooperation, and mobility of medical doctors. In A. Driouchi (Ed.), *Labor and health economics in the Mediterranean region: Migration and mobility of medical doctors* (pp. 376–395). Hershey, PA: IGI Global. doi:10.4018/978-1-4666-4723-7.ch015

Driouchi, A. (2014). Skilled human resources in the health sectors and impacts of new health technologies on health workforce in developing economies. In A. Driouchi (Ed.), *Labor and health economics in the Mediterranean region: Migration and mobility of medical doctors* (pp. 23–50). Hershey, PA: IGI Global. doi:10.4018/978-1-4666-4723-7.ch002

Duan, X., Wang, X., & Huang, Q. (2013). Medical manipulators for surgical applications. In J. Wu (Ed.), *Technological advancements in biomedicine for healthcare applications* (pp. 111–122). Hershey, PA: IGI Global. doi:10.4018/978-1-4666-2196-1.ch012

Dugdale, A. (2013). Australian patient organizations: Using digital technologies to engage health citizen communities in health policy. In I. Management Association (Ed.), User-driven healthcare: Concepts, methodologies, tools, and applications (pp. 853-869). Hershey, PA: IGI Global. doi:10.4018/978-1-4666-2770-3.ch043

Dunwell, I., & Jarvis, S. (2013). A serious game for on-the-ward infection control awareness training: Ward off infection. In S. Arnab, I. Dunwell, & K. Debattista (Eds.), *Serious games for healthcare: Applications and implications* (pp. 233–246). Hershey, PA: IGI Global. doi:10.4018/978-1-4666-1903-6.ch011

Durant, K. T., McCray, A. T., & Safran, C. (2013). Identifying temporal changes and topics that promote growth within online communities: A prospective study of six online cancer forums. In A. Gangopadhyay (Ed.), *Methods, models, and computation for medical informatics* (pp. 78–97). Hershey, PA: IGI Global. doi:10.4018/978-1-4666-2653-9.ch005

El-Farargy, N. (2013). Refresher training in clinical psychology supervision: A blended learning approach. In A. Benson, J. Moore, & S. Williams van Rooij (Eds.), *Cases on educational technology planning, design, and implementation: A project management perspective* (pp. 295–317). Hershey, PA: IGI Global. doi:10.4018/978-1-4666-4237-9.ch016

Enquist, H. (2013). From idea to use: lessons learned from a participatory ICT healthcare case study. In I. Management Association (Ed.), User-driven healthcare: Concepts, methodologies, tools, and applications (pp. 1037-1053). Hershey, PA: IGI Global. doi:10.4018/978-1-4666-2770-3.ch052

Ervin, K. (2014). Legal and ethical considerations in the implementation of electronic health records. In J. Krueger (Ed.), *Cases on electronic records and resource management implementation in diverse environments* (pp. 193–210). Hershey, PA: IGI Global. doi:10.4018/978-1-4666-4466-3.ch012

Escayola, J., Trigo, J., Martínez, I., Martínez-Espronceda, M., Aragüés, A., Sancho, D., . . . García, J. (2013). Overview of the ISO/IEEE11073 family of standards and their applications to health monitoring. In I. Management Association (Ed.), User-driven healthcare: Concepts, methodologies, tools, and applications (pp. 357-381). Hershey, PA: IGI Global. doi:10.4018/978-1-4666-2770-3.ch018

Facelli, J. C., Hurdle, J. F., & Mitchell, J. A. (2013). Medical informatics and bioinformatics. In I. Management Association (Ed.), Bioinformatics: Concepts, methodologies, tools, and applications (pp. 195-221). Hershey, PA: IGI Global. doi:10.4018/978-1-4666-3604-0.ch010

Fakhar, A. (2014). Beyond brain drain: A case study of the benefits of cooperation on medical immigration. In A. Driouchi (Ed.), *Labor and health economics in the Mediterranean region: Migration and mobility of medical doctors* (pp. 294–313). Hershey, PA: IGI Global. doi:10.4018/978-1-4666-4723-7.ch012

Falan, S. L., Han, B., Zoeller, L. H., Tarn, J. M., & Roach, D. M. (2013). Sustaining healthcare through waste elimination: A taxonomic analysis with case illustrations. In J. Tan (Ed.), *Healthcare information technology innovation and sustainability: Frontiers and adoption* (pp. 18–39). Hershey, PA: IGI Global. doi:10.4018/978-1-4666-2797-0.ch002

Farinha, C., & Mira da Silva, M. (2013). Identifying requirements for healthcare information systems with focus groups. In M. Cruz-Cunha, I. Miranda, & P. Gonçalves (Eds.), *Handbook of research on ICTs for human-centered healthcare and social care services* (pp. 491–510). Hershey, PA: IGI Global. doi:10.4018/978-1-4666-3986-7.ch026

Fernando, J. (2013). The protocols of privileged information handling in an e-health context: Australia. In I. Management Association (Ed.), User-driven healthcare: Concepts, methodologies, tools, and applications (pp. 737-759). Hershey, PA: IGI Global. doi:10.4018/978-1-4666-2770-3.ch036

Ferreira, L., Teixeira, A., & Cunha, J. P. (2013). Medical information extraction in European Portuguese. In M. Cruz-Cunha, I. Miranda, & P. Gonçalves (Eds.), *Handbook of research on ICTs for human-centered healthcare and social care services* (pp. 607–626). Hershey, PA: IGI Global. doi:10.4018/978-1-4666-3986-7.ch032

Fitzpatrick, J. (2013). An exploration of the experiences of migrant women: Implications for policy development of effective user driven health care delivery systems. In I. Management Association (Ed.), User-driven healthcare: Concepts, methodologies, tools, and applications (pp. 954-967). Hershey, PA: IGI Global. doi:10.4018/978-1-4666-2770-3.ch048

Fitzpatrick, J., & Ako, W. (2013). Developing community ontologies in user driven healthcare. In I. Management Association (Ed.), User-driven healthcare: Concepts, methodologies, tools, and applications (pp. 655-672). Hershey, PA: IGI Global. doi:10.4018/978-1-4666-2770-3.ch032

Flores, A. E., Win, K. T., & Susilo, W. (2013). Secure exchange of electronic health records. In I. Management Association (Ed.), IT policy and ethics: Concepts, methodologies, tools, and applications (pp. 1059-1079). Hershey, PA: IGI Global. doi:10.4018/978-1-4666-2919-6.ch048

Flores, A. E., Win, K. T., & Susilo, W. (2013). Secure exchange of electronic health records. In I. Management Association (Ed.), User-driven healthcare: Concepts, methodologies, tools, and applications (pp. 1403-1424). Hershey, PA: IGI Global. doi:10.4018/978-1-4666-2770-3.ch070

Forrestal, E. J., Cellucci, L. W., Zeng, X., Kennedy, M. H., & Smith, D. (2013). Health information technology collaboration in community health centers: The community partners HealthNet, Inc. In S. Sarnikar, D. Bennett, & M. Gaynor (Eds.), *Cases on healthcare information technology for patient care management* (pp. 171–196). Hershey, PA: IGI Global. doi:10.4018/978-1-4666-2671-3.ch011

Frederico, C. (2013). Nutrition games. In S. Arnab, I. Dunwell, & K. Debattista (Eds.), *Serious games for healthcare: Applications and implications* (pp. 167–190). Hershey, PA: IGI Global. doi:10.4018/978-1-4666-1903-6.ch008

Freitas, L., Pereira, R. T., Pereira, H. G., Martini, R., Mozzaquatro, B. A., Kasper, J., & Librelotto, G. (2013). Ontological representation and an architecture for homecare pervasive systems. In R. Martinho, R. Rijo, M. Cruz-Cunha, & J. Varajão (Eds.), *Information systems and technologies for enhancing health and social care* (pp. 215–234). Hershey, PA: IGI Global. doi:10.4018/978-1-4666-3667-5.ch015

Frigo, C. A., & Pavan, E. E. (2014). Prosthetic and orthotic devices. In *Assistive technologies: Concepts, methodologies, tools, and applications* (pp. 549–613). Hershey, PA: IGI Global. doi:10.4018/978-1-4666-4422-9.ch028

Fukami, T., & Wu, J. (2013). Image fusion method and the efficacy of multimodal cardiac images. In J. Wu (Ed.), *Technological advancements in biomedicine for healthcare applications* (pp. 47–54). Hershey, PA: IGI Global. doi:10.4018/978-1-4666-2196-1.ch006

Furdu, I., & Patrut, B. (2013). ICT applications and solutions in healthcare: Present and perspectives. In M. Cruz-Cunha, I. Miranda, & P. Gonçalves (Eds.), *Handbook of research on ICTs and management systems for improving efficiency in healthcare and social care* (pp. 559–576). Hershey, PA: IGI Global. doi:10.4018/978-1-4666-3990-4.ch029

Gabbrielli, F. (2013). Telemedicine R&D influencing incoming strategies and organization models. In V. Gulla, A. Mori, F. Gabbrielli, & P. Lanzafame (Eds.), *Telehealth networks for hospital services: New methodologies* (pp. 250–264). Hershey, PA: IGI Global. doi:10.4018/978-1-4666-2979-0.ch017

Gaivéo, J. M. (2013). Security of ICTs supporting healthcare activities. In M. Cruz-Cunha, I. Miranda, & P. Gonçalves (Eds.), *Handbook of research on ICTs for human-centered healthcare and social care services* (pp. 208–228). Hershey, PA: IGI Global. doi:10.4018/978-1-4666-3986-7.ch011

Gallo, C. (2013). A multichannel framework for multimedia content deployment in e-health environments. In M. Cruz-Cunha, I. Miranda, & P. Gonçalves (Eds.), *Handbook of research on ICTs and management systems for improving efficiency in healthcare and social care* (pp. 872–891). Hershey, PA: IGI Global. doi:10.4018/978-1-4666-3990-4.ch045

Gao, Y., Yang, W., Yang, J., Satoshi, T., & Wu, J. (2013). Neural mechanisms of audiovisual integration in integrated processing for verbal perception and spatial factors. In J. Wu (Ed.), *Biomedical engineering and cognitive neuroscience for healthcare: Interdisciplinary applications* (pp. 327–336). Hershey, PA: IGI Global. doi:10.4018/978-1-4666-2113-8.ch034

Garzo, A., Carmien, S. P., & Madina, X. (2013). Mapping input technology to ability. In I. Management Association (Ed.), User-driven healthcare: Concepts, methodologies, tools, and applications (pp. 480-501). Hershey, PA: IGI Global. doi:10.4018/978-1-4666-2770-3.ch024

Gatzidis, C. (2013). First-person shooter game engines and healthcare: An examination of the current state of the art and future potential. In S. Arnab, I. Dunwell, & K. Debattista (Eds.), *Serious Games for Healthcare: Applications and Implications* (pp. 76–89). Hershey, PA: IGI Global. doi:10.4018/978-1-4666-1903-6.ch004

Gaughan, M. (2013). The hybridized nature of America's health care system: Medicare as a case of both market and public failure. In M. Merviö (Ed.), *Healthcare management and economics: Perspectives on public and private administration* (pp. 154–164). Hershey, PA: IGI Global. doi:10.4018/978-1-4666-3982-9.ch012

Gavgani, V. Z. (2013). Information therapy (ix) service and patients' preference. In A. Gangopadhyay (Ed.), *Methods, models, and computation for medical informatics* (pp. 117–125). Hershey, PA: IGI Global. doi:10.4018/978-1-4666-2653-9.ch007

Gavgani, V. Z. (2013). Ubiquitous information therapy service through social networking libraries: An operational web 2.0 service model. In I. Management Association (Ed.), User-driven healthcare: Concepts, methodologies, tools, and applications (pp. 673-688). Hershey, PA: IGI Global. doi:10.4018/978-1-4666-2770-3.ch033

Germaine-McDaniel, N. S. (2013). The emerging hispanic use of online health information in the United States: Cultural convergence or dissociation? In I. Management Association (Ed.), User-driven healthcare: Concepts, methodologies, tools, and applications (pp. 1607-1621). Hershey, PA: IGI Global. doi:10.4018/978-1-4666-2770-3.ch079

Gholson, J., & Tennyson, H. (2013). One system of care, one electronic chart. In S. Sarnikar, D. Bennett, & M. Gaynor (Eds.), *Cases on healthcare information technology for patient care management* (pp. 55–69). Hershey, PA: IGI Global. doi:10.4018/978-1-4666-2671-3.ch003

Ghosh, B. (2013). Healthcare systems using clinical data: Addressing data interoperability challenges. In S. Sarnikar, D. Bennett, & M. Gaynor (Eds.), *Cases on healthcare information technology for patient care management* (pp. 208–223). Hershey, PA: IGI Global. doi:10.4018/978-1-4666-2671-3.ch013

Gibson, L., Sloan, D., & Moncur, W. (2013). E-health and digital inclusion. In I. Management Association (Ed.), User-driven healthcare: Concepts, methodologies, tools, and applications (pp. 197-210). Hershey, PA: IGI Global. doi:10.4018/978-1-4666-2770-3.ch011

Gillies, A. C., & Howard, J. (2013). Information as change agent or barrier in health care reform? In J. Tan (Ed.), *Healthcare information technology innovation and sustainability: Frontiers and adoption* (pp. 1–17). Hershey, PA: IGI Global. doi:10.4018/978-1-4666-2797-0.ch001

Glusker, A., & Hoelscher, E. (2014). Transitioning from print to online-only resources: The experience of a medium-sized healthcare organization library. In J. Krueger (Ed.), *Cases on electronic records and resource management implementation in diverse environments* (pp. 226–242). Hershey, PA: IGI Global. doi:10.4018/978-1-4666-4466-3.ch014

Gofuku, A., Fukumori, S., & Sato, K. (2013). A mirror visual feedback therapy system applying virtual reality technology. In J. Wu (Ed.), *Biomedical engineering and cognitive neuroscience for healthcare: Interdisciplinary applications* (pp. 73–80). Hershey, PA: IGI Global. doi:10.4018/978-1-4666-2113-8.ch008

Gomes, C., Sperandio, F., Peles, A., Borges, J., Brito, A. C., & Almada-Lobo, B. (2013). An operating theater planning decision support system. In R. Martinho, R. Rijo, M. Cruz-Cunha, & J. Varajão (Eds.), *Information systems and technologies for enhancing health and social care* (pp. 69–86). Hershey, PA: IGI Global. doi:10.4018/978-1-4666-3667-5.ch005

Grissom, T. E., DuKatz, A., Kordylewski, H. A., & Dutton, R. P. (2013). Bring out your data: The evolution of the national anesthesia clinical outcomes registry (NACOR). In A. Gangopadhyay (Ed.), *Methods, models, and computation for medical informatics* (pp. 126–145). Hershey, PA: IGI Global. doi:10.4018/978-1-4666-2653-9.ch008

Gudes, O., Kendall, E., Yigitcanlar, T., Han, J. H., & Pathak, V. (2013). Developing a competitive city through healthy decision-making. In I. Management Association (Ed.), User-driven healthcare: Concepts, methodologies, tools, and applications (pp. 808-822). Hershey, PA: IGI Global. doi:10.4018/978-1-4666-2770-3.ch040

Gugerty, B., & Maranda, M. J. (2013). The promises and challenges of health information technology. In I. Management Association (Ed.), User-driven healthcare: Concepts, methodologies, tools, and applications (pp. 57-76). Hershey, PA: IGI Global. doi:10.4018/978-1-4666-2770-3.ch004

Guimarães, C., Antunes, D. R., García, L. S., & Fernandes, S. (2013). Information challenges of the deaf in their health and social care needs. In M. Cruz-Cunha, I. Miranda, & P. Gonçalves (Eds.), *Handbook of research on ICTs for human-centered healthcare and social care services* (pp. 93–111). Hershey, PA: IGI Global. doi:10.4018/978-1-4666-3986-7.ch005

Guinalíu, M., Marta, J., & Subero, J. M. (2013). Social networks as a tool to improve the life quality of chronic patients and their relatives. In M. Cruz-Cunha, I. Miranda, & P. Gonçalves (Eds.), *Handbook of research on ICTs for human-centered healthcare and social care services* (pp. 172–186). Hershey, PA: IGI Global. doi:10.4018/978-1-4666-3986-7.ch009

Gullà, V. (2013). Leading the technological innovation in healthcare systems: The telematic medicine approach. In V. Gulla, A. Mori, F. Gabbrielli, & P. Lanzafame (Eds.), *Telehealth networks for hospital services: New methodologies* (pp. 134–153). Hershey, PA: IGI Global. doi:10.4018/978-1-4666-2979-0.ch009

Gullà, V., & Cancellotti, C. (2013). Telemedicine in emergency: A first aid hospital network experience. In V. Gulla, A. Mori, F. Gabbrielli, & P. Lanzafame (Eds.), *Telehealth networks for hospital services: New methodologies* (pp. 240–248). Hershey, PA: IGI Global. doi:10.4018/978-1-4666-2979-0.ch016

Guo, M., Yu, Y., Yang, J., & Wu, J. (2013). The crossmodal between the visual and tactile for motion perception. In J. Wu (Ed.), *Biomedical engineering and cognitive neuroscience for healthcare: Interdisciplinary applications* (pp. 99–108). Hershey, PA: IGI Global. doi:10.4018/978-1-4666-2113-8.ch011

Habib, M. K. (2014). Web-based multi-user distributed and collaborative environment supporting emergency and relief activities. In I. Management Association (Ed.), Crisis management: Concepts, methodologies, tools and applications (pp. 425-445). Hershey, PA: IGI Global. doi:10.4018/978-1-4666-4707-7.ch019

Hafeez-Baig, A., & Gururajan, R. (2013). Phenomena of adoption of wireless handheld devices: A case of healthcare setting. In H. Muga & K. Thomas (Eds.), *Cases on the diffusion and adoption of sustainable development practices* (pp. 20–43). Hershey, PA: IGI Global. doi:10.4018/978-1-4666-2842-7.ch002

Haida, M. (2013). Implications of NIRS brain signals. In J. Wu (Ed.), *Biomedical engineering and cognitive neuroscience for healthcare: Interdisciplinary applications* (pp. 120–128). Hershey, PA: IGI Global. doi:10.4018/978-1-4666-2113-8.ch013

Han, D., & Braun, K. L. (2013). Promoting active ageing through technology training in Korea. In *Digital literacy: Concepts, methodologies, tools, and applications* (pp. 572–589). Hershey, PA: IGI Global. doi:10.4018/978-1-4666-1852-7.ch030

Haniff, D. (2013). Usability engineering and e-health. In I. Management Association (Ed.), User-driven healthcare: Concepts, methodologies, tools, and applications (pp. 1446-1468). Hershey, PA: IGI Global. doi:10.4018/978-1-4666-2770-3.ch072

Hareva, D. H., Okada, H., & Oka, H. (2013). Ecological momentary assessment using a mobile phone. In J. Wu (Ed.), *Technological advancements in biomedicine for healthcare applications* (pp. 398–407). Hershey, PA: IGI Global. doi:10.4018/978-1-4666-2196-1.ch039

Harnett, B. (2013). Patient centered medicine and technology adaptation. In I. Management Association (Ed.), User-driven healthcare: Concepts, methodologies, tools, and applications (pp. 77-98). Hershey, PA: IGI Global. doi:10.4018/978-1-4666-2770-3.ch005

Hatton, J. D., Schmidt, T. M., & Jelen, J. (2013). Adoption of electronic health care records: Physician heuristics and hesitancy. In R. Martinho, R. Rijo, M. Cruz-Cunha, & J. Varajão (Eds.), *Information systems and technologies for enhancing health and social care* (pp. 148–165). Hershey, PA: IGI Global. doi:10.4018/978-1-4666-3667-5.ch010

Heinrichs, L., Fellander-Tsai, L., & Davies, D. (2013). Clinical virtual worlds: The wider implications for professional development in healthcare. In K. Bredl & W. Bösche (Eds.), *Serious games and virtual worlds in education, professional development, and healthcare* (pp. 221–240). Hershey, PA: IGI Global. doi:10.4018/978-1-4666-3673-6.ch014

Heinrichs, W. L., Davies, D., & Davies, J. (2013). Virtual worlds in healthcare: Applications and implications. In S. Arnab, I. Dunwell, & K. Debattista (Eds.), *Serious games for healthcare: Applications and implications* (pp. 1–22). Hershey, PA: IGI Global. doi:10.4018/978-1-4666-1903-6.ch001

Hirata, M., Yanagisawa, T., Matsushita, K., Sugata, H., Kamitani, Y., & Suzuki, T. … Yoshimine, T. (2013). Brain–machine interface using brain surface electrodes: Real-time robotic control and a fully implantable wireless system. In J. Wu (Ed.), Technological advancements in biomedicine for healthcare applications (pp. 362-374). Hershey, PA: IGI Global. doi:10.4018/978-1-4666-2196-1.ch036

Hocine, N., & Gouaïch, A. (2013). Difficulty and scenario adaptation: An approach to customize therapeutic games. In S. Arnab, I. Dunwell, & K. Debattista (Eds.), *Serious games for healthcare: Applications and implications* (pp. 107–134). Hershey, PA: IGI Global. doi:10.4018/978-1-4666-1903-6.ch006

Hoonakker, P., Cartmill, R. S., Carayon, P., & Walker, J. M. (2013). Development and psychometric qualities of the SEIPS survey to evaluate CPOE/EHR implementation in ICUs. In J. Tan (Ed.), *Healthcare information technology innovation and sustainability: Frontiers and adoption* (pp. 161–179). Hershey, PA: IGI Global. doi:10.4018/978-1-4666-2797-0.ch010

Hoshi, K. (2013). Reframing dichotomies: Human experiential design of healthcare technologies. In I. Management Association (Ed.), User-driven healthcare: Concepts, methodologies, tools, and applications (pp. 1303-1331). Hershey, PA: IGI Global. doi:10.4018/978-1-4666-2770-3.ch065

Høstgaard, A. M. (2013). End-user participation in health IT development: The EUPHIT method. In I. Management Association (Ed.), User-driven healthcare: Concepts, methodologies, tools, and applications (pp. 608-629). Hershey, PA: IGI Global. doi:10.4018/978-1-4666-2770-3.ch030

Igrejas, G., Amaral, J. S., & Rodrigues, P. J. (2013). Fall detection systems to be used by elderly people. In M. Cruz-Cunha, I. Miranda, & P. Gonçalves (Eds.), *Handbook of research on ICTs for human-centered healthcare and social care services* (pp. 449–473). Hershey, PA: IGI Global. doi:10.4018/978-1-4666-3986-7.ch024

Inomata, C., & Nitta, S. (2013). Nursing in integrative medicine and nurses' engagement in caring-healing: A discussion based on the practice and study of music therapy and nursing care for patients with neurodegenerative disorders. In J. Wu (Ed.), *Technological advancements in biomedicine for healthcare applications* (pp. 235–239). Hershey, PA: IGI Global. doi:10.4018/978-1-4666-2196-1.ch025

Ishaq, G. M., Hussain, P. T., Iqbal, M. J., & Mushtaq, M. B. (2013). Risk-benefit analysis of combination vs. unopposed HRT in post-menopausal women. In I. Management Association (Ed.), Bioinformatics: Concepts, methodologies, tools, and applications (pp. 1424-1440). Hershey, PA: IGI Global. doi:10.4018/978-1-4666-3604-0.ch073

Iwaki, S. (2013). Multimodal neuroimaging to visualize human visual processing. In J. Wu (Ed.), *Biomedical engineering and cognitive neuroscience for healthcare: Interdisciplinary applications* (pp. 274–282). Hershey, PA: IGI Global. doi:10.4018/978-1-4666-2113-8.ch028

Ji, Z., Sugi, T., Goto, S., Wang, X., & Nakamura, M. (2013). Multi-channel template extraction for automatic EEG spike detection. In J. Wu (Ed.), *Biomedical engineering and cognitive neuroscience for healthcare: Interdisciplinary applications* (pp. 255–265). Hershey, PA: IGI Global. doi:10.4018/978-1-4666-2113-8.ch026

Jiang, Y., Wang, S., Tan, R., Ishida, K., Ando, T., & Fujie, M. G. (2013). Motor cortex activation during mental imagery of walking: An fNIRS study. In J. Wu (Ed.), *Biomedical engineering and cognitive neuroscience for healthcare: Interdisciplinary applications* (pp. 29–37). Hershey, PA: IGI Global. doi:10.4018/978-1-4666-2113-8.ch004

Johnson, K., & Tashiro, J. (2013). Interprofessional care and health care complexity: Factors shaping human resources effectiveness in health information management. In I. Management Association (Ed.), User-Driven Healthcare: Concepts, Methodologies, Tools, and Applications (pp. 1273-1302). Hershey, PA: IGI Global. doi:10.4018/978-1-4666-2770-3.ch064

Jose, J. (2013). Pharmacovigilance: Basic concepts and applications of pharmacoinformatics. In I. Management Association (Ed.), Bioinformatics: Concepts, methodologies, tools, and applications (pp. 1453-1473). Hershey, PA: IGI Global. doi:10.4018/978-1-4666-3604-0.ch075

Kalina, J., & Zvárová, J. (2013). Decision support systems in the process of improving patient safety. In A. Moumtzoglou & A. Kastania (Eds.), *E-health technologies and improving patient safety: Exploring organizational factors* (pp. 71–83). Hershey, PA: IGI Global. doi:10.4018/978-1-4666-2657-7.ch005

Kalina, J., & Zvárová, J. (2013). Decision support systems in the process of improving patient safety. In I. Management Association (Ed.), Bioinformatics: Concepts, methodologies, tools, and applications (pp. 1113-1125). Hershey, PA: IGI Global. doi:10.4018/978-1-4666-3604-0.ch057

Kamath, J. R., & Donahoe-Anshus, A. L. (2013). Electronic health record: Adoption, considerations and future direction. In I. Management Association (Ed.), User-driven healthcare: Concepts, methodologies, tools, and applications (pp. 34-56). Hershey, PA: IGI Global. doi:10.4018/978-1-4666-2770-3.ch003

Karamagkioli, K. Z., & Karamagioli, E. (2013). European e-health framework: Towards more "patient-friendly" healthcare services? In I. Management Association (Ed.), User-driven healthcare: Concepts, methodologies, tools, and applications (pp. 760-775). Hershey, PA: IGI Global. doi:10.4018/978-1-4666-2770-3.ch037

Kardaras, D. K., & Karakostas, B. (2013). Case studies in customization of e-health services. In I. Management Association (Ed.), User-driven healthcare: Concepts, methodologies, tools, and applications (pp. 1018-1036). Hershey, PA: IGI Global. doi:10.4018/978-1-4666-2770-3.ch051

Kastania, A. N. (2013). Evaluation considerations for e-health systems. In I. Management Association (Ed.), User-driven healthcare: Concepts, methodologies, tools, and applications (pp. 1126-1140). Hershey, PA: IGI Global. doi:10.4018/978-1-4666-2770-3.ch057

Kato, P. M. (2013). The role of the researcher in making serious games for health. In S. Arnab, I. Dunwell, & K. Debattista (Eds.), *Serious games for healthcare: Applications and implications* (pp. 213–231). Hershey, PA: IGI Global. doi:10.4018/978-1-4666-1903-6.ch010

Katsura, S. (2013). Preservation and reproduction of human motion based on a motion-copying system. In J. Wu (Ed.), *Technological advancements in biomedicine for healthcare applications* (pp. 375–384). Hershey, PA: IGI Global. doi:10.4018/978-1-4666-2196-1.ch037

Kikuchi, T. (2013). Human-friendly mechatronics systems with functional fluids and elastomers. In J. Wu (Ed.), *Technological advancements in biomedicine for healthcare applications* (pp. 94–101). Hershey, PA: IGI Global. doi:10.4018/978-1-4666-2196-1.ch010

Kimura, T., Miura, T., Shinohara, K., & Doi, S. (2013). Visual attention in 3-D space while moving forward. In J. Wu (Ed.), *Biomedical engineering and cognitive neuroscience for healthcare: Interdisciplinary applications* (pp. 81–88). Hershey, PA: IGI Global. doi:10.4018/978-1-4666-2113-8.ch009

Kldiashvili, E. (2013). Implementation of telecytology in Georgia. In V. Gulla, A. Mori, F. Gabbrielli, & P. Lanzafame (Eds.), *Telehealth networks for hospital services: New methodologies* (pp. 341–361). Hershey, PA: IGI Global. doi:10.4018/978-1-4666-2979-0.ch022

Kolovou, L. T., & Lymberopoulos, D. K. (2013). The concept of interoperability for AAL systems. In I. Management Association (Ed.), User-driven healthcare: Concepts, methodologies, tools, and applications (pp. 1364-1385). Hershey, PA: IGI Global. doi:10.4018/978-1-4666-2770-3.ch068

Koppar, A. R., & Sridhar, V. (2013). Malaria parasite detection: Automated method using microscope color image. In J. Rodrigues (Ed.), *Digital advances in medicine, e-health, and communication technologies* (pp. 289–300). Hershey, PA: IGI Global. doi:10.4018/978-1-4666-2794-9.ch016

Kotsonis, E., & Eliakis, S. (2013). Information security standards for health information systems: The implementer's approach. In I. Management Association (Ed.), User-driven healthcare: Concepts, methodologies, tools, and applications (pp. 225-257). Hershey, PA: IGI Global. doi:10.4018/978-1-4666-2770-3.ch013

Krishnaswamy, K., & Oates, T. (2014). Pathway to independence: Past, present, and beyond via robotics. In G. Kouroupetroglou (Ed.), *Disability informatics and web accessibility for motor limitations* (pp. 153–201). Hershey, PA: IGI Global. doi:10.4018/978-1-4666-4442-7.ch005

Kuehler, M., Schimke, N., & Hale, J. (2013). Privacy considerations for electronic health records. In I. Management Association (Ed.), User-driven healthcare: Concepts, methodologies, tools, and applications (pp. 1387-1402). Hershey, PA: IGI Global. doi:10.4018/978-1-4666-2770-3.ch069

Kurita, Y., Ikeda, A., Nagata, K., Okajima, M., & Ogasawara, T. (2013). Biomedical robotics for healthcare. In J. Wu (Ed.), *Technological advancements in biomedicine for healthcare applications* (pp. 160–169). Hershey, PA: IGI Global. doi:10.4018/978-1-4666-2196-1.ch017

Lakkaraju, S., & Lakkaraju, S. (2013). Mobile device application in healthcare. In S. Sarnikar, D. Bennett, & M. Gaynor (Eds.), *Cases on healthcare information technology for patient care management* (pp. 276–307). Hershey, PA: IGI Global. doi:10.4018/978-1-4666-2671-3.ch016

Laskowski, M. (2013). A prototype agent based model and machine learning hybrid system for healthcare decision support. In J. Rodrigues (Ed.), *Digital advances in medicine, e-health, and communication technologies* (pp. 230–253). Hershey, PA: IGI Global. doi:10.4018/978-1-4666-2794-9.ch013

Lee, T. (2014). Mobile healthcare computing in the cloud. In J. Rodrigues, K. Lin, & J. Lloret (Eds.), *Mobile networks and cloud computing convergence for progressive services and applications* (pp. 275–294). Hershey, PA: IGI Global. doi:10.4018/978-1-4666-4781-7.ch015

Lelardeux, C., Alvarez, J., Montaut, T., Galaup, M., & Lagarrigue, P. (2013). Healthcare games and the metaphoric approach. In S. Arnab, I. Dunwell, & K. Debattista (Eds.), *Serious games for healthcare: Applications and implications* (pp. 23–49). Hershey, PA: IGI Global. doi:10.4018/978-1-4666-1903-6.ch002

Lhotska, L., Bursa, M., Huptych, M., Chudacek, V., & Havlik, J. (2013). Interoperability of medical devices and information systems. In M. Cruz-Cunha, I. Miranda, & P. Gonçalves (Eds.), *Handbook of research on ICTs for human-centered healthcare and social care services* (pp. 749–762). Hershey, PA: IGI Global. doi:10.4018/978-1-4666-3986-7.ch039

Li, X., Lin, Z., & Wu, J. (2013). Language processing in the human brain of literate and illiterate subjects. In J. Wu (Ed.), *Biomedical engineering and cognitive neuroscience for healthcare: Interdisciplinary applications* (pp. 201–209). Hershey, PA: IGI Global. doi:10.4018/978-1-4666-2113-8.ch021

Liao, H. (2013). Biomedical information processing and visualization for minimally invasive neurosurgery. In J. Wu (Ed.), *Technological advancements in biomedicine for healthcare applications* (pp. 36–46). Hershey, PA: IGI Global. doi:10.4018/978-1-4666-2196-1.ch005

Libreri, C., & Graffigna, G. (2014). How web 2.0 shapes patient knowledge sharing: The case of diabetes in Italy. In C. El Morr (Ed.), *Research perspectives on the role of informatics in health policy and management* (pp. 238–260). Hershey, PA: IGI Global. doi:10.4018/978-1-4666-4321-5.ch014

Lin, C., Huang, Y., Li, C., & Jalleh, G. (2013). Key health information systems outsourcing issues from six hospital cases. In I. Management Association (Ed.), User-driven healthcare: Concepts, methodologies, tools, and applications (pp. 824-837). Hershey, PA: IGI Global. doi:10.4018/978-1-4666-2770-3.ch041

Lin, L., Chen, Y., Wu, J., & Tennyson, R. D. (2013). What skill/knowledge is important to a nursing professional? In P. Ordóñez de Pablos (Ed.), *Business, technology, and knowledge management in Asia: Trends and innovations* (pp. 234–249). Hershey, PA: IGI Global. doi:10.4018/978-1-4666-2652-2.ch018

Liu, G. (2014). Using case costing data and case mix for funding and benchmarking in rehabilitation hospitals. In C. El Morr (Ed.), *Research perspectives on the role of informatics in health policy and management* (pp. 62–78). Hershey, PA: IGI Global. doi:10.4018/978-1-4666-4321-5.ch005

Lixun, Z., Dapeng, B., & Lei, Y. (2013). Design of and experimentation with a walking assistance robot. In J. Wu (Ed.), *Technological advancements in biomedicine for healthcare applications* (pp. 123–127). Hershey, PA: IGI Global. doi:10.4018/978-1-4666-2196-1.ch013

Lui, K. (2013). The health informatics professional. In I. Management Association (Ed.), User-driven healthcare: Concepts, methodologies, tools, and applications (pp. 120-141). Hershey, PA: IGI Global. doi:10.4018/978-1-4666-2770-3.ch007

Ma, X., Chen, G., & Xiao, J. (2013). Understanding weight change behaviors through online social networks. In A. Gangopadhyay (Ed.), *Methods, models, and computation for medical informatics* (pp. 189–214). Hershey, PA: IGI Global. doi:10.4018/978-1-4666-2653-9.ch012

Makikawa, M., Okada, S., Fujiwara, Y., & Esaki, M. (2013). Sleep monitoring system equipped with a flexible non-contact ECG, respiration, and body motion sensor. In J. Wu (Ed.), *Technological advancements in biomedicine for healthcare applications* (pp. 287–297). Hershey, PA: IGI Global. doi:10.4018/978-1-4666-2196-1.ch030

Malindretos, G. (2013). Distribution and logistics outsourcing in the pharmaceutical sector. In D. Folinas (Ed.), *Outsourcing management for supply chain operations and logistics service* (pp. 202–222). Hershey, PA: IGI Global. doi:10.4018/978-1-4666-2008-7.ch012

Manvi, S. S., & B., M. R. (2013). A survey on health care services using wireless sensor networks. In M. Cruz-Cunha, I. Miranda, & P. Gonçalves (Eds.), *Handbook of research on ICTs for human-centered healthcare and social care services* (pp. 587-606). Hershey, PA: IGI Global. doi:10.4018/978-1-4666-3986-7.ch031

Marshall, S., & Hogan, J. (2013). The use of medical simulation to improve patient safety. In A. Moumtzoglou & A. Kastania (Eds.), *E-health technologies and improving patient safety: Exploring organizational factors* (pp. 155–172). Hershey, PA: IGI Global. doi:10.4018/978-1-4666-2657-7.ch011

Martin, J., & McKay, E. (2013). Mental health, post-secondary education, and information communications technology. In J. Lannon & E. Halpin (Eds.), *Human rights and information communication technologies: Trends and consequences of use* (pp. 196–213). Hershey, PA: IGI Global. doi:10.4018/978-1-4666-1918-0.ch012

Martin, J., & McKay, E. (2014). Mental health, post-secondary education, and information communications technology. In *Assistive technologies: Concepts, methodologies, tools, and applications* (pp. 1209–1226). Hershey, PA: IGI Global. doi:10.4018/978-1-4666-4422-9.ch063

Martin, V. (2013). Developing a library collection in bioinformatics: Support for an evolving profession. In I. Management Association (Ed.), Bioinformatics: Concepts, methodologies, tools, and applications (pp. 130-150). Hershey, PA: IGI Global. doi:10.4018/978-1-4666-3604-0.ch007

Masayuki, K., Eiji, K., Tetsuo, T., & Nozomu, M. (2013). Evaluation of olfactory impairment in Parkinson's disease using near-infrared spectroscopy. In J. Wu (Ed.), *Biomedical engineering and cognitive neuroscience for healthcare: Interdisciplinary applications* (pp. 293–302). Hershey, PA: IGI Global. doi:10.4018/978-1-4666-2113-8.ch030

Mazzanti, I., Maolo, A., & Antonicelli, R. (2013). E-health and telemedicine in the elderly: State of the art. In V. Gulla, A. Mori, F. Gabbrielli, & P. Lanzafame (Eds.), *Telehealth Networks for Hospital Services: New Methodologies* (pp. 33–43). Hershey, PA: IGI Global. doi:10.4018/978-1-4666-2979-0.ch003

Mazzanti, I., Maolo, A., & Antonicelli, R. (2014). E-health and telemedicine in the elderly: State of the art. In *Assistive technologies: Concepts, methodologies, tools, and applications* (pp. 693–704). Hershey, PA: IGI Global. doi:10.4018/978-1-4666-4422-9.ch034

McCrossan, B. A., & Casey, F. A. (2013). The role of telemedicine in paediatric cardiology. In V. Gulla, A. Mori, F. Gabbrielli, & P. Lanzafame (Eds.), *Telehealth networks for hospital services: New methodologies* (pp. 44–88). Hershey, PA: IGI Global. doi:10.4018/978-1-4666-2979-0.ch004

McGaha, J. (2013). Implementation issues on a national electronic health record network. In I. Management Association (Ed.), User-driven healthcare: Concepts, methodologies, tools, and applications (pp. 1236-1251). Hershey, PA: IGI Global. doi:10.4018/978-1-4666-2770-3.ch062

McGinnes, S., & Burke, M. (2013). Hoping for the best: A qualitative study of information technology in primary care. In M. Cruz-Cunha, I. Miranda, & P. Gonçalves (Eds.), *Handbook of research on ICTs and management systems for improving efficiency in healthcare and social care* (pp. 1088–1108). Hershey, PA: IGI Global. doi:10.4018/978-1-4666-3990-4.ch057

Medhekar, A., Wong, H. Y., & Hall, J. (2014). Innovation in medical tourism service marketing: A case of India. In A. Goyal (Ed.), *Innovations in services marketing and management: Strategies for emerging economies* (pp. 49–66). Hershey, PA: IGI Global. doi:10.4018/978-1-4666-4671-1.ch003

Medhekar, A., Wong, H. Y., & Hall, J. (2014). Medical tourism: A conceptual framework for an innovation in global healthcare provision. In A. Goyal (Ed.), *Innovations in services marketing and management: Strategies for emerging economies* (pp. 148–169). Hershey, PA: IGI Global. doi:10.4018/978-1-4666-4671-1.ch009

Menciassi, A., & Laschi, C. (2014). Biorobotics. In I. Management Association (Ed.), Robotics: Concepts, methodologies, tools, and applications (pp. 1613-1643). Hershey, PA: IGI Global. doi:10.4018/978-1-4666-4607-0.ch079

Mendes, D., & Rodrigues, I. P. (2013). A semantic web pragmatic approach to develop clinical ontologies, and thus semantic interoperability, based in HL7 v2.xml messaging. In R. Martinho, R. Rijo, M. Cruz-Cunha, & J. Varajão (Eds.), *Information systems and technologies for enhancing health and social care* (pp. 205–214). Hershey, PA: IGI Global. doi:10.4018/978-1-4666-3667-5.ch014

Mendoza-González, R., Martin, M. V., & Rodríguez-Martínez, L. C. (2013). Identifying the essential design requirements for usable e-health communities in mobile devices. In I. Management Association (Ed.), User-driven healthcare: Concepts, methodologies, tools, and applications (pp. 533-552). Hershey, PA: IGI Global. doi:10.4018/978-1-4666-2770-3.ch027

Mettler, T. (2013). Transformation of the hospital supply chain: How to measure the maturity of supplier relationship management systems in hospitals? In J. Tan (Ed.), *Healthcare information technology innovation and sustainability: Frontiers and adoption* (pp. 180–192). Hershey, PA: IGI Global. doi:10.4018/978-1-4666-2797-0.ch011

Miesenberger, K., Nussbaum, G., & Ossmann, R. (2014). AsTeRICS: A framework for including sensor technology into AT solutions for people with motor disabilities. In G. Kouroupetroglou (Ed.), *Assistive technologies and computer access for motor disabilities* (pp. 154–179). Hershey, PA: IGI Global. doi:10.4018/978-1-4666-4438-0.ch006

Miller, K., & Sankaranarayanan, S. (2013). Applications of policy based agents in wireless body sensor mesh networks for patient health monitoring. In J. Rodrigues (Ed.), *Digital advances in medicine, e-health, and communication technologies* (pp. 85–101). Hershey, PA: IGI Global. doi:10.4018/978-1-4666-2794-9.ch005

Mohammadian, M., & Jentzsch, R. (2013). User and data classification for a secure and practical approach for patient-doctor profiling using an RFID framework in hospital. In S. Sarnikar, D. Bennett, & M. Gaynor (Eds.), *Cases on healthcare information technology for patient care management* (pp. 224–253). Hershey, PA: IGI Global. doi:10.4018/978-1-4666-2671-3.ch014

Monguet, J. M., Huerta, E., Fernández, J., Ferruzca, M., & Badillo, S. (2013). E-health business models prototyping by incremental design. In I. Management Association (Ed.), User-driven healthcare: Concepts, methodologies, tools, and applications (pp. 776-790). Hershey, PA: IGI Global. doi:10.4018/978-1-4666-2770-3.ch038

Montazemi, A. R., Pittaway, J. J., & Keshavjee, K. (2013). State of IS integration in the context of patient-centered care: A network analysis and research directions. In J. Tan (Ed.), *Healthcare information technology innovation and sustainability: Frontiers and adoption* (pp. 127–144). Hershey, PA: IGI Global. doi:10.4018/978-1-4666-2797-0.ch008

Mori, A. R., Contenti, M., & Verbicaro, R. (2013). Policies on telemedicine-enhanced hospital services: Prioritization criteria for the interventions at regional level. In V. Gulla, A. Mori, F. Gabbrielli, & P. Lanzafame (Eds.), *Telehealth networks for hospital services: New methodologies* (pp. 1–14). Hershey, PA: IGI Global. doi:10.4018/978-1-4666-2979-0.ch001

Morita, A. (2013). The quantitative EEG change in Parkinson's disease. In J. Wu (Ed.), *Biomedical engineering and cognitive neuroscience for healthcare: Interdisciplinary applications* (pp. 225–234). Hershey, PA: IGI Global. doi:10.4018/978-1-4666-2113-8.ch023

Moromugi, S., & Ishimatsu, T. (2013). A strength training machine with a dynamic resistance control function based on muscle activity level. In J. Wu (Ed.), *Technological advancements in biomedicine for healthcare applications* (pp. 102–110). Hershey, PA: IGI Global. doi:10.4018/978-1-4666-2196-1.ch011

Morrow, D., & Chin, J. (2013). Technology as a bridge between health care systems and older adults. In R. Zheng, R. Hill, & M. Gardner (Eds.), *Engaging older adults with modern technology: Internet use and information access needs* (pp. 59–79). Hershey, PA: IGI Global. doi:10.4018/978-1-4666-1966-1.ch004

Morrow, D., & Chin, J. (2013). Technology as a bridge between health care systems and older adults. In I. Management Association (Ed.), User-driven healthcare: Concepts, methodologies, tools, and applications (pp. 99-119). Hershey, PA: IGI Global. doi:10.4018/978-1-4666-2770-3.ch006

Mostafa, R., Hasan, G. M., Kabir, A. A., & Rahman, M. A. (2013). Proposed framework for the deployment of telemedicine centers in rural Bangladesh. In J. Rodrigues (Ed.), *Digital advances in medicine, e-health, and communication technologies* (pp. 254–270). Hershey, PA: IGI Global. doi:10.4018/978-1-4666-2794-9.ch014

Motoi, K., Ogawa, M., Yamakoshi, T., & Yamakoshi, K. (2013). Fusion physiological sensing system for healthcare. In J. Wu (Ed.), *Technological advancements in biomedicine for healthcare applications* (pp. 298–313). Hershey, PA: IGI Global. doi:10.4018/978-1-4666-2196-1.ch031

Motorny, S. P. (2013). Big information technology bet of a small community hospital. In S. Sarnikar, D. Bennett, & M. Gaynor (Eds.), *Cases on healthcare information technology for patient care management* (pp. 70–94). Hershey, PA: IGI Global. doi:10.4018/978-1-4666-2671-3.ch004

Moumtzoglou, A. (2013). Health 2.0 and medicine 2.0: Safety, ownership and privacy issues. In I. Management Association (Ed.), User-driven healthcare: Concepts, methodologies, tools, and applications (pp. 1508-1522). Hershey, PA: IGI Global. doi:10.4018/978-1-4666-2770-3.ch075

Moumtzoglou, A. (2013). Risk perception as a patient safety dimension. In A. Moumtzoglou & A. Kastania (Eds.), *E-health technologies and improving patient safety: Exploring organizational factors* (pp. 285–299). Hershey, PA: IGI Global. doi:10.4018/978-1-4666-2657-7.ch017

Msanjila, S. S. (2013). Emerging ICT challenges on provision of online HIV/AIDS advisory services. In M. Cruz-Cunha, I. Miranda, & P. Gonçalves (Eds.), *Handbook of research on ICTs for human-centered healthcare and social care services* (pp. 248–269). Hershey, PA: IGI Global. doi:10.4018/978-1-4666-3986-7.ch013

Müller, A. (2013). Improving the identification of medication names by increasing phonological awareness via a language-teaching computer game (medicina). In S. Arnab, I. Dunwell, & K. Debattista (Eds.), *Serious games for healthcare: Applications and implications* (pp. 283–295). Hershey, PA: IGI Global. doi:10.4018/978-1-4666-1903-6.ch014

Murakami, S., Kim, H., Tan, J. K., Ishikawa, S., & Aoki, T. (2013). The development of a quantitative method for the detection of periarticular osteoporosis using density features within ROIs from computed radiography images of the hand. In J. Wu (Ed.), *Technological advancements in biomedicine for healthcare applications* (pp. 55–67). Hershey, PA: IGI Global. doi:10.4018/978-1-4666-2196-1.ch007

Nadathur, S. G., & Warren, J. R. (2013). Formal-transfer in and out of stroke care units: An analysis using Bayesian networks. In J. Tan (Ed.), *Healthcare information technology innovation and sustainability: Frontiers and adoption* (pp. 193–207). Hershey, PA: IGI Global. doi:10.4018/978-1-4666-2797-0.ch012

Naidoo, V., & Naidoo, Y. (2014). Home telecare, medical implant, and mobile technology: Evolutions in geriatric care. In C. El Morr (Ed.), *Research perspectives on the role of informatics in health policy and management* (pp. 222–237). Hershey, PA: IGI Global. doi:10.4018/978-1-4666-4321-5.ch013

Nakagawa, S. (2013). Bone-conducted ultrasonic perception: An elucidation of perception mechanisms and the development of a novel hearing aid for the profoundly deaf. In J. Wu (Ed.), *Technological advancements in biomedicine for healthcare applications* (pp. 148–159). Hershey, PA: IGI Global. doi:10.4018/978-1-4666-2196-1.ch016

Nakai, M., & Niinomi, M. (2013). Recent progress in mechanically biocompatible titanium-based materials. In J. Wu (Ed.), *Technological advancements in biomedicine for healthcare applications* (pp. 206–212). Hershey, PA: IGI Global. doi:10.4018/978-1-4666-2196-1.ch022

Nakakuki, T., & Okada-Hatakeyama, M. (2013). Methods for the analysis of intracellular signal transduction systems. In J. Wu (Ed.), *Technological advancements in biomedicine for healthcare applications* (pp. 347–353). Hershey, PA: IGI Global. doi:10.4018/978-1-4666-2196-1.ch034

Nalin, M., Verga, M., Sanna, A., & Saranummi, N. (2013). Directions for ICT research in disease prevention. In M. Cruz-Cunha, I. Miranda, & P. Gonçalves (Eds.), *Handbook of research on ICTs for human-centered healthcare and social care services* (pp. 229–247). Hershey, PA: IGI Global. doi:10.4018/978-1-4666-3986-7.ch012

Nap, H. H., & Diaz-Orueta, U. (2013). Rehabilitation gaming. In S. Arnab, I. Dunwell, & K. Debattista (Eds.), *Serious games for healthcare: Applications and implications* (pp. 50–75). Hershey, PA: IGI Global. doi:10.4018/978-1-4666-1903-6.ch003

Narushima, T., & Ueda, K. (2013). Calcium phosphate coating on titanium by RF magnetron sputtering. In J. Wu (Ed.), *Technological advancements in biomedicine for healthcare applications* (pp. 223–233). Hershey, PA: IGI Global. doi:10.4018/978-1-4666-2196-1.ch024

Nava-Muñoz, S., & Morán, A. L. (2013). A review of notifications systems in elder care environments: Challenges and opportunities. In M. Cruz-Cunha, I. Miranda, & P. Gonçalves (Eds.), *Handbook of research on ICTs for human-centered healthcare and social care services* (pp. 407–429). Hershey, PA: IGI Global. doi:10.4018/978-1-4666-3986-7.ch022

Nganji, J. T., & Nggada, S. H. (2014). Adoption of blended learning technologies in selected secondary schools in Cameroon and Nigeria: Challenges in disability inclusion. In N. Ololube (Ed.), *Advancing technology and educational development through blended learning in emerging economies* (pp. 159–173). Hershey, PA: IGI Global. doi:10.4018/978-1-4666-4574-5.ch009

Nikolov, S., Vera, J., & Wolkenhauer, O. (2013). Bifurcation analysis of a model accounting for the 14-3-3s signalling compartmentalisation. In I. Management Association (Ed.), Bioinformatics: Concepts, methodologies, tools, and applications (pp. 851-859). Hershey, PA: IGI Global. doi:10.4018/978-1-4666-3604-0.ch046

Nishiguchi, H. (2013). Description of and applications for a motion analysis method for upper limbs. In J. Wu (Ed.), *Technological advancements in biomedicine for healthcare applications* (pp. 1–10). Hershey, PA: IGI Global. doi:10.4018/978-1-4666-2196-1.ch001

Nokata, M. (2013). Small medical robot. In J. Wu (Ed.), *Technological advancements in biomedicine for healthcare applications* (pp. 170–179). Hershey, PA: IGI Global. doi:10.4018/978-1-4666-2196-1.ch018

Noritsugu, T. (2013). Wearable power assist robot driven with pneumatic rubber artificial muscles. In J. Wu (Ed.), *Technological advancements in biomedicine for healthcare applications* (pp. 139–147). Hershey, PA: IGI Global. doi:10.4018/978-1-4666-2196-1.ch015

Noteboom, C. (2013). Physician interaction with EHR: The importance of stakeholder identification and change management. In S. Sarnikar, D. Bennett, & M. Gaynor (Eds.), *Cases on healthcare information technology for patient care management* (pp. 95–112). Hershey, PA: IGI Global. doi:10.4018/978-1-4666-2671-3.ch005

O'Hanlon, S. (2013). Avoiding adverse consequences of e-health. In A. Moumtzoglou & A. Kastania (Eds.), *E-health technologies and improving patient safety: Exploring organizational factors* (pp. 13–26). Hershey, PA: IGI Global. doi:10.4018/978-1-4666-2657-7.ch002

Ogawa, K., Nishio, S., Minato, T., & Ishiguro, H. (2013). Android robots as telepresence media. In J. Wu (Ed.), *Biomedical engineering and cognitive neuroscience for healthcare: Interdisciplinary applications* (pp. 54–63). Hershey, PA: IGI Global. doi:10.4018/978-1-4666-2113-8.ch006

Ohashi, M., Sakimura, N., Fujimoto, M., Hori, M., & Kurata, N. (2013). Technical perspective of authentication policy extension for the adaptive social services and e-health care management. In M. Cruz-Cunha, I. Miranda, & P. Gonçalves (Eds.), *Handbook of research on ICTs for human-centered healthcare and social care services* (pp. 719–726). Hershey, PA: IGI Global. doi:10.4018/978-1-4666-3986-7.ch037

Ohta, Y., & Uchida, M. (2013). Non-contact pulse monitoring using live imaging. In J. Wu (Ed.), *Technological advancements in biomedicine for healthcare applications* (pp. 240–246). Hershey, PA: IGI Global. doi:10.4018/978-1-4666-2196-1.ch026

Ohuchida, K., & Hashizume, M. (2013). Biomedical robotics for healthcare. In J. Wu (Ed.), *Technological advancements in biomedicine for healthcare applications* (pp. 200–205). Hershey, PA: IGI Global. doi:10.4018/978-1-4666-2196-1.ch021

Oikonomou, D., Moulianitis, V., Lekkas, D., & Koutsabasis, P. (2013). DSS for health emergency response: A contextual, user-centred approach. In R. Biswas (Ed.), *Clinical solutions and medical progress through user-driven healthcare* (pp. 51–69). Hershey, PA: IGI Global. doi:10.4018/978-1-4666-1876-3.ch006

Okamoto, S., Hirotomi, T., Aoki, K., & Hosomi, Y. (2013). Evaluation of walking motions with the aid of walkers using acceleration sensors. In J. Wu (Ed.), *Biomedical engineering and cognitive neuroscience for healthcare: Interdisciplinary applications* (pp. 346–354). Hershey, PA: IGI Global. doi:10.4018/978-1-4666-2113-8.ch036

Okamura, H. (2013). Rehabilitation of elderly people with dementia. In J. Wu (Ed.), *Biomedical engineering and cognitive neuroscience for healthcare: Interdisciplinary applications* (pp. 235–242). Hershey, PA: IGI Global. doi:10.4018/978-1-4666-2113-8.ch024

Olvera-Lobo, M., & Gutiérrez-Artacho, J. (2013). Searching health information in question-answering systems. In M. Cruz-Cunha, I. Miranda, & P. Gonçalves (Eds.), *Handbook of research on ICTs for human-centered healthcare and social care services* (pp. 474–490). Hershey, PA: IGI Global. doi:10.4018/978-1-4666-3986-7.ch025

Padovani, E., Orelli, R. L., Agnoletti, V., & Buccioli, M. (2013). Low cost and human-centered innovations in healthcare services: A case of excellence in Italy. In S. Saeed & C. Reddick (Eds.), *Human-centered system design for electronic governance* (pp. 239–252). Hershey, PA: IGI Global. doi:10.4018/978-1-4666-3640-8.ch014

Paninchukunnath, A. (2014). Healthcare services delivery in India: special reference to mother and child health. In A. Goyal (Ed.), *Innovations in services marketing and management: Strategies for emerging economies* (pp. 170–189). Hershey, PA: IGI Global. doi:10.4018/978-1-4666-4671-1.ch010

Paparountas, T., Nikolaidou-Katsaridou, M. N., Rustici, G., & Aidinis, V. (2013). Data mining and meta-analysis on DNA microarray data. In I. Management Association (Ed.), Bioinformatics: Concepts, methodologies, tools, and applications (pp. 1196-1236). Hershey, PA: IGI Global. doi:10.4018/978-1-4666-3604-0.ch062

Parentela, G., Mancini, P., Naccarella, F., Feng, Z., & Rinaldi, G. (2013). Telemedicine, the European space agency, and the support to the african population for infectious disease problems: Potentiality and perspectives for Asia countries and China. In V. Gulla, A. Mori, F. Gabbrielli, & P. Lanzafame (Eds.), *Telehealth networks for hospital services: New methodologies* (pp. 89–96). Hershey, PA: IGI Global. doi:10.4018/978-1-4666-2979-0.ch005

Paterson, G. I., MacDonald, J. M., & Mensink, N. N. (2014). The administrative policy quandary in Canada's health service organizations. In C. El Morr (Ed.), *Research perspectives on the role of informatics in health policy and management* (pp. 116–134). Hershey, PA: IGI Global. doi:10.4018/978-1-4666-4321-5.ch008

Penchovsky, R. (2013). Engineering gene control circuits with allosteric ribozymes in human cells as a medicine of the future. In I. Management Association (Ed.), Bioinformatics: Concepts, methodologies, tools, and applications (pp. 860-883). Hershey, PA: IGI Global. doi:10.4018/978-1-4666-3604-0.ch047

Pereira, O. R., Caldeira, J. M., & Rodrigues, J. J. (2013). An advanced and secure symbian-based mobile approach for body sensor networks interaction. In J. Rodrigues (Ed.), *Digital advances in medicine, e-health, and communication technologies* (pp. 33–48). Hershey, PA: IGI Global. doi:10.4018/978-1-4666-2794-9.ch002

Petkovic, M., & Ibraimi, L. (2013). Privacy and security in e-health applications. In I. Management Association (Ed.), User-driven healthcare: Concepts, methodologies, tools, and applications (pp. 1141-1166). Hershey, PA: IGI Global. doi:10.4018/978-1-4666-2770-3.ch058

Peyton, L., & Hu, J. (2013). Identity management and audit trail support for privacy protection in e-health networks. In I. Management Association (Ed.), User-driven healthcare: Concepts, methodologies, tools, and applications (pp. 1112-1125). Hershey, PA: IGI Global. doi:10.4018/978-1-4666-2770-3.ch056

Pham, D. V., Halgamuge, M. N., Nirmalathas, T., & Moran, B. (2013). A centralized real-time e-healthcare system for remote detection and prediction of epileptic seizures. In I. Management Association (Ed.), User-driven healthcare: Concepts, methodologies, tools, and applications (pp. 326-356). Hershey, PA: IGI Global. doi:10.4018/978-1-4666-2770-3.ch017

Phua, C., Roy, P. C., Aloulou, H., Biswas, J., Tolstikov, A., & Foo, V. S. … Xu, D. (2014). State-of-the-art assistive technology for people with dementia. In Assistive technologies: Concepts, methodologies, tools, and applications (pp. 1606-1625). Hershey, PA: IGI Global. doi:10.4018/978-1-4666-4422-9.ch085

Pino, A. (2014). Augmentative and alternative communication systems for the motor disabled. In G. Kouroupetroglou (Ed.), *Disability informatics and web accessibility for motor limitations* (pp. 105–152). Hershey, PA: IGI Global. doi:10.4018/978-1-4666-4442-7.ch004

Portela, F., Cabral, A., Abelha, A., Salazar, M., Quintas, C., Machado, J., ... Santos, M. F. (2013). Knowledge acquisition process for intelligent decision support in critical health care. In R. Martinho, R. Rijo, M. Cruz-Cunha, & J. Varajão (Eds.), *Information systems and technologies for enhancing health and social care* (pp. 55–68). Hershey, PA: IGI Global. doi:10.4018/978-1-4666-3667-5.ch004

Previtali, P. (2013). Grid technology for archive solutions in health care organizations. In A. Moumtzoglou & A. Kastania (Eds.), *E-health technologies and improving patient safety: Exploring organizational factors* (pp. 148–154). Hershey, PA: IGI Global. doi:10.4018/978-1-4666-2657-7.ch010

Purkayastha, S. (2013). Design and implementation of mobile-based technology in strengthening health information system: Aligning mhealth solutions to infrastructures. In I. Management Association (Ed.), User-driven healthcare: Concepts, methodologies, tools, and applications (pp. 689-713). Hershey, PA: IGI Global. doi:10.4018/978-1-4666-2770-3.ch034

Qi, G., & Wu, J. (2013). Functional role of the left ventral occipito-temporal cortex in reading. In J. Wu (Ed.), *Biomedical engineering and cognitive neuroscience for healthcare: Interdisciplinary applications* (pp. 192–200). Hershey, PA: IGI Global. doi:10.4018/978-1-4666-2113-8.ch020

Queirós, A., Alvarelhão, J., Silva, A. G., Teixeira, A., & Pacheco da Rocha, N. (2013). A conceptual framework for the design and development of AAL services. In M. Cruz-Cunha, I. Miranda, & P. Gonçalves (Eds.), *Handbook of research on ICTs for human-centered healthcare and social care services* (pp. 568–586). Hershey, PA: IGI Global. doi:10.4018/978-1-4666-3986-7.ch030

Ravka, N. (2014). Informatics and health services: The potential benefits and challenges of electronic health records and personal electronic health records in patient care, cost control, and health research – An overview. In C. El Morr (Ed.), *Research perspectives on the role of informatics in health policy and management* (pp. 89–114). Hershey, PA: IGI Global. doi:10.4018/978-1-4666-4321-5.ch007

Reibling, N., & Wendt, C. (2013). Regulating patients' access to healthcare services. In M. Merviö (Ed.), *Healthcare management and economics: Perspectives on public and private administration* (pp. 53–68). Hershey, PA: IGI Global. doi:10.4018/978-1-4666-3982-9.ch005

Reis, C. I., Freire, C. S., Fernández, J., & Monguet, J. M. (2013). Patient centered design: Challenges and lessons learned from working with health professionals and schizophrenic patients in e-therapy contexts. In R. Martinho, R. Rijo, M. Cruz-Cunha, & J. Varajão (Eds.), *Information systems and technologies for enhancing health and social care* (pp. 120–135). Hershey, PA: IGI Global. doi:10.4018/978-1-4666-3667-5.ch008

Remmers, H., & Hülsken-Giesler, M. (2013). e-Health technologies in home care nursing: Recent survey results and subsequent ethical issues. In I. Management Association (Ed.), User-driven healthcare: Concepts, methodologies, tools, and applications (pp. 396-420). Hershey, PA: IGI Global. doi:10.4018/978-1-4666-2770-3.ch020

Ricketts, M. (2014). Making health information personal: How anecdotes bring concepts to life. In S. Hai-Jew (Ed.), *Packaging digital information for enhanced learning and analysis: Data visualization, spatialization, and multidimensionality* (pp. 1–36). Hershey, PA: IGI Global. doi:10.4018/978-1-4666-4462-5.ch001

Rocha, Á. (2013). Evolution of information systems and technologies maturity in healthcare. In J. Tan (Ed.), *Healthcare information technology innovation and sustainability: Frontiers and adoption* (pp. 238–246). Hershey, PA: IGI Global. doi:10.4018/978-1-4666-2797-0.ch015

Rodríguez-Gómez, D., & Gairín, J. (2014). Communities of practice in the Catalan public administration: Promoting their improvement. In Y. Al-Bastaki & A. Shajera (Eds.), *Building a competitive public sector with knowledge management strategy* (pp. 383–402). Hershey, PA: IGI Global. doi:10.4018/978-1-4666-4434-2.ch018

Rodríguez-Solano, C., Lezcano, L., & Sicilia, M. (2013). Automated generation of SNOMED CT subsets from clinical guidelines. In R. Martinho, R. Rijo, M. Cruz-Cunha, & J. Varajão (Eds.), *Information systems and technologies for enhancing health and social care* (pp. 190–204). Hershey, PA: IGI Global. doi:10.4018/978-1-4666-3667-5.ch013

Rosu, S. M., & Dragoi, G. (2014). E-health sites development using open source software and OMT methodology as support for family doctors' activities: A Romanian case study. In M. Cruz-Cunha, F. Moreira, & J. Varajão (Eds.), *Handbook of research on enterprise 2.0: Technological, social, and organizational dimensions* (pp. 72–88). Hershey, PA: IGI Global. doi:10.4018/978-1-4666-4373-4.ch004

Roy, N., Das, S. K., & Julien, C. (2013). Resolving and mediating ambiguous contexts in pervasive environments. In I. Management Association (Ed.), User-driven healthcare: Concepts, methodologies, tools, and applications (pp. 630-654). Hershey, PA: IGI Global. doi:10.4018/978-1-4666-2770-3.ch031

Russo, M. R. (2014). Emergency management professional development: Linking information communication technology and social communication skills to enhance a sense of community and social justice in the 21st century. In I. Management Association (Ed.), Crisis management: Concepts, methodologies, tools and applications (pp. 651-665). Hershey, PA: IGI Global. doi:10.4018/978-1-4666-4707-7.ch031

Sabone, M. B., Mogobe, K. D., & Sabone, T. G. (2013). ICTS and their role in health promotion: A preliminary situation analysis in selected botswana rural communities. In I. Management Association (Ed.), User-driven healthcare: Concepts, methodologies, tools, and applications (pp. 211-224). Hershey, PA: IGI Global. doi:10.4018/978-1-4666-2770-3.ch012

Saha, P. (2014). Systemic enterprise architecture as future: Tackling complexity in governments in the cusp of change. In P. Saha (Ed.), *A systemic perspective to managing complexity with enterprise architecture* (pp. 1–70). Hershey, PA: IGI Global. doi:10.4018/978-1-4666-4518-9.ch001

Saijo, Y. (2013). Biomedical application of multimodal ultrasound microscope. In J. Wu (Ed.), *Technological advancements in biomedicine for healthcare applications* (pp. 27–35). Hershey, PA: IGI Global. doi:10.4018/978-1-4666-2196-1.ch004

Santos, M., Bastião, L., Costa, C., Silva, A., & Rocha, N. (2013). Clinical data mining in small hospital PACS: Contributions for radiology department improvement. In R. Martinho, R. Rijo, M. Cruz-Cunha, & J. Varajão (Eds.), *Information systems and technologies for enhancing health and social care* (pp. 236–251). Hershey, PA: IGI Global. doi:10.4018/978-1-4666-3667-5.ch016

Santos, M. F., Portela, F., Miranda, M., Machado, J., Abelha, A., Silva, Á., & Rua, F. (2013). Grid data mining strategies for outcome prediction in distributed intensive care units. In R. Martinho, R. Rijo, M. Cruz-Cunha, & J. Varajão (Eds.), *Information systems and technologies for enhancing health and social care* (pp. 87–101). Hershey, PA: IGI Global. doi:10.4018/978-1-4666-3667-5.ch006

Santos, R. J., Bernardino, J., & Vieira, M. (2013). A hypotension surveillance and prediction system for critical care. In M. Cruz-Cunha, I. Miranda, & P. Gonçalves (Eds.), *Handbook of research on ICTs and management systems for improving efficiency in healthcare and social care* (pp. 341–355). Hershey, PA: IGI Global. doi:10.4018/978-1-4666-3990-4.ch017

Sanz, P. R., Mezcua, B. R., & Pena, J. M. (2013). ICTs for orientation and mobility for blind people: A state of the art. In M. Cruz-Cunha, I. Miranda, & P. Gonçalves (Eds.), *Handbook of research on ICTs for human-centered healthcare and social care services* (pp. 646–669). Hershey, PA: IGI Global. doi:10.4018/978-1-4666-3986-7.ch034

Sarabdeen, J. (2013). Legal issues in e-healthcare systems. In I. Management Association (Ed.), User-driven healthcare: Concepts, methodologies, tools, and applications (pp. 1194-1219). Hershey, PA: IGI Global. doi:10.4018/978-1-4666-2770-3.ch060

Sarbadhikari, S. N. (2013). Unlearning and relearning in online health education. In I. Management Association (Ed.), User-driven healthcare: Concepts, methodologies, tools, and applications (pp. 1348-1363). Hershey, PA: IGI Global. doi:10.4018/978-1-4666-2770-3.ch067

Sasayama, T., Hamada, S., & Kobayashi, T. (2013). Application of prewhitening beamformer with linear constraints for correlated EEG signal source estimation. In J. Wu (Ed.), *Biomedical engineering and cognitive neuroscience for healthcare: Interdisciplinary applications* (pp. 243–254). Hershey, PA: IGI Global. doi:10.4018/978-1-4666-2113-8.ch025

Sato, T., & Minato, K. (2013). Differences in analysis methods of the human uncinate fasciculus using diffusion tensor MRI. In J. Wu (Ed.), *Biomedical engineering and cognitive neuroscience for healthcare: Interdisciplinary applications* (pp. 162–170). Hershey, PA: IGI Global. doi:10.4018/978-1-4666-2113-8.ch017

Satoh, J. (2013). Molecular network analysis of target RNAs and interacting proteins of TDP-43, a causative gene for the neurodegenerative diseases ALS/FTLD. In I. Management Association (Ed.), Bioinformatics: Concepts, methodologies, tools, and applications (pp. 964-985). Hershey, PA: IGI Global. doi:10.4018/978-1-4666-3604-0.ch052

Satoh, J. (2013). Molecular network analysis of target RNAs and interacting proteins of TDP-43, a causative gene for the neurodegenerative diseases ALS/FTLD. In J. Wu (Ed.), *Technological advancements in biomedicine for healthcare applications* (pp. 314–335). Hershey, PA: IGI Global. doi:10.4018/978-1-4666-2196-1.ch032

Schafer, S. B. (2013). Fostering psychological coherence: With ICTs. In M. Cruz-Cunha, I. Miranda, & P. Gonçalves (Eds.), *Handbook of research on ICTs for human-centered healthcare and social care services* (pp. 29–47). Hershey, PA: IGI Global. doi:10.4018/978-1-4666-3986-7.ch002

Schmeida, M., & McNeal, R. (2013). Bridging the inequality gap to accessing medicare and medicaid information online: An empirical analysis of e-government success 2002 through 2010. In J. Gil-Garcia (Ed.), *E-government success around the world: Cases, empirical studies, and practical recommendations* (pp. 60–78). Hershey, PA: IGI Global. doi:10.4018/978-1-4666-4173-0.ch004

Scholl, J. C., & Olaniran, B. A. (2013). ICT use and multidisciplinary healthcare teams. In M. Cruz-Cunha, I. Miranda, & P. Gonçalves (Eds.), *Handbook of research on ICTs for human-centered healthcare and social care services* (pp. 627–645). Hershey, PA: IGI Global. doi:10.4018/978-1-4666-3986-7.ch033

Serenko, N. (2013). The impact of genetic testing and genetic information on ethical, legal and social issues in North America: The framework. In I. Management Association (Ed.), Bioinformatics: Concepts, methodologies, tools, and applications (pp. 1317-1333). Hershey, PA: IGI Global. doi:10.4018/978-1-4666-3604-0.ch067

Serrano, M., Elmisery, A., Foghlú, M. Ó., Donnelly, W., Storni, C., & Fernström, M. (2013). Pervasive computing support in the transition towards personalised health systems. In J. Rodrigues (Ed.), *Digital advances in medicine, e-health, and communication technologies* (pp. 49–64). Hershey, PA: IGI Global. doi:10.4018/978-1-4666-2794-9.ch003

Shaw, V., & Braa, J. (2013). "Developed in the south": An evolutionary and prototyping approach to developing scalable and sustainable health information systems. In I. Management Association (Ed.), User-driven healthcare: Concepts, methodologies, tools, and applications (pp. 583-607). Hershey, PA: IGI Global. doi:10.4018/978-1-4666-2770-3.ch029

Shi, J., Upadhyaya, S., & Erdem, E. (2013). Health information exchange for improving the efficiency and quality of healthcare delivery. In I. Management Association (Ed.), User-driven healthcare: Concepts, methodologies, tools, and applications (pp. 714-736). Hershey, PA: IGI Global. doi:10.4018/978-1-4666-2770-3.ch035

Shibata, T. (2013). A human-like cognitive computer based on a psychologically inspired VLSI brain model. In J. Wu (Ed.), *Technological advancements in biomedicine for healthcare applications* (pp. 247–266). Hershey, PA: IGI Global. doi:10.4018/978-1-4666-2196-1.ch027

Shimada, S. (2013). Self-body recognition and its impairment. In J. Wu (Ed.), *Biomedical engineering and cognitive neuroscience for healthcare: Interdisciplinary applications* (pp. 156–161). Hershey, PA: IGI Global. doi:10.4018/978-1-4666-2113-8.ch016

Shimogonya, Y., Ishikawa, T., Yamaguchi, T., Kumamaru, H., & Itoh, K. (2013). Computational study of the hemodynamics of cerebral aneurysm initiation. In J. Wu (Ed.), *Technological advancements in biomedicine for healthcare applications* (pp. 267–277). Hershey, PA: IGI Global. doi:10.4018/978-1-4666-2196-1.ch028

Shimonomura, K. (2013). A neuromorphic robot vision system to predict the response of visual neurons. In J. Wu (Ed.), *Technological advancements in biomedicine for healthcare applications* (pp. 193–199). Hershey, PA: IGI Global. doi:10.4018/978-1-4666-2196-1.ch020

Shrestha, S. (2013). Clinical decision support system for diabetes prevention: An illustrative case. In S. Sarnikar, D. Bennett, & M. Gaynor (Eds.), *Cases on healthcare information technology for patient care management* (pp. 308–329). Hershey, PA: IGI Global. doi:10.4018/978-1-4666-2671-3.ch017

Siddiqui, Z. S., & Jonas-Dwyer, D. R. (2013). Mobile learning in health professions education: A systematic review. In J. Keengwe (Ed.), *Pedagogical applications and social effects of mobile technology integration* (pp. 193–205). Hershey, PA: IGI Global. doi:10.4018/978-1-4666-2985-1.ch011

Silvana de Rosa, A., Fino, E., & Bocci, E. (2014). Addressing healthcare on-line demand and supply relating to mental illness: Knowledge sharing about psychiatry and psychoanalysis through social networks in Italy and France. In A. Kapoor & C. Kulshrestha (Eds.), *Dynamics of competitive advantage and consumer perception in social marketing* (pp. 16–55). Hershey, PA: IGI Global. doi:10.4018/978-1-4666-4430-4.ch002

Siqueira, S. R., Rocha, E. C., & Nery, M. S. (2013). Brazilian occupational therapy perspective about digital games as an inclusive resource to disabled people in schools. In I. Management Association (Ed.), User-driven healthcare: Concepts, methodologies, tools, and applications (pp. 918-937). Hershey, PA: IGI Global. doi:10.4018/978-1-4666-2770-3.ch046

Sliedrecht, S., & Kotzé, E. (2013). Patients with a spinal cord injury inform and co-construct services at a spinal cord rehabilitation unit. In I. Management Association (Ed.), User-driven healthcare: Concepts, methodologies, tools, and applications (pp. 1054-1072). Hershey, PA: IGI Global. doi:10.4018/978-1-4666-2770-3.ch053

Smedberg, Å. (2013). E-health communities for learning healthy habits: How to consider quality and usability. In I. Management Association (Ed.), User-driven healthcare: Concepts, methodologies, tools, and applications (pp. 310-325). Hershey, PA: IGI Global. doi:10.4018/978-1-4666-2770-3.ch016

Smedberg, Å., & Sandmark, H. (2013). Dynamic stress management: Self-help through holistic system design. In I. Management Association (Ed.), User-driven healthcare: Concepts, methodologies, tools, and applications (pp. 1469-1486). Hershey, PA: IGI Global. doi:10.4018/978-1-4666-2770-3.ch073

Sobol, M., & Prater, E. (2013). Adoption, usage and efficiency: Benchmarking healthcare IT in private practices. In J. Tan (Ed.), *Healthcare information technology innovation and sustainability: Frontiers and adoption* (pp. 145–159). Hershey, PA: IGI Global. doi:10.4018/978-1-4666-2797-0.ch009

Sobrinho, Á. A., Dias da Silva, L., Melo de Medeiros, L., & Pinheiro, M. E. (2013). A mobile assistant to aid early detection of chronic kidney disease. In R. Martinho, R. Rijo, M. Cruz-Cunha, & J. Varajão (Eds.), *Information systems and technologies for enhancing health and social care* (pp. 309–323). Hershey, PA: IGI Global. doi:10.4018/978-1-4666-3667-5.ch020

Soomlek, C., & Benedicenti, L. (2013). Agent-based wellness indicator. In V. Gulla, A. Mori, F. Gabbrielli, & P. Lanzafame (Eds.), *Telehealth networks for hospital services: New methodologies* (pp. 300–330). Hershey, PA: IGI Global. doi:10.4018/978-1-4666-2979-0.ch020

Spadaro, L., Timpano, F., Marino, S., & Bramanti, P. (2013). Telemedicine and Alzheimer disease: ICT-based services for people with Alzheimer disease and their caregivers. In V. Gulla, A. Mori, F. Gabbrielli, & P. Lanzafame (Eds.), *Telehealth networks for hospital services: New methodologies* (pp. 191–206). Hershey, PA: IGI Global. doi:10.4018/978-1-4666-2979-0.ch013

Springer, J. A., Beever, J., Morar, N., Sprague, J. E., & Kane, M. D. (2013). Ethics, privacy, and the future of genetic information in healthcare information assurance and security. In I. Management Association (Ed.), Bioinformatics: Concepts, methodologies, tools, and applications (pp. 1405-1423). Hershey, PA: IGI Global. doi:10.4018/978-1-4666-3604-0.ch072

Stachura, M. E., Wood, J., Angjellari-Dajci, F., Grayson, J., Astapova, E. V., Tung, H., . . . Lawless, W. (2013). Representing organizational conservation of information: A review of telemedicine and e-health in Georgia. In I. Management Association (Ed.), User-driven healthcare: Concepts, methodologies, tools, and applications (pp. 1220-1235). Hershey, PA: IGI Global. doi:10.4018/978-1-4666-2770-3.ch061

Stefaniak, J. E. (2013). Resuscitating team roles within wayburn health system. In A. Ritzhaupt & S. Kumar (Eds.), *Cases on educational technology implementation for facilitating learning* (pp. 130–145). Hershey, PA: IGI Global. doi:10.4018/978-1-4666-3676-7.ch008

Sugiura, M. (2013). A cognitive neuroscience approach to self and mental health. In J. Wu (Ed.), *Biomedical engineering and cognitive neuroscience for healthcare: Interdisciplinary applications* (pp. 1–10). Hershey, PA: IGI Global. doi:10.4018/978-1-4666-2113-8.ch001

Supnithi, T., Buranarach, M., Thatphithakkul, N., Junsirimongkol, B., Wongrochananan, S., Kulnawan, N., & Jiamjarasrangsi, W. (2014). A self-management service framework to support chronic disease patients' self-management. In M. Kosaka & K. Shirahada (Eds.), *Progressive trends in knowledge and system-based science for service innovation* (pp. 425–450). Hershey, PA: IGI Global. doi:10.4018/978-1-4666-4663-6.ch023

Takahashi, K., & Watanabe, K. (2013). Crossmodal interactions in visual competition. In J. Wu (Ed.), *Biomedical engineering and cognitive neuroscience for healthcare: Interdisciplinary applications* (pp. 64–72). Hershey, PA: IGI Global. doi:10.4018/978-1-4666-2113-8.ch007

Tamiya, T., Kawanishi, M., Miyake, K., Kawai, N., & Guo, S. (2013). Neurosurgical operations using navigation microscope integration system. In J. Wu (Ed.), *Technological advancements in biomedicine for healthcare applications* (pp. 128–138). Hershey, PA: IGI Global. doi:10.4018/978-1-4666-2196-1.ch014

Tan, R., Wang, S., Jiang, Y., Ishida, K., & Fujie, M. G. (2013). Motion control of an omni-directional walker for walking support. In J. Wu (Ed.), *Biomedical engineering and cognitive neuroscience for healthcare: Interdisciplinary applications* (pp. 20–28). Hershey, PA: IGI Global. doi:10.4018/978-1-4666-2113-8.ch003

Tanaka, H., & Furutani, M. (2013). Sleep management promotes healthy lifestyle, mental health, QOL, and a healthy brain. In J. Wu (Ed.), *Biomedical engineering and cognitive neuroscience for healthcare: Interdisciplinary applications* (pp. 211–224). Hershey, PA: IGI Global. doi:10.4018/978-1-4666-2113-8.ch022

Tang, C., & Carpendale, S. (2013). Human-centered design for health information technology: A qualitative approach. In I. Management Association (Ed.), User-driven healthcare: Concepts, methodologies, tools, and applications (pp. 158-179). Hershey, PA: IGI Global. doi:10.4018/978-1-4666-2770-3.ch009

Tang, X., Gao, Y., Yang, W., Zhang, M., & Wu, J. (2013). Audiovisual integration of natural auditory and visual stimuli in the real-world situation. In J. Wu (Ed.), *Biomedical engineering and cognitive neuroscience for healthcare: Interdisciplinary applications* (pp. 337–344). Hershey, PA: IGI Global. doi:10.4018/978-1-4666-2113-8.ch035

Targowski, A. (2013). Well-being, wisdom, health, and IT: From the big-picture to the small-picture. In M. Cruz-Cunha, I. Miranda, & P. Gonçalves (Eds.), *Handbook of research on ICTs for human-centered healthcare and social care services* (pp. 1–28). Hershey, PA: IGI Global. doi:10.4018/978-1-4666-3986-7.ch001

Tayabali, S., & Martin, C. M. (2013). The need to transform the core values of medical care and health organizations. In R. Biswas (Ed.), *Clinical solutions and medical progress through user-driven healthcare* (pp. 85–92). Hershey, PA: IGI Global. doi:10.4018/978-1-4666-1876-3.ch009

Taylor, B. W. (2014). Decision-making and decision support in acute care. In C. El Morr (Ed.), *Research perspectives on the role of informatics in health policy and management* (pp. 1–18). Hershey, PA: IGI Global. doi:10.4018/978-1-4666-4321-5.ch001

Teixeira, C., Pinto, J. S., Ferreira, F., Oliveira, A., Teixeira, A., & Pereira, C. (2013). Cloud computing enhanced service development architecture for the living usability lab. In R. Martinho, R. Rijo, M. Cruz-Cunha, & J. Varajão (Eds.), *Information systems and technologies for enhancing health and social care* (pp. 33–53). Hershey, PA: IGI Global. doi:10.4018/978-1-4666-3667-5.ch003

Teixeira, L., Saavedra, V., Ferreira, C., & Santos, B. S. (2013). The role of ICTs in the management of rare chronic diseases: The case of hemophilia. In M. Cruz-Cunha, I. Miranda, & P. Gonçalves (Eds.), *Handbook of research on ICTs and management systems for improving efficiency in healthcare and social care* (pp. 635–649). Hershey, PA: IGI Global. doi:10.4018/978-1-4666-3990-4.ch033

Teoh, S. Y., Singh, M., & Chong, J. (2013). An overview of e-health development in Australia. In I. Management Association (Ed.), User-driven healthcare: Concepts, methodologies, tools, and applications (pp. 901-917). Hershey, PA: IGI Global. doi:10.4018/978-1-4666-2770-3.ch045

Tiwari, S., & Srivastava, R. (2014). Research and developments in medical image reconstruction methods and its applications. In R. Srivastava, S. Singh, & K. Shukla (Eds.), *Research developments in computer vision and image processing: Methodologies and applications* (pp. 274–312). Hershey, PA: IGI Global. doi:10.4018/978-1-4666-4558-5.ch014

Tobolcea, I. (2013). The psychosocial impact of ICT efficiency on speech disorders-treatment. In M. Cruz-Cunha, I. Miranda, & P. Gonçalves (Eds.), *Handbook of research on ICTs for human-centered healthcare and social care services* (pp. 70–92). Hershey, PA: IGI Global. doi:10.4018/978-1-4666-3986-7.ch004

Toda, T., Chen, P., Ozaki, S., Fujita, K., & Ideguchi, N. (2013). A simple web-based image database system for facilitating medical care in dermatological clinics. In I. Management Association (Ed.), User-driven healthcare: Concepts, methodologies, tools, and applications (pp. 502-513). Hershey, PA: IGI Global. doi:10.4018/978-1-4666-2770-3.ch025

Toda, T., Chen, P., Ozaki, S., Fujita, K., & Ideguchi, N. (2013). A simple web-based image database system for facilitating medical care in dermatological clinics. In J. Wu (Ed.), *Technological advancements in biomedicine for healthcare applications* (pp. 385–397). Hershey, PA: IGI Global. doi:10.4018/978-1-4666-2196-1.ch038

Trudeau, S. (2013). CoRDS registry: An HIT case study concerning setup and maintenance of a disease registry. In S. Sarnikar, D. Bennett, & M. Gaynor (Eds.), *Cases on healthcare information technology for patient care management* (pp. 197–207). Hershey, PA: IGI Global. doi:10.4018/978-1-4666-2671-3.ch012

Tseng, R., & Yi-Luen Do, E. (2013). The role of information and computer technology for children with autism spectrum disorder and the facial expression wonderland (FEW). In A. Gangopadhyay (Ed.), *Methods, models, and computation for medical informatics* (pp. 98–116). Hershey, PA: IGI Global. doi:10.4018/978-1-4666-2653-9.ch006

Uchitomi, H., Suzuki, K., Nishi, T., Hove, M. J., Miyake, Y., Orimo, S., & Wada, Y. (2013). Gait rhythm of Parkinson's disease patients and an interpersonal synchrony emulation system based on cooperative gait. In J. Wu (Ed.), *Biomedical engineering and cognitive neuroscience for healthcare: Interdisciplinary applications* (pp. 38–53). Hershey, PA: IGI Global. doi:10.4018/978-1-4666-2113-8.ch005

Usher, W., & San Too, L. (2013). E-health knowledge management by australian university students. In I. Management Association (Ed.), User-driven healthcare: Concepts, methodologies, tools, and applications (pp. 938-953). Hershey, PA: IGI Global. doi:10.4018/978-1-4666-2770-3.ch047

Van Genderen, E. (2014). Intensive care. In V. Jham & S. Puri (Eds.), *Cases on consumer-centric marketing management* (pp. 53–67). Hershey, PA: IGI Global. doi:10.4018/978-1-4666-4357-4.ch006

Van Leuven, N., Newton, D., Leuenberger, D. Z., & Esteves, T. (2014). Reaching citizen 2.0: How government uses social media to send public messages during times of calm and times of crisis. In I. Management Association (Ed.), Crisis management: Concepts, methodologies, tools and applications (pp. 839-857). Hershey, PA: IGI Global. doi:10.4018/978-1-4666-4707-7.ch041

Vasudevan, V., & Rao, H. (2013). E-discovery and health care IT: An investigation. In I. Management Association (Ed.), User-driven healthcare: Concepts, methodologies, tools, and applications (pp. 1622-1635). Hershey, PA: IGI Global. doi:10.4018/978-1-4666-2770-3.ch080

Vat, K. H. (2013). Conceiving community knowledge records as e-governance concerns in wired healthcare provision. In I. Management Association (Ed.), User-driven healthcare: Concepts, methodologies, tools, and applications (pp. 1093-1111). Hershey, PA: IGI Global. doi:10.4018/978-1-4666-2770-3.ch055

Venkatasubramanian, K. K., Nabar, S., Gupta, S. K., & Poovendran, R. (2013). Cyber physical security solutions for pervasive health monitoring systems. In I. Management Association (Ed.), User-driven healthcare: Concepts, methodologies, tools, and applications (pp. 447-465). Hershey, PA: IGI Global. doi:10.4018/978-1-4666-2770-3.ch022

Victan, H. (2013). Emerging trends in user-driven healthcare: Negotiating disclosure in online health community organizations. In I. Management Association (Ed.), User-driven healthcare: Concepts, methodologies, tools, and applications (pp. 1589-1606). Hershey, PA: IGI Global. doi:10.4018/978-1-4666-2770-3.ch078

Vidal, B., Pereira, J. M., & Santos, G. (2013). SimBody: An interactive simulator for health education. In S. Arnab, I. Dunwell, & K. Debattista (Eds.), *Serious games for healthcare: Applications and implications* (pp. 265–282). Hershey, PA: IGI Global. doi:10.4018/978-1-4666-1903-6.ch013

Vivekananda-Schmidt, P. (2013). Ethics in the design of serious games for healthcare and medicine. In S. Arnab, I. Dunwell, & K. Debattista (Eds.), *Serious games for healthcare: Applications and implications* (pp. 91–106). Hershey, PA: IGI Global. doi:10.4018/978-1-4666-1903-6.ch005

Wahbeh, A. (2013). Application of handheld computing and mobile phones in diabetes self-care. In S. Sarnikar, D. Bennett, & M. Gaynor (Eds.), *Cases on healthcare information technology for patient care management* (pp. 254–275). Hershey, PA: IGI Global. doi:10.4018/978-1-4666-2671-3.ch015

Waidyanatha, N., & Dekker, S. (2013). The RTBP – Collective intelligence driving health for the user. In R. Biswas (Ed.), *Clinical solutions and medical progress through user-driven healthcare* (pp. 70–78). Hershey, PA: IGI Global. doi:10.4018/978-1-4666-1876-3.ch007

Waidyanatha, N., Dubrawski, A. M. G., & Gow, G. (2013). Affordable system for rapid detection and mitigation of emerging diseases. In J. Rodrigues (Ed.), *Digital advances in medicine, e-health, and communication technologies* (pp. 271–288). Hershey, PA: IGI Global. doi:10.4018/978-1-4666-2794-9.ch015

Walker, D. (2013). How would a ban on prescriber-identifying information impact pharmaceutical marketing? In M. Merviö (Ed.), *Healthcare management and economics: Perspectives on public and private administration* (pp. 141–153). Hershey, PA: IGI Global. doi:10.4018/978-1-4666-3982-9.ch011

Wang, B., Yan, T., & Wu, J. (2013). Neuronal function in the cortical face perception network. In J. Wu (Ed.), *Biomedical engineering and cognitive neuroscience for healthcare: Interdisciplinary applications* (pp. 171–182). Hershey, PA: IGI Global. doi:10.4018/978-1-4666-2113-8.ch018

Wang, Y., & Wang, Q. (2013). Evaluating the IEEE 802.15.6 2.4GHz WBAN proposal on medical multi-parameter monitoring under WiFi/bluetooth interference. In J. Rodrigues (Ed.), *Digital advances in medicine, e-health, and communication technologies* (pp. 312–325). Hershey, PA: IGI Global. doi:10.4018/978-1-4666-2794-9.ch018

Watanabe, T., & Miura, N. (2013). Functional electrical stimulation (FES) control for restoration and rehabilitation of motor function. In J. Wu (Ed.), *Technological advancements in biomedicine for healthcare applications* (pp. 80–93). Hershey, PA: IGI Global. doi:10.4018/978-1-4666-2196-1.ch009

Watanabe, Y., Tanaka, H., & Hirata, K. (2013). Evaluation of cognitive function in migraine patients: A study using event-related potentials. In J. Wu (Ed.), *Biomedical engineering and cognitive neuroscience for healthcare: Interdisciplinary applications* (pp. 303–310). Hershey, PA: IGI Global. doi:10.4018/978-1-4666-2113-8.ch031

Watfa, M. K., Kaur, M., & Daruwala, R. F. (2013). RFID applications in e-healthcare. In I. Management Association (Ed.), User-driven healthcare: Concepts, methodologies, tools, and applications (pp. 259-287). Hershey, PA: IGI Global. doi:10.4018/978-1-4666-2770-3.ch014

Wesorick, B. (2013). Essential steps for successful implementation of the EHR to achieve sustainable, safe, quality care. In A. Moumtzoglou & A. Kastania (Eds.), *E-health technologies and improving patient safety: Exploring organizational factors* (pp. 27–55). Hershey, PA: IGI Global. doi:10.4018/978-1-4666-2657-7.ch003

Whitaker, R. (2013). Securing health-effective medicine in practice: A critical perspective on user-driven healthcare. In R. Biswas (Ed.), *Clinical solutions and medical progress through user-driven healthcare* (pp. 35–50). Hershey, PA: IGI Global. doi:10.4018/978-1-4666-1876-3.ch005

Wickramasinghe, N., Troshani, I., Hill, S. R., Hague, W., & Goldberg, S. (2013). A transaction cost assessment of a pervasive technology solution for gestational diabetes. In J. Tan (Ed.), *Healthcare information technology innovation and sustainability: Frontiers and adoption* (pp. 109–126). Hershey, PA: IGI Global. doi:10.4018/978-1-4666-2797-0.ch007

Wilkowska, W., & Ziefle, M. (2013). User diversity as a challenge for the integration of medical technology into future smart home environments. In I. Management Association (Ed.), User-driven healthcare: Concepts, methodologies, tools, and applications (pp. 553-582). Hershey, PA: IGI Global. doi:10.4018/978-1-4666-2770-3.ch028

Willis, E., Wang, Y., & Rodgers, S. (2013). Online health communities and health literacy: Applying a framework for understanding domains of health literacy. In I. Management Association (Ed.), User-driven healthcare: Concepts, methodologies, tools, and applications (pp. 180-196). Hershey, PA: IGI Global. doi:10.4018/978-1-4666-2770-3.ch010

Wu, Q., Li, C., Takahashi, S., & Wu, J. (2013). Visual-tactile bottom-up and top-down attention. In J. Wu (Ed.), *Biomedical engineering and cognitive neuroscience for healthcare: Interdisciplinary applications* (pp. 183–191). Hershey, PA: IGI Global. doi:10.4018/978-1-4666-2113-8.ch019

Yamaguchi, S., Onoda, K., & Abe, S. (2013). Feedback-related negativity and its clinical implications. In J. Wu (Ed.), *Biomedical engineering and cognitive neuroscience for healthcare: Interdisciplinary applications* (pp. 283–292). Hershey, PA: IGI Global. doi:10.4018/978-1-4666-2113-8.ch029

Yan, B., Lei, Y., Tong, L., & Chen, K. (2013). Functional neuroimaging of acupuncture: A systematic review. In J. Wu (Ed.), *Biomedical engineering and cognitive neuroscience for healthcare: Interdisciplinary applications* (pp. 142–155). Hershey, PA: IGI Global. doi:10.4018/978-1-4666-2113-8.ch015

Yang, J. (2014). Towards healthy public policy: GIS and food systems analysis. In C. El Morr (Ed.), *Research perspectives on the role of informatics in health policy and management* (pp. 135–152). Hershey, PA: IGI Global. doi:10.4018/978-1-4666-4321-5.ch009

Yang, J., Li, Q., Gao, Y., & Wu, J. (2013). Temporal dependency of multisensory audiovisual integration. In J. Wu (Ed.), *Biomedical engineering and cognitive neuroscience for healthcare: Interdisciplinary applications* (pp. 320–326). Hershey, PA: IGI Global. doi:10.4018/978-1-4666-2113-8.ch033

Yang, J. J., Liu, J. F., Kurokawa, T., Kitamura, N., Yasuda, K., & Gong, J. P. (2013). Tough double-network hydrogels as scaffolds for tissue engineering: Cell behavior in vitro and in vivo test. In J. Wu (Ed.), *Technological advancements in biomedicine for healthcare applications* (pp. 213–222). Hershey, PA: IGI Global. doi:10.4018/978-1-4666-2196-1.ch023

Yang, W., Gao, Y., & Wu, J. (2013). Effects of selective and divided attention on audiovisual interaction. In J. Wu (Ed.), *Biomedical engineering and cognitive neuroscience for healthcare: Interdisciplinary applications* (pp. 311–319). Hershey, PA: IGI Global. doi:10.4018/978-1-4666-2113-8.ch032

Yano, Y. (2013). An EMG control system for an ultrasonic motor using a PSoC microcomputer. In J. Wu (Ed.), *Technological advancements in biomedicine for healthcare applications* (pp. 11–17). Hershey, PA: IGI Global. doi:10.4018/978-1-4666-2196-1.ch002

Yap, K. Y. (2013). The evolving role of pharmacoinformatics in targeting drug-related problems in clinical oncology practice. In I. Management Association (Ed.), User-driven healthcare: Concepts, methodologies, tools, and applications (pp. 1541-1588). Hershey, PA: IGI Global. doi:10.4018/978-1-4666-2770-3.ch077

Yokoi, H., Kato, R., Mori, T., Yamamura, O., & Kubota, M. (2013). Functional electrical stimulation based on interference-driven PWM signals for neuro-rehabilitation. In J. Wu (Ed.), *Technological advancements in biomedicine for healthcare applications* (pp. 180–192). Hershey, PA: IGI Global. doi:10.4018/978-1-4666-2196-1.ch019

York, A. M., & Nordengren, F. R. (2013). E-learning and web 2.0 case study: The role of gender in contemporary models of health care leadership. In H. Yang & S. Wang (Eds.), *Cases on formal and informal e-learning environments: Opportunities and practices* (pp. 292–313). Hershey, PA: IGI Global. doi:10.4018/978-1-4666-1930-2.ch016

Yu, W. D., & Bhagwat, R. (2013). Modeling emergency and telemedicine health support system: A service oriented architecture approach using cloud computing. In J. Rodrigues (Ed.), *Digital advances in medicine, e-health, and communication technologies* (pp. 187–213). Hershey, PA: IGI Global. doi:10.4018/978-1-4666-2794-9.ch011

Yu, Y., Yang, J., & Wu, J. (2013). Cognitive functions and neuronal mechanisms of tactile working memory. In J. Wu (Ed.), *Biomedical engineering and cognitive neuroscience for healthcare: Interdisciplinary applications* (pp. 89–98). Hershey, PA: IGI Global. doi:10.4018/978-1-4666-2113-8.ch010

Zaheer, S. (2014). Implementation of evidence-based practice and the PARIHS framework. In C. El Morr (Ed.), *Research perspectives on the role of informatics in health policy and management* (pp. 19–36). Hershey, PA: IGI Global. doi:10.4018/978-1-4666-4321-5.ch002

Zalzala, A., Chia, S., Zalzala, L., Sahu, S., Vaghasiya, S., & Karimi, A. (2013). Rural e-health infrastructure development. In I. Management Association (Ed.), User-driven healthcare: Concepts, methodologies, tools, and applications (pp. 870-900). Hershey, PA: IGI Global. doi:10.4018/978-1-4666-2770-3.ch044

Zapirain, B. G., & Zorrilla, A. M. (2013). Independent living support for disabled and elderly people using cell phones. In M. Cruz-Cunha, I. Miranda, & P. Gonçalves (Eds.), *Handbook of research on ICTs for human-centered healthcare and social care services* (pp. 379–397). Hershey, PA: IGI Global. doi:10.4018/978-1-4666-3986-7.ch020

Zgodavová, K., & Bourek, A. (2013). Potential of web based learning in managing for the sustained success of a healthcare organization based on IMPROHEALTH® project. In I. Management Association (Ed.), User-driven healthcare: Concepts, methodologies, tools, and applications (pp. 1523-1540). Hershey, PA: IGI Global. doi:10.4018/978-1-4666-2770-3.ch076

Zhao, X., Zuo, M. J., & Moghaddass, R. (2013). Generating indicators for diagnosis of fault levels by integrating information from two or more sensors. In I. Management Association (Ed.), User-driven healthcare: Concepts, methodologies, tools, and applications (pp. 288-309). Hershey, PA: IGI Global. doi:10.4018/978-1-4666-2770-3.ch015

Zhou, X., & Ren, X. (2013). Speed-accuracy tradeoff models of target-based and trajectory-based movements. In J. Wu (Ed.), *Biomedical engineering and cognitive neuroscience for healthcare: Interdisciplinary applications* (pp. 355–368). Hershey, PA: IGI Global. doi:10.4018/978-1-4666-2113-8.ch037

Zouag, N., & Driouchi, A. (2014). Trends and prospects of the Moroccan health system: 2010-2030. In A. Driouchi (Ed.), *Labor and health economics in the mediterranean region: Migration and mobility of medical doctors* (pp. 314–336). Hershey, PA: IGI Global. doi:10.4018/978-1-4666-4723-7.ch013

Zvikhachevskaya, A., & Mihaylova, L. (2013). Advanced video distribution for wireless e-healthcare systems. In I. Management Association (Ed.), User-driven healthcare: Concepts, methodologies, tools, and applications (pp. 421-446). Hershey, PA: IGI Global. doi:10.4018/978-1-4666-2770-3.ch021

Compilation of References

Abdollahzade, H., Bagher Pour, M., BoujMehrani, S., & Lotfi, M. (2000). Spritual intelligence (Concepts, Assessment and Applications). Tehran: Psychometric Publications.

Abdullah, A. A., Subasi, A., & Qaisar, S. M. (2017). Surface EMG Signal Classification by Using WPD and Ensemble Tree Classifiers. In CMBEBIH 2017 (pp. 475-481). Springer. doi:10.1007/978-981-10-4166-2_73

Acharya, U. R., Molinari, F., Sree, S. V., Chattopadhyay, S., Ng, K. H., & Suri, J. S. (2012). Automated diagnosis of epileptic EEG using entropies. *Biomedical Signal Processing and Control*, *7*(4), 401–408. doi:10.1016/j.bspc.2011.07.007

Addison, P. S. (2017). *The illustrated wavelet transform handbook: introductory theory and applications in science, engineering, medicine and finance*. CRC Press.

Addison, P. S., Watson, J. N., Clegg, G. R., Holzer, M., Sterz, F., & Robertson, C. E. (2000). Evaluating arrhythmias in ECG signals using wavelet transforms. *IEEE Engineering in Medicine and Biology Magazine*, *19*(5), 104–109. doi:10.1109/51.870237 PMID:11016036

Afarideh, M., Aryan, Z., Ghajar, A., Noshad, S., Nakhjavani, M., Baber, U., ... Esteghamati, A. (2016). Complex association of serum alanine aminotransferase with the risk of future cardiovascular disease in type 2 diabetes. *Atherosclerosis*, *254*, 42–51. doi:10.1016/j.atherosclerosis.2016.09.009 PMID:27684605

Aguiar-Conraria, L., & Soares, M. J. (2014). The continuous wavelet transform: Moving beyond uni-and bivariate analysis. *Journal of Economic Surveys*, *28*(2), 344–375. doi:10.1111/joes.12012

Ahmad, A., & Hashmi, S. (2016). K-Harmonic means type clustering algorithm for mixed datasets. *Applied Soft Computing*, *48*, 39–49. doi:10.1016/j.asoc.2016.06.019

Ahmad, F., Isa, N. A. M., Hussain, Z., & Osman, M. K. (2013). Intelligent medical disease diagnosis using improved hybrid genetic algorithm-multilayer perceptron network. *Journal of Medical Systems*, *37*(2), 9934. doi:10.100710916-013-9934-7 PMID:23479268

Ait-Sahalia, Y., & Yu, J. (2008). *High frequency market microstructure noise estimates and liquidity measures*. National Bureau of Economic Research. doi:10.3386/w13825

Akay. (2009). Support vector machines combined with feature selection for breast cancer diagnosis. *Expert Syst. With Applicat., 36*(2), 3240–3247. 10.1016/j.eswa.2008.01.009

Akbarizadeh, F., Hajivandi, A., Bagheri, F., & Hatami, H. (2012). Relationship between nurses spiritual intelligence with hardiness and general health. *Majallah-i Danishgah-i Ulum-i Pizishki-i Kirmanshah, 15*(6).

Alagumariappan, P., Krishnamurthy, K., Kandiah, S., & Ponnuswamy, M. J. (2017). Effect of electrode contact area on the information content of the recorded electrogastrograms: An analysis based on Renyi entropy and Teager-Kaiser Energy. *Polish Journal of Medical Physics and Engineering, 23*(2), 37–42. doi:10.1515/pjmpe-2017-0007

Alagumariappan, P., Rajagopal, A., & Krishnamurthy, K. (2016). Complexity Analysis on Normal and Abnormal Electrogastrograms Using Tsallis Entropy. In *3rd International Electronic and Flipped Conference on Entropy and Its Applications*. Multidisciplinary Digital Publishing Institute. 10.3390/ecea-3-A003

Aldape-Pérez, M., Yáñez-Márquez, C., Camacho-Nieto, O., & Argüelles-Cruz, A. J. (2012). An associative memory approach to medical decision support systems. *Computer Methods and Programs in Biomedicine, 106*(3), 287–307. doi:10.1016/j.cmpb.2011.05.002 PMID:21703713

Alexakis, C., Nyongesa, H., Saatchi, R., Harris, N., Davies, C., & Emery, C. (2003). *Feature extraction and classification of electrocardiogram (ECG) signals related to hypoglycaemia.* Paper presented at the Computers in Cardiology.

Alfaouri, M., & Daqrouq, K. (2008). ECG signal denoising by wavelet transform thresholding. *American Journal of Applied Sciences, 5*(3), 276–281. doi:10.3844/ajassp.2008.276.281

Al-Obeidat, F., Belacel, N., Carretero, J. A., & Mahanti, P. (2011). An evolutionary framework using particle swarm optimization for classification method PROAFTN. *Applied Soft Computing, 11*(8), 4971–4980. doi:10.1016/j.asoc.2011.06.003

Al-Subari, K., Al-Baddai, S., Tome, A. M., Goldhacker, M., Faltermeier, R., & Lang, E. W. (2015). EMDLAB: A toolbox for analysis of single-trial EEG dynamics using empirical mode decomposition. *Journal of Neuroscience Methods, 253*, 193–205. doi:10.1016/j.jneumeth.2015.06.020 PMID:26162614

Amato, F., López, A., Peña-Méndez, E. M., Vaňhara, P., Hampl, A., & Havel, J. (2013). *Artificial neural networks in medical diagnosis*. Academic Press.

American College of Radiology (ACR) Breast Imaging Reporting and Data System Atlas. (2003). *BI-RADS Atlas*. Reston, VA: American College of Radiology.

Amin, M. F., Islam, M. M., & Murase, K. (2009). Ensemble of single-layered complex-valued neural networks for classification tasks. *Neurocomputing, 72*(10), 2227–2234. doi:10.1016/j.neucom.2008.12.028

Amin, M. F., & Murase, K. (2009). Single-layered complex-valued neural network for real-valued classification problems. *Neurocomputing, 72*(4), 945–955. doi:10.1016/j.neucom.2008.04.006

Amram, J. Y. (2009). *The contribution of emotional and spiritual intelligence to effective business leadership*. Institute of Transpersonal Psychology.

Anderhill, E. (1993). The Spiritual Life. *Australian Journal of Psychology*, 23.

Antoniadis, A., & Oppenheim, G. (2012). *Wavelets and statistics* (Vol. 103). Springer Science & Business Media.

Arunachalam, K., Jacob, L. V., & Kamalanand, K. (2014). Design and analysis of finite element based sensors for diagnosis of liver disorders using biocompatible metals. *Technology and Health Care*, *22*(6), 867–875. PMID:25391529

Assender, H., Bliznyuk, V., & Porfyrakis, K. (2002). How surface topography relates to materials' properties. *Science*, *297*(5583), 973–976. doi:10.1126cience.1074955 PMID:12169724

Asuncion, A., & Newman, D. (2007). *UCI machine learning repository*. Academic Press.

Aubert, A. E., Ramaekers, D., Beckers, F., Breem, R., Denef, C., Van de Werf, F., & Ector, H. (1999). The analysis of heart rate variability in unrestrained rats. Validation of method and results. *Computer Methods and Programs in Biomedicine*, *60*(3), 197–213. doi:10.1016/S0169-2607(99)00017-6 PMID:10579513

Aydın, S., Saraoğlu, H. M., & Kara, S. (2009). Log energy entropy-based EEG classification with multilayer neural networks in seizure. *Annals of Biomedical Engineering*, *37*(12), 2626–2630. doi:10.100710439-009-9795-x PMID:19757057

Babu, R. V., Suresh, S., & Savitha, R. (2012). Human action recognition using a fast learning fully complex-valued classifier. *Neurocomputing*, *89*, 202–212. doi:10.1016/j.neucom.2012.03.003

Baert, A., Reiser, M., Hricak, H., & Kanuth, M. (2010). *Digital Mammography*. Springer.

Bag heri, F., Akbarizadeh, F., & Hatami, H. (2010). The relationship between nurses' spiritual intelligence and happiness in Iran. *Procardia Social and Behavioral Sciences, 5*, 1556–1561.

Barhatte, A. S., Ghongade, R., & Tekale, S. V. (2016). *Noise analysis of ECG signal using fast ICA*. Paper presented at the Advances in Signal Processing (CASP), Conference on. 10.1109/CASP.2016.7746149

Barroso-Alvarado, A. J., Tovar-Corona, B., Contreras-Uribe, T. J., Santiago-Godoy, R., González-Navarro, Y. E., Solís-Villela, J. G., . . . Garay-Jiménez, L. I. (2011, October). Wavelet analysis of an electrogastrogram database. In *Electrical Engineering Computing Science and Automatic Control (CCE), 2011 8th International Conference on* (pp. 1-5). IEEE. 10.1109/ICEEE.2011.6106644

Bascil, M. S., & Oztekin, H. (2012). A study on Hepatitis disease diagnosis using probabilistic neural network. *Journal of Medical Systems*, *36*(3), 1603–1606. doi:10.100710916-010-9621-x PMID:21057884

Bascil, M. S., & Temurtas, F. (2011). A study on Hepatitis disease diagnosis using multilayer neural network with levenbergmarquardt training algorithm. *Journal of Medical Systems*, *35*(3), 433–436. doi:10.100710916-009-9378-2 PMID:20703548

Bashir, S., Qamar, U., & Khan, F. H. (2016). IntelliHealth: A medical decision support application using a novel weighted multi-layer classifier ensemble framework. *Journal of Biomedical Informatics*, *59*, 185–200. doi:10.1016/j.jbi.2015.12.001 PMID:26703093

Ben Hassen, D., Ben Zakour, S., & Taleb, H. (2016). A Hybrid Fuzzy-SVM classifier for automated lung diseases diagnosis. *Polish Journal of Medical Physics and Engineering*, *22*(4), 97–103. doi:10.1515/pjmpe-2016-0017

Berradja, K., & Boughanmi, N. (2016). Assessment of myocardial metabolic rate of glucose by means of Bayesian ICA and Markov Chain Monte Carlo methods in small animal PET imaging. *Polish Journal of Medical Physics and Engineering*, *22*(3), 69–75. doi:10.1515/pjmpe-2016-0012

Bezdek, J. C. (1981). *Pattern Recognition with Fuzzy Objective Function Algorithms*. Norwell, MA: Kluwer Academic Publishers. doi:10.1007/978-1-4757-0450-1

Billman, G. E. (2013). The LF/HF ratio does not accurately measure cardiac sympatho-vagal balance. *Frontiers in Physiology*, 4. PMID:23431279

Bilous, R., & Donnelly, R. (2010). *Handbook of diabetes*. John Wiley & Sons. doi:10.1002/9781444391374

Bland, J. M., & Altman, D. G. (1996). Statistics notes: Measurement error. *BMJ (Clinical Research Ed.)*, *313*(7059), 744. doi:10.1136/bmj.313.7059.744 PMID:8819450

Bradshaw, L. A., Cheng, L. K., Chung, E., Obioha, C. B., Erickson, J. C., Gorman, B. L., ... Richards, W. O. (2016). Diabetic gastroparesis alters the biomagnetic signature of the gastric slow wave. *Neurogastroenterology and Motility*, *28*(6), 837–848. doi:10.1111/nmo.12780 PMID:26839980

Breiman, L. (1996). Bagging predictors. *Machine Learning*, *24*(2), 123–140. doi:10.1007/BF00058655

Breiman, L. (2001). Random forests. *Machine Learning*, *45*(1), 5–32. doi:10.1023/A:1010933404324

Bude, R. O., & Adler, R. S. (1995). An easily made, low-cost, tissue-like ultrasound phantom material. *Journal of Clinical Ultrasound*, *23*(4), 271–273. doi:10.1002/jcu.1870230413 PMID:7797668

Calder, S., Cheng, L. K., & Du, P. (2014, August). A theoretical analysis of the electrogastrogram (EGG). In *Engineering in Medicine and Biology Society (EMBC), 2014 36th Annual International Conference of the IEEE* (pp. 4330-4333). IEEE.

Camm, A. J., Malik, M., Bigger, J., Breithardt, G., Cerutti, S., Cohen, R. J., & .... (1996). Heart rate variability: Standards of measurement, physiological interpretation and clinical use. Task Force of the European Society of Cardiology and the North American Society of Pacing and Electrophysiology. *Circulation*, *93*(5), 1043–1065. doi:10.1161/01.CIR.93.5.1043 PMID:8598068

Cancer Fact SheetsW. H. O. (2009). Available: http://www.who.int/mediacentre/factsheets/fs297/en/index.html

Carl, F. G., Jr., & De Rouffignac, E. P. (1993). *Current to power crossover heater control.* Google Patents.

Castaldo, R., Melillo, P., Bracale, U., Caserta, M., Triassi, M., & Pecchia, L. (2015). Acute mental stress assessment via short term HRV analysis in healthy adults: A systematic review with meta-analysis. *Biomedical Signal Processing and Control, 18*, 370–377. doi:10.1016/j.bspc.2015.02.012

Center, E. I., Center, C. R., & Center, P. F. (2005). *Music therapy*. Academic Press.

Cha, S. H., Choi, S., & Tappert, C. C. (2009). Anomaly between jaccard and tanimoto coefficients. *Proceedings of Student-Faculty Research Day, CSIS.* Pace University.

Cha, S. H. (2007). Comprehensive survey on distance/similarity measures between probability density functions. *City*, *1*(2), 1.

Chen, K.-C. J., Ni, Y.-S., & Wang, J.-Y. (2016). *Electrocardiogram diagnosis using wavelet-based artificial neural network.* Paper presented at the Consumer Electronics, 2016 IEEE 5th Global Conference on. 10.1109/GCCE.2016.7800547

Cheng, H. D., Wu, C. Y., & Li, J. (1998). VLSI architectures for moments and their applications to pattern recognition. In C. H. Chen, L. F. Pau, & P. S. P. Wang (Eds.), *Handbook of Pattern Recognition and Computer Vision* (2nd ed.). Singapore: World Scientific.

Cheng, H. D., & Xu, H. (2002). A novel fuzzy logic approach to mammogram contrast enhancement. *Information Sciences, 148*(1-4), 167–184. doi:10.1016/S0020-0255(02)00293-1

Cheng-Yu, H., Yi-Fan, Z., Guo-Wei, L., Meng-Xi, Z., & Zi-Xiong, L. (2017). Recent progress of using Brillouin distributed fiber sensors for geotechnical health monitoring. *Sensors and Actuators. A, Physical.*

Chen, L. F., Su, C. T., Chen, K. H., & Wang, P. C. (2012). Particle swarm optimization for feature selection with application in obstructive sleep apnea diagnosis. *Neural Computing & Applications, 21*(8), 2087–2096. doi:10.100700521-011-0632-4

Chen, S., Hong, X., Harris, C. J., & Hanzo, L. (2008). Fully complex-valued radial basis function networks: Orthogonal least squares regression and classification. *Neurocomputing*, *71*(16), 3421–3433. doi:10.1016/j.neucom.2007.12.003

Chen, S., McLaughlin, S., & Mulgrew, B. (1994). Complex-valued radial basis function network, Part II: Application to digital communications channel equalisation. *Signal Processing*, *36*(2), 175–188. doi:10.1016/0165-1684(94)90206-2

Chen, W., Wang, Y., Cao, G., Chen, G., & Gu, Q. (2014). A random forest model based classification scheme for neonatal amplitude-integrated EEG. *Biomedical Engineering Online*, *13*(2Suppl 2), S4. doi:10.1186/1475-925X-13-S2-S4 PMID:25560269

Cheung, N. (2001). *Machine learning techniques for medical analysis* (Doctoral dissertation). University of Queensland.

Cheung, Y. M. (2003). k*-Means: A new generalized k-means clustering algorithm. *Pattern Recognition Letters*, *24*(15), 2883–2893. doi:10.1016/S0167-8655(03)00146-6

Chévez, P., Barbero, D., Martini, I., & Discoli, C. (2017). *Application of the k-means clustering method for the detection and analysis of areas of homogeneous residential electricity consumption at the Great La Plata region*. Buenos Aires, Argentina: Sustainable Cities and Society.

Chiang, C. C., Lin, C. C. K., & Ju, M. S. (2007). An implantable capacitive pressure sensor for biomedical applications. *Sensors and Actuators. A, Physical*, *134*(2), 382–388. doi:10.1016/j.sna.2006.06.007

Choubey, D. K., & Paul, S. (2016). Classification techniques for diagnosis of diabetes: A review. *International Journal of Biomedical Engineering and Technology*, *21*(1), 15–39. doi:10.1504/IJBET.2016.076730

Chuang, K.-S., Tzeng, H.-L., Chen, S., Wu, J., & Chen, T. J. (2006). Fuzzy c-means clustering with spatial information for image segmentation. *Computerized Medical Imaging and Graphics, Elsevier*, *30*(1), 9–15. doi:10.1016/j.compmedimag.2005.10.001 PMID:16361080

Clark, A. J. (2015). *Comparative physiology of the heart*. Cambridge University Press.

Contreras, T. J., Mayen, M. A., Servin, A., & Garay, L. I. (2010, September). System for acquisition and analysis of multichannel electrogastrogram. In *Electrical Engineering Computing Science and Automatic Control (CCE), 2010 7th International Conference on* (pp. 220-224). IEEE. 10.1109/ICEEE.2010.5608577

Cook, J. R., Bouchard, R. R., & Emelianov, S. Y. (2011). Tissue-mimicking phantoms for photoacoustic and ultrasonic imaging. *Biomedical Optics Express*, *2*(11), 3193–3206. doi:10.1364/BOE.2.003193 PMID:22076278

Cueva, M., Kuhnley, R., Stueckemann, C., Lanier, A. P., & McMahon, P. (2010). *Understanding Cancer*. Alaska Native Tribal Health Consortium.

Cyran, K. A., Kawulok, J., Kawulok, M., Stawarz, M., Michalak, M., Pietrowska, M., & Polańska, J. (2013). Support Vector Machines in Biomedical and Biometrical Applications. Emerging Paradigms in Machine Learning, 13, 379–417. doi:10.1007/978-3-642-28699-5_15

Das, A., & Bhattacharya, M. (2008). GA based Neuro Fuzzy Techniques for Breast Cancer Identification. *Proc. of Int. Machine Vision and Image Processing Conference (IMVIP-08)*, 136-141. 10.1109/IMVIP.2008.19

Das, A., & Bhattacharya, M. (2011). Computerized Decision Support System for Mass Identification in Breast Using Digital Mammogram: A Study on GA Based Neuro Fuzzy Approaches. *Advances in Experimental Medicine and Biology*, *696*(6), 523–533. doi:10.1007/978-1-4419-7046-6_53

Das, R. (2010). A comparison of multiple classification methods for diagnosis of Parkinson disease. *Expert Systems with Applications*, *37*(2), 1568–1572. doi:10.1016/j.eswa.2009.06.040

Das, R., & Sengur, A. (2010). Evaluation of ensemble methods for diagnosing of valvular heart disease. *Expert Systems with Applications*, *37*(7), 5110–5115. doi:10.1016/j.eswa.2009.12.085

Das, R., Turkoglu, I., & Sengur, A. (2009). Diagnosis of valvular heart disease through neural networks ensembles. *Computer Methods and Programs in Biomedicine*, *93*(2), 185–191. doi:10.1016/j.cmpb.2008.09.005 PMID:18951649

Datla, N. V., Konh, B., Koo, J. J., Choi, D. J., Yu, Y., Dicker, A. P., ... Hutapea, P. (2014). Polyacrylamide phantom for self-actuating needle–tissue interaction studies. *Medical Engineering & Physics*, *36*(1), 140–145. doi:10.1016/j.medengphy.2013.07.004 PMID:23932314

De Bock, K. W., Coussement, K., & Van den Poel, D. (2010). Ensemble classification based on generalized additive models. *Computational Statistics & Data Analysis*, *54*(6), 1535–1546. doi:10.1016/j.csda.2009.12.013

De Chazal, P., Celler, B., & Reilly, R. (2000). Using wavelet coefficients for the classification of the electrocardiogram. *Paper presented at the Engineering in Medicine and Biology Society, 2000. Proceedings of the 22nd Annual International Conference of the IEEE.* 10.1109/IEMBS.2000.900669

De Jong, G. W., & Meijer, G. C. (1997). An efficient retrieving algorithm for accurate capacitive position sensors. *Sensors and Actuators. A, Physical*, *58*(1), 75–84. doi:10.1016/S0924-4247(97)80227-0

De Mello, W. C. (2013). *Electrical phenomena in the heart*. Academic Press.

DeCarlo, L. T. (1997). On the meaning and use of kurtosis. *Psychological Methods*, *2*(3), 292–307. doi:10.1037/1082-989X.2.3.292

Deering, R., & Kaiser, J. F. (2005). The use of masking signal to improve empirical mode decomposition. *IEEE Int. Conf. Acoustics, Speech Signal Processing (ICASSP '05)*, 4, 485-488. 10.1109/ICASSP.2005.1416051

Dehuri, S., Roy, R., Cho, S. B., & Ghosh, A. (2012). An improved swarm optimized functional link artificial neural network (ISO-FLANN) for classification. *Journal of Systems and Software*, *85*(6), 1333–1345. doi:10.1016/j.jss.2012.01.025

Demšar, J., Curk, T., Erjavec, A., Gorup, Č., Hočevar, T., Milutinovič, M., ... Štajdohar, M. (2013). Orange: Data mining toolbox in Python. *Journal of Machine Learning Research*, *14*(1), 2349–2353.

Ding, W., Qin, S., Miao, L., Xi, N., Li, H., & Wang, Y. (2010, December). Processing and analysis of bio-signals from human stomach. In *Robotics and Biomimetics (ROBIO), 2010 IEEE International Conference on* (pp. 769-772). IEEE. 10.1109/ROBIO.2010.5723423

Dougherty, E. R., Hua, J., & Bittner, M. L. (2007). Validation of computational methods in genomics. *Current Genomics*, *8*(1), 1–19. doi:10.2174/138920207780076956 PMID:18645624

Duch, W., Adamczak, R., & Grabczewski, K. (2001). A new methodology of extraction, optimization and application of crisp and fuzzy logical rules. *IEEE Transactions on Neural Networks*, *12*(2), 277–306. doi:10.1109/72.914524 PMID:18244384

Durna, Z. (2002). DiyabetinSınıflandırılmasıveTanıKriteleri.İçinde: Edit. Erdoğan S. DiyabetH emşireliğiTemelBilgiler. YüceYayım, İstanbul, 11-21.

Earle, M., De Portu, G., & DeVos, E. (2016). Agar ultrasound phantoms for low-cost training without refrigeration. *African Journal of Emergency Medicine*, *6*(1), 18–23. doi:10.1016/j.afjem.2015.09.003

El-Sherif, M., Bansal, L., & Yuan, J. (2007). Fiber optic sensors for detection of toxic and biological threats. *Sensors (Basel)*, *7*(12), 3100–3118. doi:10.33907123100 PMID:28903282

Emmons, R. A. (2000). Spirituality and intelligence: Problems and prospects. *The International Journal for the Psychology of Religion*, *10*(1), 57–64. doi:10.1207/S15327582IJPR1001_6

Emmons, R. A. (2000). *The Psychology of Ultimate Concerns: Motivation and Spirituality in Personality*. New York: Guilford Publication.

Emmons, R. A. (2000a). Is Spirituality an Intelligence? Motivation, Cognition, and the Psychology of Ultimate Concern. *The International Journal for the Psychology of Religion*, *10*(1), 3–26. doi:10.1207/S15327582IJPR1001_2

Engin, M. (2004). ECG beat classification using neuro-fuzzy network. *Pattern Recognition Letters*, *25*(15), 1715–1722. doi:10.1016/j.patrec.2004.06.014

Erkamp, R. Q., Skovoroda, A. R., Emelianov, S. Y., & O'Donnell, M. (2004). Measuring the nonlinear elastic properties of tissue-like phantoms. *IEEE Transactions on Ultrasonics, Ferroelectrics, and Frequency Control*, *51*(4), 410–419. doi:10.1109/TUFFC.2004.1295426 PMID:15139542

Familoni, B. O., Abell, T. L., & Bowes, K. L. (1995). A model of gastric electrical activity in health and disease. *IEEE Transactions on Biomedical Engineering*, *42*(7), 647–657. doi:10.1109/10.391163 PMID:7622148

Farrer, A. I., Odéen, H., de Bever, J., Coats, B., Parker, D. L., Payne, A., & Christensen, D. A. (2015). Characterization and evaluation of tissue-mimicking gelatin phantoms for use with MRgFUS. *Journal of Therapeutic Ultrasound*, *3*(1), 9. doi:10.118640349-015-0030-y PMID:26146557

Fidanboylu, K. A., & Efendioglu, H. S. (2009, May). Fiber optic sensors and their applications. *5th International Advanced Technologies Symposium (IATS'09)*, 6.

Freund, Y., & Schapire, R. E. (1995, March). A desicion-theoretic generalization of on-line learning and an application to boosting. In *European conference on computational learning theory* (pp. 23-37). Springer. 10.1007/3-540-59119-2_166

Friedl, M. A., & Brodley, C. E. (1997). Decision tree classification of land cover from remotely sensed data. *Remote Sensing of Environment*, *61*(3), 399–409. doi:10.1016/S0034-4257(97)00049-7

Fujita, H., Sudarshan, V. K., Adam, M., Oh, S. L., Tan, J. H., & Hagiwara, Y. (2017). *Characterization of Cardiovascular Diseases Using Wavelet Packet Decomposition and Nonlinear Measures of Electrocardiogram Signal.* Paper presented at the International Conference on Industrial, Engineering and Other Applications of Applied Intelligent Systems. 10.1007/978-3-319-60042-0_30

Galar, M., Fernandez, A., Barrenechea, E., Bustince, H., & Herrera, F. (2012). A review on ensembles for the class imbalance problem: Bagging-, boosting-, and hybrid-based approaches. *IEEE Transactions on Systems, Man, and Cybernetics*, *42*(4), 463–484. doi:10.1109/TSMCC.2011.2161285

Gang, R., Jiapin, X., HongHui, W., & Lu, J. (2004). *A new quadrature sampling and reconstruction technique and computer simulation of its performances.* Paper presented at the Communications, Circuits and Systems, 2004. ICCCAS 2004. 2004 International Conference on.

Gardner, H. (1999). *Intelligence reframes: multiple intelligence for 21st century*. New York: Basic Books.

Gardner, L., & Stough, C. (2003). Assessing the Relationship between Workplace Emotional Intelligence, Job Satisfaction and Organizational Commitment. *Australian Journal of Psychology*, *55*, 1–5.

Ghabaribanab, B, & Salim, M., Seliani, L., & NuriMoghadam, S. (2007). Spiritual intelligence. *Scientific-Research Journal of New Religious Thinking*, *3*(10), 125–147.

Ghaffari, A., Homaeinezhad, M., Khazraee, M., & Daevaeiha, M. (2010). Segmentation of holter ECG waves via analysis of a discrete wavelet-derived multiple skewness–kurtosis based metric. *Annals of Biomedical Engineering*, *38*(4), 1497–1510. doi:10.100710439-010-9919-3 PMID:20087769

Gharibans, A. A., Kim, S., Kunkel, D. C., & Coleman, T. P. (2017). High-Resolution Electrogastrogram: A Novel, Noninvasive Method for Determining Gastric Slow-Wave Direction and Speed. *IEEE Transactions on Biomedical Engineering*, *64*(4), 807–815. doi:10.1109/TBME.2016.2579310 PMID:27305668

Gonçalves, L. B., Vellasco, M. M. B. R., Pacheco, M. A. C., & de Souza, F. J. (2006). Inverted hierarchical neuro-fuzzy BSP system: A novel neuro-fuzzy model for pattern classification and rule extraction in databases. *IEEE Transactions on Systems, Man and Cybernetics. Part C, Applications and Reviews*, *36*(2), 236–248. doi:10.1109/TSMCC.2004.843220

Gonzalez, R., & Woods, R. (2002). Digital Image Processing (2nd ed.). PHI.

González-Barajas, J. E. (2014). Threshold calculation for R wave detection in complex cardiac. *Tecno Lógicas*, *17*(32), 47–55.

Goodall, D. W. (1966). A new similarity index based on probability. *Biometrics*, *22*(4), 882–907. doi:10.2307/2528080

Gopu, G., Neelaveni, R., & Porkumaran, K. (2008). Investigation of digestive system disorders using Electrogastrogram. In *Computer and Communication Engineering, 2008. ICCCE 2008. International Conference on* (pp. 201-205). IEEE. 10.1109/ICCCE.2008.4580596

Gopu, G., Neelaveni, R., & Porkumaran, K. (2008). Acquisition and analysis of electrogastrogram for digestive system disorders using a novel approach. *Proceedings of International Conference on Electrical and Computer Engineering*, 65–69. 10.1109/ICECE.2008.4769174

Graupe, D. (2013). *Principles of artificial neural networks* (Vol. 7). World Scientific. doi:10.1142/8868

Gray, K. R., Aljabar, P., Heckemann, R. A., Hammers, A., & Rueckert, D. (2013). Random forest-based similarity measures for multi-modal classification of Alzheimer's disease. *NeuroImage*, *65*, 167–175. doi:10.1016/j.neuroimage.2012.09.065 PMID:23041336

Guha, S., Rastogi, R., & Shim, K. (2000). ROCK: A robust clustering algorithm for categorical attributes. *Information Systems*, *25*(5), 345–366. doi:10.1016/S0306-4379(00)00022-3

Guzik, P., Piskorski, J., Krauze, T., Schneider, R., Wesseling, K. H., Wykretowicz, A., & Wysocki, H. (2007). Correlations between the Poincare plot and conventional heart rate variability parameters assessed during paced breathing. *The Journal of Physiological Sciences; JPS*, *57*(1), 63–71. doi:10.2170/physiolsci.RP005506 PMID:17266795

Haddab, S., & Laghrouche, M. (2009). Microcontroller-based system for electrogastrography monitoring through wireless transmission. *Measurement Science Review*, *9*(5), 122–126. doi:10.2478/v10048-009-0022-6

Hammer, D., Romashchenko, A., Shen, A., & Vereshchagin, N. (2000). Inequalities for Shannon entropy and Kolmogorov complexity. *Journal of Computer and System Sciences*, *60*(2), 442–464. doi:10.1006/jcss.1999.1677

Handlon, R. L. (2009). Departure Of The Insurance Agent: The Impact Organizational Commitment, Organizational Justice, And Job Satisfaction Have On Intent To Leave In The Insurance Industry (PhD thesis). Capella University.

Haque, A., Ali, M. H., Kiber, M. A., & Hasan, M. T. (2009). Detection of small variations of ECG features using wavelet. *Journal of Engineering and Applied Sciences (Asian Research Publishing Network)*, *4*(6), 27–30.

Hare, T. A., Schultz, W., Camerer, C. F., O'Doherty, J. P., & Rangel, A. (2011). Transformation of stimulus value signals into motor commands during simple choice. *Proceedings of the National Academy of Sciences of the United States of America*, *108*(44), 18120–18125. doi:10.1073/pnas.1109322108 PMID:22006321

Haus, A. G., & Yaffe, M. J. (Eds.). (1993). *A categorical course in physics, technical aspects of breast imaging*. Presented at the *79 Scientific Assembly and Annual Meeting of RSNA*.

He, Q.-H., Yu, B., Hong, X., Lv, B., Liu, T., & Ran, J. (2016). An Improved Lung Sound De-noising Method by Wavelet Packet Transform with Pso-Based Threshold Selection. *Intelligent Automation & Soft Computing*, 1-7.

Heydari, M., Teimouri, M., Heshmati, Z., & Alavinia, S. M. (2016). Comparison of various classification algorithms in the diagnosis of type 2 diabetes in Iran. *International Journal of Diabetes in Developing Countries*, *36*(2), 167–173. doi:10.100713410-015-0374-4

HeydariTafreshi, G., & Darbayegan, A. (2011). Studying the Relationship between Job Satisfaction, Organizational Commitment and Organizational Citizenship Behavioral in the Employees of a Half-private Company in Hormozgan Province. *Scientific Journal of Educational Management Researches*.

Hildebrant, L. S. (2011). *Spiritual intelligence: Is it related to a leader's level of ethical development?* (Doctoral dissertation). Capella University.

Holzapfel, G. A. (2001). Biomechanics of soft tissue. The handbook of materials behavior models, 3, 1049-1063.

Houshyarifar, V., & Amirani, M. C. (2017). Early detection of sudden cardiac death using Poincaré plots and recurrence plot-based features from HRV signals. *Turkish Journal of Electrical Engineering and Computer Sciences*, *25*(2), 1541–1553. doi:10.3906/elk-1509-149

Hu, D., Li, W., & Chen, X. (2011). *Feature extraction of motor imagery EEG signals based on wavelet packet decomposition.* Paper presented at the Complex Medical Engineering (CME), 2011 IEEE/ICME International Conference on. 10.1109/ICCME.2011.5876829

Inoue, M., Iwamura, S., & Yoshida, M. (2001). EGG measurement under various situations. In *Engineering in Medicine and Biology Society, 2001. Proceedings of the 23rd Annual International Conference of the IEEE* (*Vol. 4*, pp. 3356-3358). IEEE.

Jaganathan, P., & Kuppuchamy, R. (2013). A threshold fuzzy entropy based feature selection for medical database classification. *Computers in Biology and Medicine*, *43*(12), 2222–2229. doi:10.1016/j.compbiomed.2013.10.016 PMID:24290939

Jain, A. K., Mao, J., & Mohiuddin, K. M. (1996). Artificial neural networks: A tutorial. *Computer*, *29*(3), 31–44. doi:10.1109/2.485891

Jain, A., Singh, S., & Bhateja, V. (2013). A Robust approach for denoising and enhancement of mammographic breast masses. *Int. J. Converg. Comput*, *1*, 38–49. doi:10.1504/IJCONVC.2013.054659

James, C. (1984). Bezdek, Robert Ehrlich, William Full, 'FCM: The Fuzzy C-Means Clustering Algorithm'. *Computers & Geosciences*, *10*(2-3), 191–203. doi:10.1016/0098-3004(84)90020-7

Jegan, R., Anusuya, K., & George, E. M. (2015). Real-time ECG peak detection for heart rate measurement using wavelet packet transform. *International Journal of Biomedical Engineering and Technology*, *19*(3), 244–254. doi:10.1504/IJBET.2015.072994

Ji, B., & Gao, H. (2004). Mechanical properties of nanostructure of biological materials. *Journal of the Mechanics and Physics of Solids*, *52*(9), 1963–1990. doi:10.1016/j.jmps.2004.03.006

Jin, B., Tang, Y. C., & Zhang, Y. Q. (2007). Support vector machines with genetic fuzzy feature transformation for biomedical data classification. *Information Sciences*, *177*(2), 476–489. doi:10.1016/j.ins.2006.03.015

Jin, X., Katsuura, T., Iwanaga, K., Shimomura, Y., & Inoie, M. (2007). The influence of taste stimuli and illumination on electrogastrogram measurements. *Journal of Physiological Anthropology*, *26*(2), 191–195. doi:10.2114/jpa2.26.191 PMID:17435364

Johnston, J. W. (1976). *Similarity Indices I: What Do They Measure?* Academic Press.

Jonderko, K., Kasicka-jonderko, A., Krusiec-świdergoł, B., Dzielicki, M., Strój, L., Doliński, M., ... Błońska-fajfrowska, B. (2005). How reproducible is cutaneous electrogastrography? An in-depth evidence-based study1. *Neurogastroenterology and Motility*, *17*(6), 800–809. doi:10.1111/j.1365-2982.2005.00707.x PMID:16336495

Juslin, P. N., & Sloboda, J. A. (2001). *Music and emotion: Theory and research.* Oxford University Press.

Kahramanli, H., & Allahverdi, N. (2008). Design of a hybrid system for the diabetes and heart diseases. *Expert Systems with Applications*, *35*(1), 82–89. doi:10.1016/j.eswa.2007.06.004

Kalantarkousheha, S., Sharghib, N., Soleimanic, M., & Ramezanid, S. (2013). The Role of Spiritual Intelligence on Organizational Commitment in Employees of Universities in Tehran Province, Iran. *Social and Behavioral Sciences.*, *140*, 499–505.

Kale, S. H., & Shrivastava, S. (2003). The Enneagram System for Enhancing Workplace Spirituality. *Journal of Management Development*, *22*(4), 318–328. doi:10.1108/02621710310467596

Kamalanand, K., & Jawahar, P. M. (2012). Coupled jumping frogs/particle swarm optimization for estimating the parameters of three dimensional HIV model. *BMC Infectious Diseases*, *12*(1Suppl 1), 82. doi:10.1186/1471-2334-12-S1-P82 PMID:22471518

Kamalanand, K., & Jawahar, P. M. (2013). Particle swarm optimization based estimation of HIV-1 viral load in resource limited settings. *African Journal of Microbiological Research*, *7*(20), 2297–2304. doi:10.5897/AJMR12.1924

Kamalanand, K., & Jawahar, P. M. (2015). Prediction of Human Immunodeficiency Virus-1 Viral Load from CD4 Cell Count Using Artificial Neural Networks. *Journal of Medical Imaging and Health Informatics*, *5*(3), 641–646. doi:10.1166/jmihi.2015.1430

Kamalanand, K., & Mannar Jawahar, P. (2016). Comparison of particle swarm and bacterial foraging optimization algorithms for therapy planning in HIV/AIDS patients. *International Journal of Biomathematics*, *9*(02), 1650024. doi:10.1142/S1793524516500248

Kamalanand, K., Sridhar, B. T. N., Rajeshwari, P. M., & Ramakrishnan, S. (2010). Correlation of Dielectric Permittivity with Mechanical Properties in Soft Tissue-Mimicking Polyacrylamide Phantoms. *Journal of Mechanics in Medicine and Biology*, *10*(02), 353–360. doi:10.1142/S0219519410003411

Kanungo, T., Mount, D. M., Netanyahu, N. S., Piatko, C. D., Silverman, R., & Wu, A. Y. (2002). An efficient k-means clustering algorithm: Analysis and implementation. *IEEE Transactions on Pattern Analysis and Machine Intelligence*, *24*(7), 881–892. doi:10.1109/TPAMI.2002.1017616

Karabulut, E. M., & İbrikçi, T. (2012). Effective diagnosis of coronary artery disease using the rotation forest ensemble method. *Journal of Medical Systems*, *36*(5), 3011–3018. doi:10.100710916-011-9778-y PMID:21912972

Kaur, M. (2013). Spiritual intelligence of secondary school teachers in relation to their job satisfaction. *International Journal of Educational Research and Technology*, *4*(3), 104–109.

Kawabata, K. I., Waki, Y., Matsumura, T., & Umemura, S. I. (2004, August). Tissue mimicking phantom for ultrasonic elastography with finely adjustable elastic and echographic properties. In *Ultrasonics Symposium*, 2004 *IEEE* (*Vol. 2*, pp. 1502-1505). IEEE. 10.1109/ULTSYM.2004.1418087

Keméņy, V., Droste, D. W., Hermes, S., Nabavi, D. G., Schulte-Altedorneburg, G., Siebler, M., & Ringelstein, B. (1999). Automatic embolus detection by a neural network. *Stroke*, *30*(4), 807–810. doi:10.1161/01.STR.30.4.807 PMID:10187883

Kemp, A. H., Brunoni, A. R., Santos, I. S., Nunes, M. A., Dantas, E. M., Carvalho de Figueiredo, R., ... Lotufo, P. A. (2014). Effects of depression, anxiety, comorbidity, and antidepressants on resting-state heart rate and its variability: An ELSA-Brasil cohort baseline study. *The American Journal of Psychiatry*, *171*(12), 1328–1334. doi:10.1176/appi.ajp.2014.13121605 PMID:25158141

Kennedy, M. H. (2002). Spirituality in the Workplace: An Empirical Study of this Phenomenon. Nova Southeastern University.

Kersey, A. D., Davis, M. A., Patrick, H. J., LeBlanc, M., Koo, K. P., Askins, C. G., & Friebele, E. J. (1997). Fiber grating sensors. *Journal of Lightwave Technology*, *15*(8), 1442–1463. doi:10.1109/50.618377

Khanmohammadi, S., Adibeig, N., & Shanehbandy, S. (2017). An improved overlapping k-means clustering method for medical applications. *Expert Systems with Applications*, *67*, 12–18. doi:10.1016/j.eswa.2016.09.025

Kim, D., & Economou, D. J. (2002). Plasma molding over surface topography: Simulation of ion flow, and energy and angular distributions over steps in RF high-density plasmas. *IEEE Transactions on Plasma Science*, *30*(5), 2048–2058. doi:10.1109/TPS.2002.805326

King, U. (2008). *The search for spirituality: Our global quest for a spiritual life*. BlueBridge.

King, D. B. (2007). The Spiritual Intelligence Project: Extracting Cognitive Ability from the Psycho Spiritual Realm. *Netherlands Journal of Happiness Studies*, *2*, 329–330.

Kinoshita, O., Fontaine, G., Rosas, F., Elias, J., Iwa, T., Tonet, J., ... Frank, R. (1995). Time-and frequency-domain analyses of the signal-averaged ECG in patients with arrhythmogenic right ventricular dysplasia. *Circulation, 91*(3), 715–721. doi:10.1161/01.CIR.91.3.715 PMID:7828298

Koch, K. L., & Stern, R. M. (2004). *Handbook of electrogastrography*. Oxford University Press.

Koerdel, M., Alatas, F., Schick, A., Rupitsch, S. J., & Lerch, R. (2011). Contactless inspection of planar electronic devices by capacitive coupling: Development of a model describing the sensor signal and its impact on signal post-processing. *Sensors and Actuators. A, Physical, 172*(1), 88–97. doi:10.1016/j.sna.2011.02.040

Kolev, V. (2000). Compressed time and frequency recording of the electrogastrogram by individual wave detection. *Physiological Measurement, 21*(1), N1–N10. doi:10.1088/0967-3334/21/1/401 PMID:10720016

Komorowski, D., & Tkacz, E. (2015, August). A new method for attenuation of respiration artifacts in electrogastrographic (EGG) signals. In *Engineering in Medicine and Biology Society (EMBC), 2015 37th Annual International Conference of the IEEE* (pp. 6006-6009). IEEE.

Komorowski, D., Pietraszek, S., Tkacz, E., & Provaznik, I. (2015). The extraction of the new components from electrogastrogram (EGG), using both adaptive filtering and electrocardiographic (ECG) derived respiration signal. *Biomedical Engineering Online, 14*(1), 60. doi:10.118612938-015-0054-0 PMID:26099312

Kononenko, I. (1994). Estimating attributes: analysis and extensions of RELIEF. In *European conference on machine learning* (pp. 171-182). Springer. 10.1007/3-540-57868-4_57

Koprowski, R., Zieleźnik, W., Wróbel, Z., Małyszek, J., Stepien, B., & Wójcik, W. (2012). Assessment of significance of features acquired from thyroid ultrasonograms in Hashimoto's disease. *Biomedical Engineering Online, 11*(1), 48. doi:10.1186/1475-925X-11-48 PMID:22898180

Krishnamurthy, K., Sridhar, B. T. N., Rajeshwari, P. M., & Swaminathan, D. R. (2009). Correlation of Electrical Impedance with Mechanical Properties in Models of Tissue Mimicking Phantoms. In *13th International Conference on Biomedical Engineering* (pp. 1708-1711). Springer Berlin Heidelberg. 10.1007/978-3-540-92841-6_424

Kumar, M., Pachori, R. B., & Acharya, U. R. (2017). Characterization of coronary artery disease using flexible analytic wavelet transform applied on ECG signals. *Biomedical Signal Processing and Control, 31*, 301–308. doi:10.1016/j.bspc.2016.08.018

Kuru, E. A., Orakdogen, N., & Okay, O. (2007). Preparation of homogeneous polyacrylamide hydrogels by free-radical crosslinking copolymerization. *European Polymer Journal, 43*(7), 2913–2921. doi:10.1016/j.eurpolymj.2007.04.019

Kutlu, Y., & Kuntalp, D. (2012). Feature extraction for ECG heartbeats using higher order statistics of WPD coefficients. *Computer Methods and Programs in Biomedicine, 105*(3), 257–267. doi:10.1016/j.cmpb.2011.10.002 PMID:22055998

Lafon, C., Kaczkowski, P. J., Vaezy, S., Noble, M., & Sapozhnikov, O. A. (2001). Development and characterization of an innovative synthetic tissue-mimicking material for high intensity focused ultrasound (HIFU) exposures. In *Ultrasonics Symposium*, 2001 *IEEE* (*Vol. 2*, pp. 1295-1298). IEEE. 10.1109/ULTSYM.2001.991957

Lai, H.-L. (2001). *The Effects of Music Therapy on Sleep Quality in Elderly Peopl.* Case Western Reserve University. Retrieved from http://onlinestatbook.com/Online_Statistics_Education.pdf

Laine, A., Fan, J., & Yang, W. (1995). *Wavelet For Contrast Enhancement of Digital Mammography.* IEEE Engineering in Medicine & Biology.

Lakshmi, V. S., Tebby, S. G., Shriranjani, D., & Rajinikanth, V. (2016). Chaotic cuckoo search and Kapur/Tsallis approach in segmentation of T. cruzi from blood smear images. *International Journal of Computer Science and Information Security*, *14*, 51–56.

Lazebnik, M., Madsen, E. L., Frank, G. R., & Hagness, S. C. (2005). Tissue-mimicking phantom materials for narrowband and ultrawideband microwave applications. *Physics in Medicine and Biology*, *50*(18), 4245–4258. doi:10.1088/0031-9155/50/18/001 PMID:16148391

Leahy, A., Besherdas, K., Clayman, C., Mason, I., & Epstein, O. (1999). Abnormalities of the electrogastrogram in functional gastrointestinal disorders. *The American Journal of Gastroenterology*, *94*(4), 1023–1028. doi:10.1111/j.1572-0241.1999.01007.x PMID:10201477

Lee, T. (2003). *Design, fabrication and characterization of fiber optic sensors for physical and chemical applications* (Doctoral dissertation). Cochin University.

Lee, C., & Lee, G. G. (2006). Information gain and divergence-based feature selection for machine learning-based text categorization. *Information Processing & Management*, *42*(1), 155–165. doi:10.1016/j.ipm.2004.08.006

Leema, N., Nehemiah, H. K., & Kannan, A. (2016). Neural network classifier optimization using differential evolution with global information and back propagation algorithm for clinical datasets. *Applied Soft Computing*, *49*, 834–844. doi:10.1016/j.asoc.2016.08.001

Lee, Y. J., & Mangasarian, O. L. (2001). SSVM: A smooth support vector machine for classification. *Computational Optimization and Applications*, *20*(1), 5–22. doi:10.1023/A:1011215321374

Levenson, R. W. (2014). The autonomic nervous system and emotion. *Emotion Review*, *6*(2), 100–112. doi:10.1177/1754073913512003

Li, Z., Guan, F., Ren, C., Liu, S., Sha, H., Zhao, S., . . . Wang, Y. (2008, May). Bio-Impedance and Synchronous Electrogastrogram to Evaluate Gastric Motility. In *Bioinformatics and Biomedical Engineering, 2008. ICBBE 2008. The 2nd International Conference on* (pp. 689-692). IEEE. 10.1109/ICBBE.2008.168

Liang, H. (2005). Extraction of gastric slow waves from electrogastrograms: Combining independent component analysis and adaptive signal enhancement. *Medical & Biological Engineering & Computing*, *43*(2), 245–251. doi:10.1007/BF02345962 PMID:15865135

Liang, H., Lin, Z., & McCallum, R. W. (2000). Artifact reduction in electrogastrogram based on empirical mode decomposition method. *Medical & Biological Engineering & Computing*, *38*(1), 35–41. doi:10.1007/BF02344686 PMID:10829388

Liang, J. I. E., & Chen, J. D. Z. (1997). What can be measured from surface electrogastrography (computer simulations). *Digestive Diseases and Sciences*, *42*(7), 1331–1343. doi:10.1023/A:1018869300296 PMID:9246026

Li, D. C., Liu, C. W., & Hu, S. C. (2011). A fuzzy-based data transformation for feature extraction to increase classification performance with small medical data sets. *Artificial Intelligence in Medicine*, *52*(1), 45–52. doi:10.1016/j.artmed.2011.02.001 PMID:21493051

Li, H., Ray Liu, K. J., & Lo Shih-Chung, B. (1997). Fractal Modeling and Segmentation for the Enhancement of Microcalcifications in Digital Mammograms. *IEEE Transactions on Medical Imaging*, *16*(6), 785–798. doi:10.1109/42.650875 PMID:9533579

Li, M. B., Huang, G. B., Saratchandran, P., & Sundararajan, N. (2006). Complex-valued growing and pruning RBF neural networks for communication channel equalisation. *IEE Proceedings. Vision Image and Signal Processing*, *153*(4), 411–418. doi:10.1049/ip-vis:20050217

Lim, C. K., & Chan, C. S. (2015). A weighted inference engine based on interval-valued fuzzy relational theory. *Expert Systems with Applications*, *42*(7), 3410–3419. doi:10.1016/j.eswa.2014.12.025

Ling, S. H., San, P. P., & Nguyen, H. T. (2016). Non-invasive hypoglycemia monitoring system using extreme learning machine for Type 1 diabetes. *ISA Transactions*, *64*, 440–446. doi:10.1016/j.isatra.2016.05.008 PMID:27311357

Linnemann, A., Kappert, M. B., Fischer, S., Doerr, J. M., Strahler, J., & Nater, U. M. (2015). The effects of music listening on pain and stress in the daily life of patients with fibromyalgia syndrome. *Frontiers in Human Neuroscience*, 9. PMID:26283951

Lin, Z., Sarosiek, I., Forster, J., Damjanov, I., Hou, Q., & McCallum, R. W. (2010). Association of the status of interstitial cells of Cajal and electrogastrogram parameters, gastric emptying and symptoms in patients with gastroparesis. *Neurogastroenterology and Motility*, *22*(1), 56–e10. PMID:19614868

Li, T., & Zhou, M. (2016). ECG classification using wavelet packet entropy and random forests. *Entropy (Basel, Switzerland)*, *18*(8), 285. doi:10.3390/e18080285

Liu, Z., Su, J., Qin, C., & Li, Z. (2016). *Wavelet packet decomposition and grey relational analysis application in fault diagnosis of aero hydraulic pump.* Paper presented at the Aircraft Utility Systems (AUS), IEEE International Conference on. 10.1109/AUS.2016.7748150

Li, X., & Meijer, G. C. (2002). An accurate interface for capacitive sensors. *IEEE Transactions on Instrumentation and Measurement*, *51*(5), 935–939. doi:10.1109/TIM.2002.807793

Li, Z., & Ren, C. (2008). Gastric motility measurement and evaluation of functional dyspepsia by a bio-impedance method. *Physiological Measurement*, *29*(6), S373–S382. doi:10.1088/0967-3334/29/6/S31 PMID:18544817

Locke, E. A. (1969). What is job satisfaction? *Organizational Behavior and Human Performance*, *4*(4), 309–336. doi:10.1016/0030-5073(69)90013-0

Lopez-de-Andres, A., Hernandez-Barrera, V., Lopez, R., Martin-Junco, P., Jimenez-Trujillo, I., Alvaro-Meca, A., ... Jimenez-Garcia, R. (2016). Predictors of in-hospital mortality following major lower extremity amputations in type 2 diabetic patients using artificial neural networks. *BMC Medical Research Methodology*, *16*(1), 160. doi:10.118612874-016-0265-5 PMID:27876006

López, F. M., Puertas, S. M., & Arriaza, J. T. (2014). Training of support vector machine with the use of multivariate normalization. *Applied Soft Computing*, *24*, 1105–1111. doi:10.1016/j.asoc.2014.08.020

Luz, E. J. D. S., Merschmann, L. H., Menotti, D., & Moreira, G. J. (2017). Evaluating a hierarchical approach for heartbeat classification from ECG. *International Journal of Bioinformatics Research and Applications*, *13*(2), 146–160. doi:10.1504/IJBRA.2017.083148

Luz, E. J. D. S., Nunes, T. M., De Albuquerque, V. H. C., Papa, J. P., & Menotti, D. (2013). ECG arrhythmia classification based on optimum-path forest. *Expert Systems with Applications*, *40*(9), 3561–3573. doi:10.1016/j.eswa.2012.12.063

MacDonald, R., Kreutz, G., & Mitchell, L. (2013). *Music, health, and wellbeing*. Oxford University Press.

Madsen, E. L., Hobson, M. A., Shi, H., Varghese, T., & Frank, G. R. (2005). Tissue-mimicking agar/gelatin materials for use in heterogeneous elastography phantoms. *Physics in Medicine and Biology*, *50*(23), 5597–5618. doi:10.1088/0031-9155/50/23/013 PMID:16306655

Madsen, E. L., Zagzebski, J. A., & Frank, G. R. (1982). Oil-in-gelatin dispersions for use as ultrasonically tissue-mimicking materials. *Ultrasound in Medicine & Biology*, *8*(3), 277–287. doi:10.1016/0301-5629(82)90034-5 PMID:7101576

Mahmoodabadi, S., Ahmadian, A., & Abolhasani, M. (2005). ECG feature extraction using Daubechies wavelets. *Proceedings of the fifth IASTED International conference on Visualization, Imaging and Image Processing.*

Malcolm, R. (2001). *Cancer*. London, UK: Imperial College School of Medicine.

Malik, M. E., & Naeem, B. (2011). Role of spirituality in job satisfaction and organizational commitment among faculty of institutes of higher learning in Pakistan. *African Journal of Business Management*, *5*(4), 1236–1244.

Mallat, S. G. (1989). A theory for multiresolution signal decomposition: The wavelet representation. *IEEE Transactions on Pattern Analysis and Machine Intelligence*, *11*(7), 674–693. doi:10.1109/34.192463

Manetje, O., & Martins, N. (2009). The Relation between Organizational Culture and Organizational Commitment. *Southern African Business Review*, *13*(1), 120–142.

Manickavasagam, K., Sutha, S., & Kamalanand, K. (2014). An automated system based on 2 d empirical mode decomposition and k-means clustering for classification of Plasmodium species in thin blood smear images. *BMC Infectious Diseases*, *14*(S3), 13. doi:10.1186/1471-2334-14-S3-P13 PMID:24405683

Manickavasagam, K., Sutha, S., & Kamalanand, K. (2014). Development of systems for classification of different plasmodium species in thin blood smear microscopic images. *Journal of Advanced Microscopy Research*, *9*(2), 86–92. doi:10.1166/jamr.2014.1194

Mantas, C. J., & Abellán, J. (2014). Credal-C4. 5: Decision tree based on imprecise probabilities to classify noisy data. *Expert Systems with Applications*, *41*(10), 4625–4637. doi:10.1016/j.eswa.2014.01.017

Mardia, K. V. (1970). Measures of multivariate skewness and kurtosis with applications. *Biometrika*, *57*(3), 519–530. doi:10.1093/biomet/57.3.519

Marieb, E. N. (2000). *Essentials of human anatomy & physiology*. Benjamin Cummings.

Matiss, I. (2014). Multi-element capacitive sensor for non-destructive measurement of the dielectric permittivity and thickness of dielectric plates and shells. *NDT & E International*, *66*, 99–105. doi:10.1016/j.ndteint.2014.05.003

Meharrar, A., Tioursi, M., Hatti, M., & Stambouli, A. B. (2011). A variable speed wind generator maximum power tracking based on adaptative neuro-fuzzy inference system. *Expert Systems with Applications*, *38*(6), 7659–7664. doi:10.1016/j.eswa.2010.12.163

Meng, A., Ge, J., Yin, H., & Chen, S. (2016). Wind speed forecasting based on wavelet packet decomposition and artificial neural networks trained by crisscross optimization algorithm. *Energy Conversion and Management*, *114*, 75–88. doi:10.1016/j.enconman.2016.02.013

Menter, P. (2000). Acrylamide Polymerization— A Practical Approach. *Bio-Rad Tech Note, 1156.*

Merino, M., Gómez, I. M., & Molina, A. J. (2015). Envelopment filter and K-means for the detection of QRS waveforms in electrocardiogram. *Medical Engineering & Physics*, *37*(6), 605–609. doi:10.1016/j.medengphy.2015.03.019 PMID:25922210

Meyer, J. P., & Allen, N. J. (1991). A three-component conceptualization of organizational commitment. *Human Resource Management Review*, *1*(1), 61–89. doi:10.1016/1053-4822(91)90011-Z

Meyer, J. P., & Herscovitch, L. (2001). Commitment in the Workplace: Toward A General Model. *Human Resource Management Review*, *11*(3), 70–83. doi:10.1016/S1053-4822(00)00053-X

Milind Kumar, Sarode, Ladhake, & Deshmukh. (2008). Fuzzy system for color image enhancement. *Proceedings of World Academy Of science, Engineering and Technology, 36*.

Mitroff, I. A., & Denton, E. A. (1999). A Study of Spirituality in the Workplace. *Journal Sloan Management Review*, 83-92.

Moradi, P., & Rostami, M. (2015). Integration of graph clustering with ant colony optimization for feature selection. *Knowledge-Based Systems*, *84*, 144–161. doi:10.1016/j.knosys.2015.04.007

Mordacq, J. C., & Ellington, R. W. (1994). Polyacrylamide gel electrophoresis (PAGE) of blood proteins. *Tested Studies for Laboratory Teaching, 15*, 15-44.

Mottaz, C. J. (1988). Work satisfaction among hospital nurses. *Hospital & Health Services Administration, 33*(1), 57–74. PMID:10286427

Myers, J. E. (1995). *Wellness throughout the Lifespan*. Guidepost.

Myers, J. E., & Allen, N. J. (1984). Testing The Side-bet Theory of Organizational commitment. *The Journal of Applied Psychology, 69*, 327–378.

Nasel, D. D. (2004). *Spiritual orientation in relation to spiritual intelligence: Anew consideration of traditional Christianity and New Age/individualistic spirituality* (Doctoral Dissertation). University of South Australia.

Nassif, H., Woods, R., Burnside, E., Ayvaci, M., Shavlik, J., & Page, D. (2009). *Information Extraction for Clinical Data Mining: A Mammography Case Study*. IEEE International Conference on Data Mining (ICDM'09) Workshops, Miami, FL.

Nayak, S. K., Shukla, R. D., Panda, I., Champaty, B., Thakur, G., Mohapatra, B., et al. (2016). Effect of Slow and Fast Music on the Autonomic Nervous System and Cardiac Health: A Preliminary Investigation. *Classification and Clustering in Biomedical Signal Processing*, 198.

Nayakam, G. N. (2013). Study of Similarity Coefficients Using MapReduce Programming Model. *Circulation, 701*, 8888.

Nazeer, K. A., & Sebastian, M. P. (2009, July). Improving the Accuracy and Efficiency of the k-means Clustering Algorithm. In *Proceedings of the World Congress on Engineering* (*Vol. 1*, pp. 1-3). Academic Press.

Nemat-Nasser, S., & Hori, M. (2013). *Micromechanics: overall properties of heterogeneous materials* (Vol. 37). Elsevier.

Neuman, M. R. (1998). Biopotential amplifiers. *Medical instrumentation: Application and design*, 292-296.

Ning, Y., Zhu, X., Zhu, S., & Zhang, Y. (2015). Surface EMG decomposition based on K-means clustering and convolution kernel compensation. *IEEE Journal of Biomedical and Health Informatics, 19*(2), 471–477. doi:10.1109/JBHI.2014.2328497 PMID:25486655

Niskanen, J.-P., Tarvainen, M. P., Ranta-Aho, P. O., & Karjalainen, P. A. (2004). Software for advanced HRV analysis. *Computer Methods and Programs in Biomedicine*, *76*(1), 73–81. doi:10.1016/j.cmpb.2004.03.004 PMID:15313543

Niwattanakul, S., Singthongchai, J., Naenudorn, E., & Wanapu, S. (2013, March). Using of Jaccard coefficient for keywords similarity. *Proceedings of the International MultiConference of Engineers and Computer Scientists*, *1*, 6.

Nodehi, H., & Nehardani, H. (2013). Relation between spiritual intelligence and job satisfaction. *Journal of Social Issues and Humanities*, *1*(5), 67–72.

Nymeyer, H., & Zhou, H. X. (2008). A method to determine dielectric constants in nonhomogeneous systems: Application to biological membranes. *Biophysical Journal*, *94*(4), 1185–1193. doi:10.1529/biophysj.107.117770 PMID:17951302

Obioha, C., Erickson, J., Suseela, S., Hajri, T., Chung, E., Richards, W., & Bradshaw, L. A. (2013). Effect of Body Mass Index on the sensitivity of Magnetogastrogram and Electrogastrogram. *Journal of Gastroenterology and Hepatology Research*, *2*(4), 513. PMID:27077053

Oksel, C., Ma, C. Y., Liu, J. L., Wilkins, T., & Wang, X. Z. (2015). (Q) SAR modelling of nano-material toxicity: A critical review. *Particuology*, *21*, 1–19. doi:10.1016/j.partic.2014.12.001

Orhan, U., Hekim, M., & Ozer, M. (2011). EEG signals classification using the K-means clustering and a multilayer perceptron neural network model. *Expert Systems with Applications*, *38*(10), 13475–13481. doi:10.1016/j.eswa.2011.04.149

Ortega, J. P., Del, M., Rojas, R. B., & Somodevilla, M. J. Research issues on k-means algorithm: An experimental trial using matlab. *CEUR Workshop Proceedings: Semantic Web and New Technologies*.

Padala, S. R. (2011). Employees' Job Satisfactions and Organisational Commitment in Nagarjuna Fertilizers and Chemicals Limited, India. *Journal of Research in International Business and Management, 1*(1), 17-27.

Pal & Kin. (1981). Image Enhancement Using Smoothing with Fuzzy Sets. *IEEE Trans. Systems, Man, And Cybernetics, 11*(7), 494-501.

Pal, M. (2005). Random forest classifier for remote sensing classification. *International Journal of Remote Sensing*, *26*(1), 217–222. doi:10.1080/01431160412331269698

Pandya, A. S., & Macy, R. B. (1995). *Pattern recognition with neural networks in C*. CRC press.

Pan, X., Luo, Y., & Xu, Y. (2015). K-nearest neighbor based structural twin support vector machine. *Knowledge-Based Systems*, *88*, 34–44. doi:10.1016/j.knosys.2015.08.009

Parkman, H. P., Hasler, W. L., Barnett, J. L., & Eaker, E. Y. (2003). Electrogastrography: A document prepared by the gastric section of the American Motility Society Clinical GI Motility Testing Task Force. *Neurogastroenterology and Motility*, *15*(2), 89–102. doi:10.1046/j.1365-2982.2003.00396.x PMID:12680908

Parzen, E. (1962). On estimation of a probability density function and mode. *Annals of Mathematical Statistics*, *33*(3), 1065–1076. doi:10.1214/aoms/1177704472

Patterson, M., Rintala, R., Lloyd, D., Abernethy, L., Houghton, D., & Williams, J. (2001). Validation of electrode placement in neonatal electrogastrography. *Digestive Diseases and Sciences*, *46*(10), 2245–2249. doi:10.1023/A:1011931502985 PMID:11680604

Peker, M. (2016). An efficient sleep scoring system based on EEG signal using complex-valued machine learning algorithms. *Neurocomputing*, *207*, 165–177. doi:10.1016/j.neucom.2016.04.049

Peng, R., Varshney, P. K., Chen, H., & Michels, J. H. (2008). Digital mammogram enhancement based on ROI enhancement and background suppression. In *Medical Imaging 2008: Image Processing*. San Diego, CA: SPIE. doi:10.1117/12.770649

Podolak, E., Kinn, J. B., & Westura, E. E. (1969). Biomedical applications of a commercial capacitance transducer. *IEEE Transactions on Biomedical Engineering*, *BME-16*(1), 40–44. doi:10.1109/TBME.1969.4502601 PMID:5775604

Puers, R. (1993). Capacitive sensors: When and how to use them. *Sensors and Actuators. A, Physical*, *37*, 93–105. doi:10.1016/0924-4247(93)80019-D

Puri, D., Ingle, R., Kachare, P., Patil, M., & Awale, R. (2017). *Wavelet Packet Sub-band Based Classification of Alcoholic and Controlled State EEG Signals*. Academic Press.

Raeiatibanadkooki, M., Quchani, S. R., KhalilZade, M. M., & Bahaadinbeigy, K. (2016). Compression and encryption of ECG signal using wavelet and chaotically Huffman code in telemedicine application. *Journal of Medical Systems*, *40*(3), 73. doi:10.100710916-016-0433-5 PMID:26779641

Rajesh, K., & Sangeetha, V. (2012). Application of data mining methods and techniques for diabetes diagnosis. *International Journal of Engineering and Innovative Technology*, *2*(3).

Rajinikanth, V., & Couceiro, M. S. (2014, October). Multilevel Segmentation of Color Image using Lévy driven BFO Algorithm. In *Proceedings of the 2014 International Conference on Interdisciplinary Advances in Applied Computing* (p. 19). ACM. 10.1145/2660859.2660925

Rajinikanth, V., Satapathy, S. C., Fernandes, S. L., & Nachiappan, S. (2017). Entropy based Segmentation of Tumor from Brain MR Images–A study with Teaching Learning Based Optimization. *Pattern Recognition Letters*, *94*, 87–95. doi:10.1016/j.patrec.2017.05.028

Rau, H. H., Hsu, C. Y., Lin, Y. A., Atique, S., Fuad, A., Wei, L. M., & Hsu, M. H. (2016). Development of a web-based liver cancer prediction model for type II diabetes patients by using an artificial neural network. *Computer Methods and Programs in Biomedicine*, *125*, 58–65. doi:10.1016/j.cmpb.2015.11.009 PMID:26701199

Real, R., & Vargas, J. M. (1996). The probabilistic basis of Jaccard's index of similarity. *Systematic Biology*, *45*(3), 380–385. doi:10.1093ysbio/45.3.380

Ribeiro, L., Ruano, A. E., Graça Ruano, M., & Pedro, M. (2007). Neural networks assisted diagnosis of ischemic CVA's through CT scan. *Proceedings of the IEEE International Symposium on Intelligent Signal Processing*, 223–227. 10.1109/WISP.2007.4447507

Rilling, G., Flandrin, P., & Goncalves, P. (2003). On empirical decomposition and its algorithms. *IEEE-EURASIP Workshop on Nonlinear Signal Image Process Grado.*

Rowan, M., & Pedersen, P. (2006, October). P2C-3 an injury mimicking ultrasound phantom as a training tool for diagnosis of internal trauma. In *Ultrasonics Symposium, 2006. IEEE* (pp. 1612-1617). IEEE.

Sabelli, H., & Lawandow, A. (2010). Homeobios: The pattern of heartbeats in newborns, adults, and elderly patients. *Nonlinear Dynamics Psychology and Life Sciences*, *14*(4), 381. PMID:20887687

Sabelli, H., Messer, J., Kovacevic, L., & Walthall, K. (2011). Biotic patterns of heart rate variation in depressed and psychotic subjects. *Nonlinear Dynamics Psychology and Life Sciences*, *15*(1), 11–28. PMID:21176437

Sabelli, H., Sugerman, A., Kovacevic, L., Kauffman, L., Carlson-Sabelli, L., Patel, M., & ... . (2005). Bios data analyzer. *Nonlinear Dynamics Psychology and Life Sciences*, *9*(4), 505–538. PMID:16194304

Sahiner, B., Chan, H. P., Petrick, N., Helvie, M. A., & Hadjiiski, L. M. (2001). Improvement of mammographic mass characterization using speculation measures and morphological features. *Medical Physics*, *28*(7), 1455–1465. doi:10.1118/1.1381548 PMID:11488579

Salimpoor, V. N., Benovoy, M., Longo, G., Cooperstock, J. R., & Zatorre, R. J. (2009). The rewarding aspects of music listening are related to degree of emotional arousal. *PLoS One*, *4*(10), e7487. doi:10.1371/journal.pone.0007487 PMID:19834599

Sampat, Markey, & Bovik. (2003). Computer-Aided Detection and Diagnosis in Mammography. In *Handbook of Image and Video Processing*. London, UK: Elsevier.

Sarosiek, I., Song, G., Sun, Y., Sandoval, H., Sands, S., Chen, J., & McCallum, R. W. (2017). Central and Peripheral Effects of Transcutaneous Acupuncture Treatment for Nausea in Patients with Diabetic Gastroparesis. *Journal of Neurogastroenterology and Motility*, *23*(2), 245–253. doi:10.5056/jnm16097 PMID:28163260

Sartakhti, J. S., Zangooei, M. H., & Mozafari, K. (2012). Hepatitis disease diagnosis using a novel hybrid method based on support vector machine and simulated annealing (SVM-SA). *Computer Methods and Programs in Biomedicine*, *108*(2), 570–579. doi:10.1016/j.cmpb.2011.08.003 PMID:21968203

Savitha, R., Suresh, S., Sundararajan, N., & Kim, H. J. (2012). A fully complex-valued radial basis function classifier for real-valued classification problems. *Neurocomputing*, *78*(1), 104–110. doi:10.1016/j.neucom.2011.05.036

Scheffe, H. (1999). *The analysis of variance* (Vol. 72). John Wiley & Sons.

Schlenker, J., & Nedělka, T. (2013). Recurrence Analysis in Patients with Vasovagal Syncopes. *Measurement*, 145–148.

Schulz, W. (2007). *Molecular Biology of Human Cancers*. New York: Springer.

Seifoddini, H., & Djassemi, M. (1991). The production data-based similarity coefficient versus Jaccard's similarity coefficient. *Computers & Industrial Engineering*, *21*(1-4), 263–266. doi:10.1016/0360-8352(91)90099-R

Seo, Y., Kim, S., Kisi, O., Singh, V. P., & Parasuraman, K. (2016). River stage forecasting using wavelet packet decomposition and machine learning models. *Water Resources Management*, *30*(11), 4011–4035. doi:10.100711269-016-1409-4

Sepulveda, A. T., Fachin, F., de Villoria, R. G., Wardle, B. L., Viana, J. C., Pontes, A. J., & Rocha, L. A. (2011). Nanocomposite flexible pressure sensor for biomedical applications. *Procedia Engineering*, *25*, 140–143. doi:10.1016/j.proeng.2011.12.035

Sérgio Matos, A. E., Ruano, M., Ruano, G., & Evans, D. H. (2001). Neural network classification of cerebral embolic signals. *23rd Annual International Conference of the IEEE Engineering in Medicine and Biology Society.*

Shao, Y. H., Chen, W. J., Wang, Z., Li, C. N., & Deng, N. Y. (2015). Weighted linear loss twin support vector machine for large-scale classification. *Knowledge-Based Systems*, *73*, 276–288. doi:10.1016/j.knosys.2014.10.011

Shao, Y. H., & Deng, N. Y. (2012). A coordinate descent margin based-twin support vector machine for classification. *Neural Networks*, *25*, 114–121. doi:10.1016/j.neunet.2011.08.003 PMID:21890319

Sheskin, D. J. (2003). *Handbook of parametric and nonparametric statistical procedures*. CRC Press. doi:10.1201/9781420036268

Shikalgar, N. R., & Dixit, A. M. (2014). JIBCA: Jaccard Index based Clustering Algorithm for Mining Online Review. *International Journal of Computers and Applications*, *105*(15).

Shiuan, C. B., Yn, I. D., & Relley, J. H. (2003). Organizational Commitment: The Chinese Super Visionary Commitment and Employee Outcomes in Context Proximal Hypothesis or Global Hypothesis. *Journal of Organizational Behavior*, *24*(3), 14–45.

Shivaramakrishna, R., Obuchowski, N., & Cardenosa, W. (2000). Comparing the performance of Mammographic Enhancement Algorithms. *AJR*, *175*(1), 45–51. doi:10.2214/ajr.175.1.1750045 PMID:10882244

Soltani, Z., & Jafarian, A. (2016). A New Artificial Neural Networks Approach for Diagnosing Diabetes Disease Type II. *International Journal of Advanced Computer Science and Applications*, *7*(6), 89–94. doi:10.14569/IJACSA.2016.070611

Speybroeck, N. (2012). Classification and regression trees. *International Journal of Public Health*, *57*(1), 243–246. doi:10.100700038-011-0315-z PMID:22015650

Speybroeck, N., Berkvens, D., Mfoukou-Ntsakala, A., Aerts, M., Hens, N., Van Huylenbroeck, G., & Thys, E. (2004). Classification trees versus multinomial models in the analysis of urban farming systems in Central Africa. *Agricultural Systems*, *80*(2), 133–149. doi:10.1016/j.agsy.2003.06.006

Stamps, P. L., & Piedmonte, E. B. (1986). *Nurses and Work Satisfaction: An Index for Measurement*. Chicago: Health Administration Press.

Subbulakshmi, C. V., Deepa, S. N., & Malathi, N. (2012, August).Extreme learning machine for two category data classification. In *Advanced Communication Control and Computing Technologies (ICACCCT), 2012 IEEE International Conference on* (pp. 458-461). IEEE. 10.1109/ICACCCT.2012.6320822

Suckling, J., Parker, J., Dance, D. R., Astley, S., Hutt, I., Boggis, C. R. M., ... Savage, J. (1994). The mammographic image analysis society mammogram database. *Proc. 2nd Int. Workshop Digital Mammography*, 375–378.

Sumathi, M., & Pratheep, R. (2012, October). *Intensity Based Fiber Optic Deflection Sensor*. ICOP-2009-International Conference on Optics and Photonics, CSIO, Chandigarh.

Surry, K. J. M., Austin, H. J. B., Fenster, A., & Peters, T. M. (2004). Poly (vinyl alcohol) cryogel phantoms for use in ultrasound and MR imaging. *Physics in Medicine and Biology*, *49*(24), 5529–5546. doi:10.1088/0031-9155/49/24/009 PMID:15724540

Susan Tee Suan Chin, R. N., Anantharaman, & Kin Tong, D.Y. (2011). The Roles of Emotional Intelligence and Spiritual Intelligence at the Workplace. *Journal of Human Resource Management Research.*

Takegami, K., Kaneko, Y., Watanabe, T., Maruyama, T., Matsumoto, Y., & Nagawa, H. (2004). Polyacrylamide gel containing egg white as new model for irradiation experiments using focused ultrasound. *Ultrasound in Medicine & Biology*, *30*(10), 1419–1422. doi:10.1016/j.ultrasmedbio.2004.07.016 PMID:15582242

Tang, J., Liu, X., & Sun, Q. (2009). A Direct Image Contrast Enhancement Algorithm in the Wavelet Domain for Screening Mammograms. *IEEE Journal of Selected Topics in Signal Processing*, *3*(1), 74–80. doi:10.1109/JSTSP.2008.2011108

Tantra, R., Oksel, C., Puzyn, T., Wang, J., Robinson, K. N., Wang, X. Z., ... Wilkins, T. (2015). Nano(Q)SAR: Challenges, pitfalls and perspectives. *Nanotoxicology*, *9*(5), 636–642. doi:10.3109/17435390.2014.952698 PMID:25211549

Tan, Y. Z., Ozdemir, S., Temiz, A., & Celik, F. (2015). The effect of relaxing music on heart rate and heart rate variability during ECG GATED-myocardial perfusion scintigraphy. *Complementary Therapies in Clinical Practice*, *21*(2), 137–140. doi:10.1016/j.ctcp.2014.12.003 PMID:25747187

Taralunga, D. D., Ungureanu, M., Hurezeanu, B., Gussi, I., & Strungaru, R. (2015, August). Empirical mode decomposition applied for non-invasive electrohysterograhic signals denoising. In *Engineering in Medicine and Biology Society (EMBC), 2015 37th Annual International Conference of the IEEE* (pp. 4134-4137). IEEE. 10.1109/EMBC.2015.7319304

Tarvainen, M. P., Niskanen, J.-P., Lipponen, J. A., Ranta-Aho, P. O., & Karjalainen, P. A. (2014). Kubios HRV–heart rate variability analysis software. *Computer Methods and Programs in Biomedicine*, *113*(1), 210–220. doi:10.1016/j.cmpb.2013.07.024 PMID:24054542

Teixeira, C. A., Graça Ruano, M., & Ruano, A. E. (2004). Emboli classification using RBF neural networks. *Proceedings of CONTROL 2004*, 630–635.

Teixeira, C. A., Graça Ruano, M., Ruano, A. E., & Pereira, W. C. A. (2008a). A soft-computing methodology for non-invasive time-spatial temperature estimation. *IEEE Transactions on Biomedical Engineering*, *55*(2), 572–580. doi:10.1109/TBME.2007.901029 PMID:18269992

Teixeira, C. A., Graça Ruano, M., Ruano, A. E., & Pereira, W. C. A. (2008b). Neuro-genetic non-invasive temperature estimation: Intensity and spatial prediction. *Artificial Intelligence in Medicine*, *43*(2), 127–139. doi:10.1016/j.artmed.2008.03.008 PMID:18468870

Teixeira, C. A., Pereira, W. C. A., Ruano, A. E., & Graça Ruano, M. (2010). On non-invasive multi-layer temperature estimation using soft-computing methods. *Ultrasonics*, *50*(1), 32–43. doi:10.1016/j.ultras.2009.07.005 PMID:19695653

Teixeira, C. A., Ruano, A. E., Graça Ruano, M., & Pereira, W. C. A. (2007). Generalization assessment of non-invasive data-driven temperature estimators from therapeutic ultrasound. *Brazilian Journal of Biomedical Engineering*, *23*(2), 143–151.

Teixeira, C. A., Ruano, A. E., Ruano, M. G., Pereira, W. C. A., & Negreira, C. (2006). Non-invasive Temperature prediction of in-vitro therapeutic ultrasound signals using neural networks. *Medical & Biological Engineering & Computing*, *44*(1-2), 111–116. doi:10.100711517-005-0004-2 PMID:16929928

Thada, V., & Jaglan, V. (2013). Comparison of jaccard, dice and cosine similarity coefficient to find best fitness value for web retrieved documents using genetic algorithm. *International Journal of Innovations in Engineering and Technology*, *2*(4), 202–205.

Thangavel, K., Karnan, M., & Sivakumar, R. (2005). *Automatic Detection of Microcalcification in Mammogram - A Review*. ICGST.

Thangavel, K., Karnan, M., Sivakumar, R., & Kaja Mohideen, A. (1998). Automatic detection of microcalcification in mammograms - a review. *Journal on Graphics Vision and Image Processing*, *5*(5), 31–61.

Tian, J., Li, M., & Chen, F. (2009). A hybrid classification algorithm based on coevolutionary EBFNN and domain covering method. *Neural Computing & Applications*, *18*(3), 293–308. doi:10.100700521-008-0182-6

Tizhoosh, H. R. (2000). Fuzzy Image Enhancement: An Overview. In Fuzzy Techniques in Image Processing. Springer.

Tokmakçi, M. (2007). Analysis of the electrogastrogram using discrete wavelet transform and statistical methods to detect gastric dysrhythmia. *Journal of Medical Systems*, *31*(4), 295–302. doi:10.100710916-007-9069-9 PMID:17685154

Torabi, M., & Javadi, S. (2013). Studying the impact of spiritual intelligence on job engagement. *International Journal of Economy Management and Social Sciences*, *2*(9), 752–756.

Tortora, G. J., & Derrickson, B. H. (2008). *Principles of anatomy and physiology*. John Wiley & Sons.

Torun, Y., & Tohumoğlu, G. (2011). Designing simulated annealing and subtractive clustering based fuzzy classifier. *Applied Soft Computing*, *11*(2), 2193–2201. doi:10.1016/j.asoc.2010.07.020

Tsang, K. M., & Chan, W. L. (2011). Dual capacitive sensors for non-contact AC voltage measurement. *Sensors and Actuators. A, Physical*, *167*(2), 261–266. doi:10.1016/j.sna.2011.02.019

Vakil, B. J. (1960). The pattern of certain gastro-intestinal diseases in India. *Postgraduate Medical Journal*, *36*(420), 614–618. doi:10.1136/pgmj.36.420.614 PMID:13779649

Van Fleet, P. J. (2011). *Discrete wavelet transformations: An elementary approach with applications*. John Wiley & Sons.

Van Gestel, T., Suykens, J. A., Lanckriet, G., Lambrechts, A., De Moor, B., & Vandewalle, J. (2002). Bayesian framework for least-squares support vector machine classifiers, Gaussian processes, and kernel Fisher discriminant analysis. *Neural Computation*, *14*(5), 1115–1147. doi:10.1162/089976602753633411 PMID:11972910

Vargas, F., Lettnin, D., de Castro, M. C. F., & Macarthy, M. (2002). Electrocardiogram pattern recognition by means of MLP network and PCA: A case study on equal amount of input signal types. *Paper presented at the Neural Networks, 2002. SBRN 2002. Proceedings. VII Brazilian Symposium on.* 10.1109/SBRN.2002.1181474

Viljoen, J. P., & Rothmann, S. (2009). Occupational Stress, Ill Health and Organisational Commitment Of Employees At A University Of Technology. *SA Journal of Industrial Psychology*, *35*(1), 1–11. doi:10.4102ajip.v35i1.730

Wang, B., Lv, Z., Zhao, J., Wang, X., & Zhang, T. (2016, December). An Adaptively Disperse Centroids K-Means Algorithm Based on MapReduce Model. In *Computational Intelligence and Security (CIS), 2016 12th International Conference on* (pp. 142-146). IEEE. 10.1109/CIS.2016.0041

Wang, C., Li, L., Wang, L., Ping, Z., Flory, M. T., Wang, G., ... Li, W. (2013). Evaluating the risk of type 2 diabetes mellitus using artificial neural network: An effective classification approach. *Diabetes Research and Clinical Practice*, *100*(1), 111–118. doi:10.1016/j.diabres.2013.01.023 PMID:23453177

Wang, J., Belatreche, A., Maguire, L., & Mcginnity, T. M. (2014). An online supervised learning method for spiking neural networks with adaptive structure. *Neurocomputing*, *144*, 526–536. doi:10.1016/j.neucom.2014.04.017

Wang, J.-S., Chiang, W.-C., Hsu, Y.-L., & Yang, Y.-T. C. (2013). ECG arrhythmia classification using a probabilistic neural network with a feature reduction method. *Neurocomputing*, *116*, 38–45. doi:10.1016/j.neucom.2011.10.045

Weisstein, E. W. (2002). *Skewness*. Academic Press.

Wojewnik, P., & Żmigrodzki, J. (2013). An infrared-based device for non-invasive monitoring of eyelid movement during sleep. *Polish Journal of Medical Physics And Engineering*, *19*(2), 85–91.

World Health Organization. (2016). *Global report on diabetes*. World Health Organization.

Xia, Y., Han, J., & Wang, K. (2015). Quick detection of QRS complexes and R-waves using a wavelet transform and K-means clustering. *Bio-Medical Materials and Engineering*, *26*(s1), S1059–S1065. doi:10.3233/BME-151402 PMID:26405862

Yadav, J., & Sharma, M. (2013). A Review of K-mean Algorithm. *International Journal of Engineering Trends and Technology*, *4*(7), 2972–2975.

Yadav, S. K., Sinha, R., & Bora, P. K. (2015). Electrocardiogram signal denoising using non-local wavelet transform domain filtering. *IET Signal Processing*, *9*(1), 88–96. doi:10.1049/iet-spr.2014.0005

Yaman, A., Pamir, I., Yarali, N., Karademir, S., Cetinkaya, S., & Ali, B. (2013). Common complications in beta-thalassemia patients. *International Journal of Hematologic Oncology*, *27*(1), 193–199. doi:10.4999/uhod.12005

Yang, C. (2006). Image enhancement by modified contrast-stretching manipulation. *Optic & Laser Technology (Elmsford, N.Y.)*, *38*, 196–201.

Yang, C. Y., Chou, J. J., & Lian, F. L. (2013). Robust classifier learning with fuzzy class labels for large-margin support vector machines. *Neurocomputing*, *99*, 1–14. doi:10.1016/j.neucom.2012.04.009

Yang, S., & Naiman, D. Q. (2014). Multiclass cancer classification based on gene expression comparison. *Statistical Applications in Genetics and Molecular Biology*, *13*(4), 477–496. PMID:24918456

Yazdani, M., & Javad Parsa, M. (2014). The moderating effect of spiritual intelligence on the relationship between organizational commitment and organizational citizenship behavior in ZobAhan factory of Isfahan. *International Journal of Scientific Management and Development*, *2*(8), 399–403.

Yedla, M., Pathakota, S. R., & Srinivasa, T. M. (2010). Enhancing K-means clustering algorithm with improved initial center. *International Journal of Computer Science and Information Technologies*, *1*(2), 121-125.

Yen, B. S., Wang, H.-M., Hou, M. C., Tcm, D., Huang, S.-C., & Chou, L.-C. (2010). The relationship between music processing and electrocardiogram (ECG) in vegetative state (VS). *Circuits and Systems (ISCAS), Proceedings of 2010 IEEE International Symposium on*. 10.1109/ISCAS.2010.5537211

Yin, J., & Chen, J. D. (2013). Electrogastrography: Methodology, validation and applications. *Journal of Neurogastroenterology and Motility*, *19*(1), 5–17. doi:10.5056/jnm.2013.19.1.5 PMID:23350042

Yuan, Y., Wyatt, C., Maccarini, P., Stauffer, P., Craciunescu, O., MacFall, J., & Das, S. K. (2012). A heterogeneous human tissue mimicking phantom for RF heating and MRI thermal monitoring verification. *Physics in Medicine and Biology*, *57*(7), 2021–2037. doi:10.1088/0031-9155/57/7/2021 PMID:22430012

Zadeh, L. A. (1965). Fuzzy sets. *Information and Control*, *8*(3), 338–353. doi:10.1016/S0019-9958(65)90241-X

Zare, H., Pedram, A., & Shirvanian, A. (2011). The prediction of students' spiritual intelligence of their personality attributes. *Behavioral Sciences Researches, 10*(1), 59-67.

Zeng, S.-d., & Zhong, Q.-h. (2015). Heart-rate Measurement via Face-video Base on FastICA and Wavelet Packet Decomposition. *Laser Journal, 11*, 13.

Zhang, J., Ji, N., Liu, J., Pan, J., & Meng, D. (2015). Enhancing performance of the backpropagation algorithm via sparse response regularization. *Neurocomputing*, *153*, 20–40. doi:10.1016/j.neucom.2014.11.055

Zhao, S., Sha, H., Li, Z. Y., & Ren, C. S. (2012). Electrical bioimpedance gastric motility measurement based on an electrical-mechanical composite mechanism. *World Journal of Gastroenterology*, *18*(25), 3282–3287. PMID:22783053

Zheng, T., Xie, W., Xu, L., He, X., Zhang, Y., You, M., ... Chen, Y. (2017). A machine learning-based framework to identify type 2 diabetes through electronic health records. *International Journal of Medical Informatics*, *97*, 120–127. doi:10.1016/j.ijmedinf.2016.09.014 PMID:27919371

Zhou, M. X., Huang, Q. A., & Qin, M. (2005). Modeling, design and fabrication of a triple-layered capacitive pressure sensor. *Sensors and Actuators. A, Physical*, *117*(1), 71–81. doi:10.1016/j.sna.2004.05.036

Zhu, F., Spronck, J. W., & Heerens, W. C. (1991). A simple capacitive displacement sensor. *Sensors and Actuators. A, Physical*, *26*(1-3), 265–269. doi:10.1016/0924-4247(91)87003-L

Zohar, D., Marshall, I. N., & Marshall, I. (2000). *Connecting with our spiritual intelligence*. Bloomsbury Publishing USA.

Zohar, D. (1997). *Rewiring the Corporate Brain: Using the New Science to Rethink How We Structure and Lead Organizations*. San Francisco: Berrett-Koehler Publishers, Inc.

Zohar, D. M. (2000). *Spiritual Intelligence: The Ultimate Intelligence*. London: Bloomsbury.

Zurek, S., & Meydan, T. (2006). A novel capacitive flux density sensor. *Sensors and Actuators. A, Physical*, *129*(1), 121–125. doi:10.1016/j.sna.2005.11.027

About the Contributors

Prasant Kumar Pattnaik, Ph.D. (Computer Science), Fellow IETE, Senior Member IEEE is Professor at the School of Computer Engineering, KIIT University, Bhubaneswar. He has more than a decade of teaching research experience. Dr. Pattnaik has published numbers of Research papers in peer reviewed international journals and conferences. His researches areas are Cloud Computing, Mobile Computing and Brain Computer Interface. He authored many computer science books in field of Robotics, Turing Machine, Cloud Computing, and Mobile Computing.

Aleena Swetapadma, Ph.D., is working as Assistant Professor at the School of Computer Engineering, KIIT University, Bhubaneswar. She did her B. Tech from CET, Bhubaneswar, Odisha, India), M. Tech and Ph. D from NIT, Raipur, India. Her field of interest includes Power System Protection, Data Mining, Brain Computer Interface and Artificial Intelligence Application

Jay Sarraf, M. Tech (Computer Sc. and Engineering), is working as Assistant Professor at the School of Computer Engineering, KIIT University. His field of interest includes Brain Computer interface.

* * *

Mohammad Abdolshah received his B.Sc. and M.Sc in Industrial Engineering from Amirkabir University of Technology, Tehran, Iran. Later, he obtained his Ph.D. from University of Putra Malaysia, Malaysia in Industrial Engineering. Dr. Mohammad Abdolshah's current research interests are Industrial Engineering, Quality Engineering, Organizational behaviour, and Human resource management.

Paramasivam Alagumariappan completed his M.E. at Karpaga Vinayaga College of Engineering and Technology in the field of Power Electronics and Drives. At present, he is a Ph.D. Research Scholar at the Department of Instrumentation Engineering, Madras Institute of Technology Campus, Anna University, Chennai.

He is a student member of Bernoulli Society for Mathematical Statistics and Probability and ASTM, and has authored 6 research papers in journals and conferences.

Sahana Apparsamy received her B.E. degree in Electrical engineering from Sri Sivasubramaniya Nadar College of Engineering, Kalavakkam, Chennai, India, and M.E. degree in Instrumentation Engineering from Madras Institute of Technology campus, Anna university, Chennai, India. Her current research interests include sensor development, capacitive imaging and machine learning algorithms. She has also worked on a funded project on Fire Fighter Locator using FPGA.

Arpita Das is an Assistant Professor of the Institute of Radio Physics and Electronics, University of Calcutta. She obtained her Ph.D. from University of Calcutta in 2012. Her research interests include medical image processing, pattern recognition, artificial intelligence etc. She published many research articles in the international journals and conferences.

Hüseyin Gürüler is working an Assistant Professor in the department of information systems engineering in Muğla Sıtkı Koçman University, Turkey. MSc Thesis deals with data mining on university students' database. PhD research is about diagnosing sleep apnea using ECG recordings. His research interests are data mining, biomedical computing, knowledge based systems and human computer interactions.

Ayhan Istanbullu is working as an Associate Professor in Computer Engineering Department of Balikesir University, Turkey. He received his undergraduate degree (1993) and his Ph.D from the Electronic and Computer Science Education Department of the Gazi University (2003), Turkey He worked as an instructor at the University of Mugla, Turkey in the Department of Electronic and Computer Science Education between 2001 and 2006. His research interests include the investigation of information technologies to support electronic and computer engineering education, mobile learning, machine learning, and biomedical instrumentation.

Amir Mohammad Khatibi is a PhD student in operation management, Department of Management, University of Isfahan.

Kamalanand Krishnamurthy is an Assistant Professor at the Department of Instrumentation Engineering, Madras Institute of Technology Campus, Anna University, Chennai. His research focuses on mathematical modeling and analysis of physical and biological systems. He has authored several papers and book chapters and is a Guest Editor for the European Journal for Biomedical Informatics and Current Bioinformatics.

Suraj Kumar Nayak received his B. Tech. in Electrical Engineering from Government College of Engineering Keonjhar, Odisha, India (formerly known as OSME Keonjhar) and M. Tech. in Biomedical Engineering from National Institute of Technology Rourkela, Odisha, India. Currently, he is pursuing his Ph.D. degree in Biomedical Engineering from National Institute of Technology Rourkela, Odisha, India. His research interests include Biomedical Instrumentation, Biomedical Signal Processing, and Drug Delivery.

Kunal Pal pursued his graduation in Pharmacy from University of Delhi, New Delhi, India in the year 2002 followed by post-graduation in Biomedical Engineering from Jadavpur University, Kolkata, India in the year 2004. Later, he did his Ph.D. in Materials Science from Indian Institute of Technology, Kharagpur, India in the year 2006. Subsequently, he joined Ryerson University, Toronto, Canada as a post-doctoral fellow in the year 2007. During his tenure at Ryerson University, he served as Vice-Chair (Elect), HQPA, AFMNet Network of Excellence, Canada. He joined National Institute of Technology, Rourkela, India in the year 2009 as an Assistant Professor in Biomedical Engineering. He is currently the Professor-in-Charge of Medical Electronics and Instrumentation Laboratory in the Department of Biotechnology and Medical Engineering, National Institute of Technology, Rourkela, India. His major research interests revolve around Biomedical Signal Processing and Biomedical Equipment Design. He is also working in the fields of soft materials and controlled drug delivery. He has more than 150 publications in SCI cited journals of high repute, Book Chapters, and peer-reviewed conferences. He is a very well cited researcher having more than 2000 citations.

Debasisha Panigrahi is an undergraduate at NIT Rourkela working on Bio signal acquisition and analysis.

Musa Peker is working an Assistant Professor in the department of information systems engineering in Muğla Sıtkı Koçman University, Turkey. MSc degree in Computer Systems Education from Sakarya University, Turkey, in 2009, and the Ph.D. degree in Computer Engineering from Karabük University, Turkey, in 2010. His research interests are in machine learning, data mining, decision support systems, artificial intelligence and biomedical signal processing.

Arivarasu Rajagopal completed his M.E. (Instrumentation Engineering) at Madras Institute of Technology Campus, Anna University, Chennai, in 2016. His major area of research is Biomedical Engineering.

Index

J

K

L

M

N

O

P

R

S

T

U

W

www.ingramcontent.com/pod-product-compliance
Lightning Source LLC
LaVergne TN
LVHW061540290926
849162LV00004B/856